PRINCIPLES OF
MANUAL MEDICINE

Third Edition

PRINCIPLES OF MANUAL MEDICINE

Third Edition

Philip E. Greenman, D.O., F.A.A.O.
Emeritus Professor
Departments of Osteopathic Manipulative Medicine &
Physical Medicine & Rehabilitation
College of Osteopathic Medicine
Michigan State University
East Lansing, Michigan

LIPPINCOTT WILLIAMS & WILKINS
A **Wolters Kluwer** Company

Philadelphia · Baltimore · New York · London
Buenos Aires · Hong Kong · Sydney · Tokyo

Acquisitions Editor: Timothy Y. Hiscock
Developmental Editor: Jenny Kim
Project Editor: Erica Woods Tucker
Manufacturing Manager: Colin Warnock
Cover Designer: Karen Quigley
Compositor: Graphic World
Printer: Maple Press

Library of Congress Cataloging-in-Publication Data

Greenman, Ph. E., 1928-
    Principles of manual medicine / Philip E. Greenman.-- 3rd ed.
        p. ; cm.
    Includes bibliographical references and index.
    ISBN 0-7817-4187-4
        1. Manipulation (Therapeutics) 2. Medicine, Physical. I. Title.
    [DNLM: 1. Manipulation, Orthopedic. 2. Physical Medicine. WB 460 G814p 2003]
    RM724.G74 2003
    615.8'2--dc21

                                                                            2003047694

Care has been taken to confirm the accuracy of the information presented and to describe generally accepted practices. However, the author and publisher are not responsible for errors or omissions or for any consequences from application of the information in this book and make no warranty, expressed or implied, with respect to the currency, completeness, or accuracy of the contents of the publication. Application of this information in a particular situation remains the professional responsibility of the practitioner.

The author and publisher have exerted every effort to ensure that drug selection and dosage set forth in this text are in accordance with current recommendations and practice at the time of publication. However, in view of ongoing research, changes in government regulations, and the constant flow of information relating to drug therapy and drug reactions, the reader is urged to check the package insert for each drug for any change in indications and dosage and for added warnings and precautions. This is particularly important when the recommended agent is a new or infrequently employed drug.

Some drugs and medical devices presented in this publication have Food and Drug Administration (FDA) clearance for limited use in restricted research settings. It is the responsibility of the health care provider to ascertain the FDA status of each drug or device planned for use in their clinical practice.

10 9 8 7 6 5 4 3 2 1

The first edition was dedicated to my long time friend and colleague E. DeVer Tucker, D.O., who was an exemplary osteopathic physician in Western New York for over 50 years.

The second edition was dedicated in memory of John F. Bourdillon, M.D., a friend and continuing medical education colleague who was a major contributor to the field of manual medicine worldwide.

This third edition is dedicated to the memory of another long time friend and colleague, Vladimir Janda, M.U.Dr., D.Sc. Dr. Janda was internationally well known for his basic and clinical research into muscle function in relation to problems of the locomotor system. He chaired the Department of Rehabilitation at Charles University in Prague, Czech Republic for many years. He traveled worldwide lecturing and teaching his principles of assessment and treatment of problems of motor control. Dr. Janda and I had a great deal in common. We were both born in the same year, both graduated from medical school in the same year, both have two sons, each 5 years apart, and were both elected to honorary membership in the International Federation of Manual Medicine at the Congress in Chicago, Illinois in 2001. The only difference between us is that my two sons are 20 years older than his. He married his beloved Jana at age 43.

Vlad had a life long interest in muscle after being ill with poliomyelitis as a teenager. While left with significant impairment, he was never disabled. He was a master at the visual assessment of muscle behavior. After being a student in one of my courses on muscle energy manual medicine he remarked, "Phil, what we need to do is put your hands and my eyes together!" He taught me, as well as many others, his concepts of motor control. They have been most helpful to many of my patients. In fact, the longer I practice manual medicine, the more I find I spend the time with my patient prescribing exercise. Thank you Vlad.

Dr. Janda passed away in November 25, 2002. He will be missed by his many friends, students, colleagues, and patients.

CONTENTS

SECTION III.   CLINICAL INTEGRATION AND CORRELATION

Manual medicine continues to be one of the oldest continuing forms of health care. In the late twentieth century the field was examined by over fifty controlled clinical trials, and many meta-analyses. The conclusions reached were that there was a role for manual medicine in acute and chronic back pain. The role of the discipline in systemic disease has been found to be useful, mainly in conjunction with other medical and surgical therapies. This is valuable in today's world of evidence-based medicine. However, medicine is still the art of applying the current scientific knowledge for the betterment of our patients. Manual medicine is a component part of a number of health professionals who practice some form of "hands on" treatment. It is found within the scope of practice of allopathic physicians, osteopathic physicians, chiropractors, physical therapists, massage therapists, and other "body workers".

The first edition of this book was originally designed to support the Continuing Medical Education's courses offered through Michigan State University and its Colleges of Osteopathic Medicine and Human Medicine. Since that time it has been used in a number of colleges of osteopathic medicine, chiropractic colleges, schools of physical therapy, and schools of massage therapy. The second edition has been translated into seven foreign languages.

This third edition attempts to bring current new information, as well as answers to many of the questions I have received when teaching this material. This edition also adds newer techniques and visuals and clarification to some of the concepts presented. As an art form, manual medicine cannot be mastered by reading a text and requires considerable practice using the hands as a diagnostic and therapeutic instrument. For the beginner, be diligent and not discouraged. For the experienced, continue to explore this fascinating field. Our patients are always grateful for the personalized nature of manual medicine. Happy voyage.

Philip E. Greenman, D.O., F.A.A.O.

ACKNOWLEDGMENTS

The third edition of *Principles of Manual Medicine* is still a single authored attempt to convey over fifty years experience in the use of manual medicine to assist patient's recovery from the effects of illness and trauma. I am deeply indebted to the many giants in the field with whom I have had the privilege to study and learn. I again acknowledge my osteopathic mentors, C.G. Beckwith, Angus Cathie, David Heilig, Paul Kimberly, Fred L Mitchell, Sr., Paul T. Lloyd, R.M. Tilley, E.DeVer Tucker, and Perrin T. Wilson. In the allopathic profession in the United States and internationally the list includes John Bourdillon, John Mennell, Johannes Fossgreen, Hans-Dieter Neumann, Robert Maigne, Karel Lewit, Vladimer Janda, and Scott Haldeman.

My colleagues at Michigan State University College of Osteopathic Medicine have long been a source of continued stimulation and the traditions are now in the hands of many of my previous students and residents. I wish them the best in their careers.

Again my thanks go to John Williamson for his photographic assistance and to Jacob Rowan for serving as the model after a sojourn in the United States Army and now embarking upon a career in Physical Medicine and Rehabilitation.

My thanks go to Jenny Kim of Lippincott Williams & Wilkins for editorial assistance and keeping me on schedule.

To my wife of fifty three years go my love and gratitude for her support throughout this current effort.

Section **1**   *PRINCIPLES AND CONCEPTS*

1

STRUCTURAL DIAGNOSIS AND MANIPULATIVE MEDICINE HISTORY

HISTORY

Manual medicine is as old as the science and art of medicine itself. There is strong evidence of the use of manual medicine procedures in ancient Thailand, as shown in statuary at least 4,000 years old. The ancient Egyptians practiced the use of the hands in treatment of injury and disease. Even Hippocrates, the father of modern medicine, was known to use manual medicine procedures, particularly traction and leverage techniques, in the treatment of spinal deformity. The writings of such notable historical figures in medicine as Galen, Celisies, and Oribasius refer to the use of manipulative procedures. There is a void in the reported use of manual medicine procedures corresponding to the approximate time of the split of physicians and barber-surgeons. As physicians became less involved in patient contact, and as direct hands-on patient care became the province of the barber-surgeons, the role of manual medicine in the healing art seems to have declined. This period also represents the time of the plagues and perhaps physicians were reticent to come in close personal contact with their patients.

The 19th century found a renaissance of interest in this field. Early in the 19th century Doctor Edward Harrison, a 1784 graduate of Edinburgh University, developed a sizable reputation in London utilizing manual medicine procedures. Like many other proponents of manual medicine in the 19th century, he became alienated from his colleagues by his continued use of these procedures. The 19th century was a popular period for "bone-setters" both in England and in the United States. The work of Mr. Hutton, a skilled and famous bonesetter, led such eminent physicians as James Paget and Wharton Hood to report in such prestigious medical journals as the British Medical Journal and Lancet that the medical community should pay attention to the successes of the unorthodox practitioners of bone setting. In the United States, the Sweet family practiced skilled bone setting in the New England region of Rhode Island and Connecticut. It has also been reported that some of the descendants of the Sweet family emi-

grated west in the mid 19th century. Sir Herbert Barker was a well-known British bonesetter who practiced well into the first quarter of the 20th century and was of such eminence that he was knighted by the crown.

The 19th century was also a time of turmoil and controversy in medical practice. Medical history of the day is replete with many unorthodox systems of healing. Two individuals who would profoundly influence the field of manual medicine were products of this period of medical turmoil. Andrew Taylor Still, M.D., was a medical physician trained in the preceptor fashion of the day, and D.D. Palmer was a grocer turned self-educated manipulative practitioner.

Osteopathic Medicine

Still (1828 to 1917) first proposed his philosophy and practice of osteopathy in 1874. His disenchantment with the medical practice of the day led to his formulation of a new medical philosophy that he termed "osteopathic medicine." He appeared to have been a great synthesizer of medical thought and built his new philosophy on both ancient medical truths and current medical successes, while being most vocal in denouncing what he viewed as poor medical practice, primarily the inappropriate use of medications then in current use.

Still's strong position against the drug therapy of his day was not well received by his medical colleagues and is certainly not supported by contemporary osteopathic physicians. However, he was not alone in expressing concern about the abuse of drug therapy. In 1861 Oliver Wendell Holmes said, "If all of the MATERIA MEDICA were thrown into the oceans, it will be all the better for mankind, and worse for the fishes." Sir William Osler, one of Still's contemporaries, stated: "One of the first duties of the physician is to educate the masses not to take medicine. Man has an inborn craving for medicine. Heroic dosing for several generations has given his tissues a thirst for drugs. The desire to take medicine is one feature which distinguishes man, the animal, from his fellow creatures."

Still's new philosophy of medicine in essence consisted of the following:

1. The unity of the body.
2. The healing power of nature. He held that the body had within itself all those things necessary for the maintenance of health and recovery from disease. The role of the physician was to enhance this capacity.
3. The somatic component of disease. He felt that the musculoskeletal system was an integral part of the total body and alterations within the musculoskeletal system affected total body health and the ability of the body to recover from injury and disease.
4. Structure–function interrelationship. The interrelationship of structure–function had been espoused by Virchow early in the 19th century and Still applied this principle within his concept of total body integration. He strongly felt that structure governed function and that function influenced structure.
5. The use of manipulative therapy. This became an integral part of Still's philosophy because he believed that restoration of the body's maximal functional capacity would enhance the level of wellness and assist in recovery from injury and disease.

It is unclear when and how Dr. Still added manipulation to his philosophy of osteopathy. It was not until 1879, some five years after his announcement of the development of osteopathy, that he became known as the "lightning bonesetter." There is no recorded history that he met or knew members of the Sweet family as they migrated west. Still never wrote a book on manipulative technique. His writings were extensive, but they focused on the philosophy, principles, and practice of osteopathy.

Still's attempt to interest his medical colleagues in these concepts was rebuffed, particularly when he took them to Baker University in Kansas.

As he became more clinically successful, and nationally and internationally well known, many individuals came to study with him and learn the new science of osteopathy. This led to the establishment in 1892 of the first college of osteopathic medicine at Kirksville, Missouri. In 2002, there were 20 colleges of osteopathic medicine in the United States graduating more than 2,000 students per year. Osteopathy in other parts of the world, particularly in the United Kingdom and in the commonwealth countries of Australia and New Zealand, is a school of practice limited to structural diagnosis and manipulative therapy, although strongly espousing some of the fundamental concepts and principles of Still. Osteopathic medicine in the United States has from its inception, and continues to be, a total school of medicine and surgery while retaining the basis of osteopathic principles and concepts and continuing the use of structural diagnosis and manipulative therapy in total patient care.

Chiropractic

Daniel David Palmer (1845–1913) was, like Still, a product of the midwestern portion of the United States in the mid 19th century. Although not schooled in medicine, he was known to practice as a magnetic healer and became a self-educated manipulative therapist. Controversy continues as to whether Palmer was ever a patient or student of Still's at Kirksville, Missouri, but it is known that Palmer and Still met in Clinton, Iowa early in the 20th century. Palmer moved about the country a great deal and founded his first college in 1896. The early colleges were at Davenport, Iowa and Oklahoma City, Oklahoma.

Although Palmer is given credit for the origin of chiropractic, it was his son Bartlett Joshua Palmer (1881–1961) who gave the chiropractic profession its momentum. Palmer's original concepts were that the cause of disease was a variation in the expression of normal neural function. He believed in the "innate intelligence" of the brain and central nervous system and believed that alterations in the spinal column (subluxations) altered neural function, causing disease. Removal of the subluxation by chiropractic adjustment was viewed to be the treatment. Chiropractic has never professed to be a total school of medicine and does not teach surgery or the use of medication beyond vitamins and simple analgesics. There remains a split within the chiropractic profession between the "straights," who continue to espouse and adhere to the original concepts of Palmer, and the "mixers," who believe in a broadened scope of chiropractic that includes other therapeutic interventions such as exercise, physiotherapy, electrotherapy, diet, and vitamins.

In the mid 1970s, the Council on Chiropractic Education (CCE) petitioned the United States Department of Education for recognition as the accrediting agency for chiropractic education. The CCE was strongly influenced by the colleges with a "mixer" orientation, which has led to increased educational requirements both before and during chiropractic education. Chiropractic is practiced throughout the world, but the vast majority of chiropractic training continues to be in the United States. The late 1970s found increased recognition of chiropractic in both Australia and New Zealand, and their registries are participants in the health programs in these countries.

MEDICAL MANIPULATORS

The 20th century has found renewed interest in manual medicine in the traditional medical profession. In the first part of the 20th century James Mennell and Edgar Cyriax brought joint manipulation recognition within the London medical community. John Mennell continued the work of his father and contributed extensively to the manual medicine literature and its teaching worldwide. As one of the founding members of the North American Academy of Manipulative Medicine (NAAMM), he was instrumental in opening the membership in NAAMM to osteopathic physicians in 1977. He has strongly advocated the expanded role of appropriately trained physical therapists to work with the medical profession in providing joint manipulation in patient care.

James Cyriax is well known for his textbooks in the field and also fostered the expanded education and scope of physical therapists. He incorporated manual medicine procedures in the practice of "orthopedic medicine" and founded the Society for Orthopedic Medicine. In his later years, Cyriax came to believe that manipulation restored function to derangements of the intervertebral discs and spoke less and less about specific arthrodial joint effects. He had no use for "osteopaths" or other manipulating groups and the influence of his dynamic personality will be felt long after his death in 1985.

John Bourdillon, a British-trained orthopedic surgeon, was first attracted to manual medicine as a student at Oxford University. During his training, he learned to perform manipulation while the patient was under general anesthesia and subsequently used the same techniques without anesthesia. He observed the successful results of non–medically qualified manipulators and began a study of their techniques. A lifelong student and teacher in the field, he published five editions of a text *Spinal Manipulation*. Subsequent to his death in 1992, a sixth edition of *Spinal Manipulation* was published with Edward Isaacs, M.D., and Mark Bookhout, M.S., P.T., as coauthors.

The NAAMM merged with the American Association of Orthopedic Medicine in 1992 and continues to represent the United States in the International Federation of Manual Medicine (FIMM). Canada is represented in FIMM by the American Academy of Osteopathy.

THE PRACTICE OF MANUAL MEDICINE

Manual medicine should not be viewed in isolation nor separate from "regular medicine," and clearly is not the panacea for all ills of humans. Manual medicine considers the functional capacity of the human organism, and its practitioners are as interested in the dynamic processes of disease as those who look at the disease process from the static perspective of laboratory data, tissue pathology, and the results of autopsy. Manual medicine focuses on the musculoskeletal system, which comprises more than 60% of the human organism, and through which evaluation of the other organ systems must be made. Structural diagnosis not only evaluates the musculoskeletal system for its particular diseases and dysfunctions, but also can be used to evaluate the somatic manifestations of disease and derangement of the internal viscera. Manipulative procedures are used primarily to increase mobility in restricted areas of musculoskeletal function and to reduce pain. Some practitioners focus on the concept of pain relief, whereas others are more interested in the influence of increased mobility in restricted areas of the musculoskeletal system. When appropriately used, manipulative procedures can be clinically effective in reducing pain within the musculoskeletal system, in increasing the level of wellness of the patient, and in helping patients with a myriad of disease processes.

GOAL OF MANIPULATION

In 1983, in Fischingen, Sweden, a 6-day workshop was held that included approximately 35 experts in manual medicine from throughout the world. They represented many different countries and schools of manual medicine with considerable diversity in clinical experience. The proceedings of this workshop (Dvorak J, Dvorak V, Schneider W, eds. *Manual medicine* 1984, Heidelberg: Springer-Verlag, 1985) represented the state of the art of manual medicine of the day. That workshop reached a consensus on the goal of manipulation: The goal of manipulation is to restore maximal, pain-free movement of the musculoskeletal system in postural balance.

This definition is comprehensive but specific and is well worth consideration by all students in the field.

ROLE OF THE MUSCULOSKELETAL SYSTEM IN HEALTH AND DISEASE

It is indeed unfortunate that much of the medical thinking and teaching look at the musculoskeletal system only as the coat rack on which the other organ systems are held and not as an organ system that is susceptible to its own unique injuries and disease processes. The field of manual medicine looks at the musculoskeletal system in a much broader context, particularly as an integral and interrelated part of the total human organism. Although most physicians would accept the concept of integration of the total body including the musculoskeletal system, specific and usable concepts of how that integration occurs and its relationship in structural diagnosis and manipulative therapy seem to be limited.

There are five basic concepts that this author has found useful. Since the hand is an integral part of the practice of manual medicine, and includes five digits, it is easy to recall one concept for each digit in the palpating hand. These concepts are as follows:

1. Holism;
2. Neurologic control;
3. Circulatory function;
4. Energy expenditure; and
5. Self-regulation.

Concept of Holism

The concept of holism has different meanings and usage by different practitioners. In manual medicine, the concept emphasizes that the musculoskeletal system deserves thoughtful and complete evaluation, wherever and whenever the patient is seen, regardless of the nature of the presenting complaint. It is just as inappropriate to avoid evaluating the cardiovascular system in a patient presenting with a primary musculoskeletal complaint as it is to avoid evaluation of the musculoskeletal system in a patient presenting with acute chest pain thought to be cardiac in origin. The concept is one of a sick patient who needs to be evaluated. The musculoskeletal system comprises most of the human body and alterations within it influence the rest of the human organism; diseases within the internal organs manifest themselves in alterations in the musculoskeletal system, frequently in the form of pain. It is indeed fortunate that holistic concepts have gained increasing popularity in the medical community recently, but the concept expressed here is one that speaks to the integration of the total human organism rather than a summation of parts. We must all

remember that our role as health professionals is to treat patients and not to treat disease.

Concept of Neural Control

The concept of neurologic control is based on the fact that humans have the most highly developed and sophisticated nervous system in the animal kingdom. All functions of the body are under some form of control by the nervous system. A patient is constantly responding to stimuli from the internal and external body environment through complex mechanisms within the central and peripheral nervous systems. As freshmen in medical school, we all studied the anatomy and physiology of the nervous system. Let us briefly review a segment of the spinal cord (Fig. 1.1). On the left side are depicted the classic somatosomatic reflex pathways with afferent impulses coming from skin, muscle, joint, and tendon. Afferent stimuli from the nociceptors, mechanoreceptors, and proprioceptors all feed in through the dorsal root and ultimately synapse, either directly or through a series of interneurons, with an anterior horn cell from which an efferent fiber extends to the skeletal muscle. It is through multiple permutations of the central reflex arc that we respond to external stimuli, including injury, orient our bodies in space, and accomplish many of the physical activities of daily living. The right-hand side of the figure represents the classical viscerovisceral reflex arc wherein afferents from the visceral sensory system synapse in the intermediolateral cell column and then to the sympathetic lateral chain ganglion or collateral ganglia to synapse with a postgan-

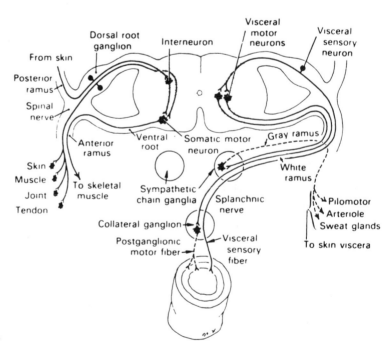

Figure 1.1.
Cross-section spinal cord segment.

glionic motor fiber to the target end organ viscera. Note that the skin viscera also receive efferent stimulation from the lateral chain ganglion.

These sympathetic reflex pathways innervate the pilomotor activity of the skin, the vasomotor tone of the vascular tree, and the secretomotor activity of the sweat glands. Alteration in the sympathetic nervous system activity to the skin viscera results in palpatory changes that are identifiable by structural diagnostic means. Although this figure separates these two pathways, they are in fact interrelated so that somatic afferents influence visceral efferents and visceral afferents can manifest themselves in somatic efferents. This figure represents the spinal cord in horizontal section and it must be recalled that ascending and descending pathways—from spinal cord segment to spinal cord segment, as well as from the higher centers of the brain—are occurring as well.

Another neurologic concept worth recalling is that of the autonomic nervous system (ANS). The ANS is made up of two divisions, the parasympathetic and sympathetic. The parasympathetic division includes cranial nerves III, VII, VIII, IX, X and the S2, S3, and S4 levels of the spinal cord. The largest and most extensive nerve of the parasympathetic division is the vagus. The vagus innervates all of the viscera from the root of the neck to the midportion of the descending colon and all glands and smooth muscle of these organs. The vagus nerve (Fig. 1.2) is the primary driving force of the cardiovascular, pulmonary, and gastrointestinal systems and has an extensive distribution. Many pharmaceutical agents alter parasympathetic nervous activity, particularly that of the vagus.

The sympathetic division of the autonomic nervous system (Fig. 1.3) is represented by preganglionic neurons originating in the spinal cord from T-1 to L-3, and the lateral chain ganglion including the superior, middle, and inferior cervical ganglia; the thoracolumbar ganglia from T-1 to L-3; and the collateral ganglia. Sympathetic fibers innervate all of the internal viscera as do the parasympathetic division but are organized differently. The sympathetic division is organized segmentally. It is interesting to note that all of the viscera above the diaphragm receive their sympathetic innervation from preganglionic fibers above T-4 and T-5, and all of the viscera below the diaphragm receive their sympathetic innervation preganglionic fibers from below T-5. It is through this segmental organization that the relationships of certain parts of the musculoskeletal system and certain internal viscera are correlated. Remember that the musculoskeletal system receives only sympathetic division innervation and receives no parasympathetic innervation. Control of all glandular and vascular activity in the musculoskeletal system is mediated through the sympathetic division of the ANS.

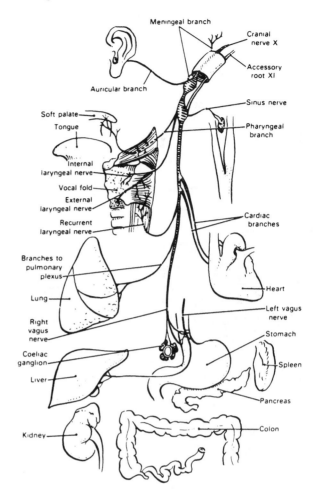

Figure 1.2.
Vagus nerve distribution.

Remember that all these reflex mechanisms are constantly under the local and central modifying control of excitation and inhibition. Conscious and subconscious control mechanisms from the brain constantly modify activity throughout the nervous system, responding to stimuli. The nervous system is intimately related to another control system, the endocrine system, and it is useful to think in terms of neuroendocrine control. Recent advances in the knowledge of neurotransmitters, endorphins, enkephalins, and materials such as substance P have enlightened us as to the detail of many of the mechanisms previously not understood, and have begun to provide answers for some of the mechanisms through which biomechanical alteration of the musculoskeletal system can alter bodily function.

Emphasis has been placed on the reflex and neural transmission activities of the nervous system, but the nervous system has a powerful trophic function as well. Highly complex protein and lipid substances are transported antegrade and retrograde along neurons and cross over the synapse of the neuron to the

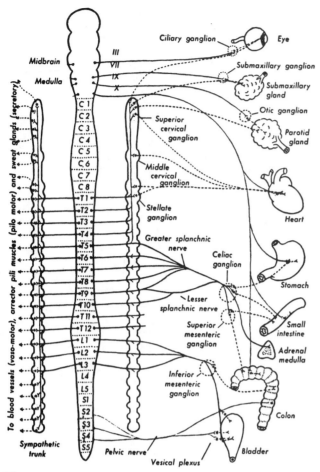

Figure 1.3.
Autonomic nervous system.

target end organ. Alteration in neurotrophin transmission can be detrimental to the health of the target end organ.

Circulatory Function

The third concept is that of circulatory function. The concept can be simply described as the maintenance of an appropriate cellular milieu for each cell of the body (Fig. 1.4). Picture a cell, a group of cells making up a tissue, or a group of tissues making up an organ resting in the middle of the "cellular milieu." That cell is dependent for its function, whatever its function is, upon the delivery of oxygen, glucose, and all other substances necessary for its metabolism being supplied by the arterial side of the circulation. The arterial system has a powerful pump, the myocardium of the heart, to propel blood forward. Cardiac pumping function is intimately controlled by the central nervous system, particularly the autonomic nervous system, through the cardiac plexus. The vascular tree receives its vasomotor tone control through the sympathetic division of the autonomic nervous system. Anything that interferes with sympathetic autonomic

nervous system outflow, segmentally mediated, can influence vasomotor tone to a target end organ.

The arteries are also encased in the fascial compartments of the body and are subject to compressive and torsional stress that can interfere with the delivery of arterial blood flow to the target organ cell. Once the cell has received its nutrients and proceeded through its normal metabolism, the end products must be removed. The low-pressure circulatory systems, the venous and the lymphatic systems, are responsible for the transport of metabolic waste products. Both the venous and lymphatic systems are much thinner-walled than the arteries, and they lack the driving force of the pumping action of the heart, depending instead on the musculoskeletal system for their propelling action. The large muscles of the extremities contribute greatly to this activity, but the major pump of the low-pressure systems is the diaphragm (Fig. 1.5).

The diaphragm has an extensive attachment to the musculoskeletal system, including the upper lumbar vertebra; the lower six ribs; the xiphoid process of the sternum; and through myofascial connections with the lower extremities, the psoas and quadratus lumborum muscles. The activity of the diaphragm modulates the negative intrathoracic pressure that provides a sucking action on venous and lymphatic return through the vena cava and the cisterna chyli. Because of the extensive attachment of the diaphragm with the musculoskeletal system, and from its innervation via the phrenic nerve from the cervical spine, alterations in the musculoskeletal system at a number of levels can alter diaphragmatic function and, consequently venous and lymphatic return. Accumulation of metabolic end products in the cellular milieu interferes with the health of the cell and its recovery from disease or injury. It should be pointed out that the foramen for the inferior vena cava is at the apex of the dome of the diaphragm. There is some evidence that diaphragmatic excursion has a direct squeezing and propelling activity on the inferior vena cava.

Another circulatory concept related to musculoskeletal function concerns the lymphatic system (Fig. 1.6), and the location where it empties into the venous system. The lymph from the right side of the head, right side of the neck, and right upper extremity enters into the right subclavian vein at the thoracic inlet just behind the anterior end of the first rib and the medial end of the clavicle. The lymph from the rest of the body empties into the left subclavian vein at the thoracic inlet behind the anterior extremity of the left first rib and the medial end of the left clavicle. Alteration in the biomechanics of the thoracic inlet, particularly its fascial continuity, can affect the thin-walled lymph vessels as they empty into the venous system. Maximal function of the musculoskeletal system is an

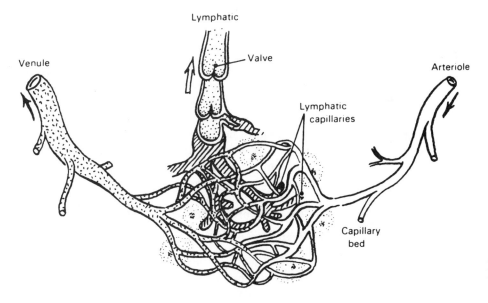

Figure 1.4.
The cellular milieu.

A

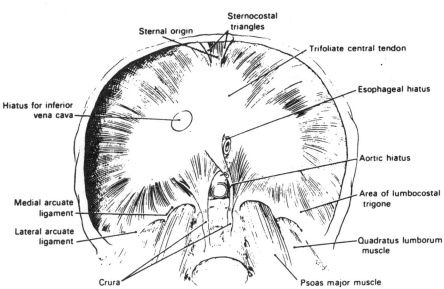

B

Figure 1.5.
Thoracoabdominal diaphragm.

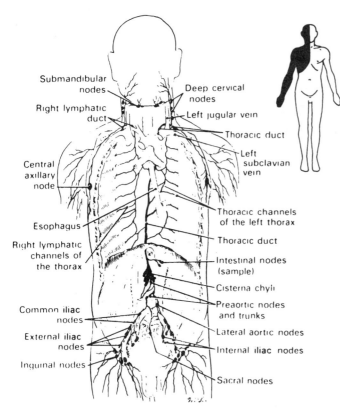

Figure 1.6.
Lymphatic system.

important factor in the efficiency of the circulatory system and the maintenance of a normal cellular milieu throughout the body.

Energy Expenditure

The fourth concept is that of energy expenditure primarily through the musculoskeletal system. The musculoskeletal system not only comprises more than 60% of the human organism but also is the major expender of body energy. Any increase in activity of the musculoskeletal system calls on the internal viscera to develop and deliver energy to sustain that physical activity. The greater the activity of the musculoskeletal system, the greater is the demand. If dysfunction alters the efficiency of the musculoskeletal system, there is an increase in demand for energy, not only for increased activity, but for normal activity as well. If we have a patient with compromised cardiovascular and pulmonary systems who has chronic congestive heart failure, any increase in demand for energy delivery to the musculoskeletal system can be detrimental. For example, a well-compensated chronic congestive heart failure patient who happens to sprain an ankle and attempts to continue normal activity might well have a rapid deterioration of the compensation because of the increased energy demand by the altered gait of the sprained ankle. Obviously, it would make

more sense to treat the altered musculoskeletal system by attending to the ankle sprain than to increase the dosage of medications controlling the congestive heart failure. Restriction of one major joint in a lower extremity can increase the energy expenditure of normal walking by as much as 40% and, if two major joints are restricted in the same extremity, it can increase as much as 300%. Multiple minor restrictions of movement of the musculoskeletal system, particularly in the maintenance of normal gait, can also have a detrimental effect on total body function.

Self-Regulation

The fifth concept is that of self-regulation. There are literally thousands of self-regulating mechanisms operative within the body at all times. These homeostatic mechanisms are essential for the maintenance of health, and if altered by disease or injury, they need to be restored. All physicians are dependent on these self-regulating mechanisms within the patient for successful treatment. The goal of the physician should be to enhance all of the body's self-regulating mechanisms to assist in the recovery from disease. Physicians should not interfere with self-regulating mechanisms more than absolutely necessary during the treatment process. All things that are done to or placed within the human body alter these mechanisms in some fashion. When any foreign substance is given to a patient, the beneficial and detrimental potentials of the substance must be considered. As modern pharmacology grows with evermore-potent pharmacological effects, we must recognize the potential for iatrogenic disease. Many patients are on multiple medications, particularly in the hospital environment, and the actions and interactions of each must be clearly understood to avoid iatrogenic problems. Only physicians cause iatrogenic disease. Reportedly, 1 in 7 hospital days in the United States is due to adverse reaction to pharmacological intervention.

THE MANIPULABLE LESION

Manual medicine deals with the identification of the manipulable lesion and the appropriate use of a manual medicine procedure to resolve the condition. The field of manual medicine has suffered from multiple, divergent, and sometimes confusing definitions of the entity amenable to manipulative intervention. It has been called the "osteopathic lesion," "chiropractic subluxation," "joint blockage," "loss of joint play," "joint dysfunction," and other names. The acceptable term for this entity is somatic dysfunction. It is defined as impaired or altered function of related components of the somatic (body framework) system; skeletal, arthrodial, and myofascial structures; and related vascular, lymphatic, and neural elements (*Hospital Adaptation of the International Classification of Disease*, 2nd ed.

1973). Notice that the emphasis is on altered function of the musculoskeletal system and not on a disease state or pain syndrome. Obviously, if a somatic dysfunction is present that alters vascular, lymphatic, and neural functions, a myriad of symptoms might well be present, including painful conditions and disease entities. The diagnosis of somatic dysfunction can accompany many other diagnoses or can be present as an independent entity. The art of structural diagnosis is to define the presence of somatic dysfunction(s) and determine any significance to the patient's complaint or disease process presenting at the time. If significant, it should be treated by manual medicine intervention just as other diagnostic findings might also need appropriate treatment.

DIAGNOSTIC TRIAD FOR SOMATIC DYSFUNCTION

The mnemonic ART can express the diagnostic criteria for identification of somatic dysfunction. "A" stands for asymmetry of related parts of the musculoskeletal system, either structural or functional. Examples are altered shoulder height, height of iliac crest, and contour and function of the thoracic cage, usually identified by palpation and observation. "R" stands for range of motion of a joint, several joints, or region of the musculoskeletal system. The range of motion could be abnormal either by being increased (hypermobility) or restricted (hypomobility). The usual finding in somatic dysfunction is restricted mobility, identified by observation and palpation using both active and passive patient cooperation. "T" stands for tissue texture abnormality of the soft tissues of the musculoskeletal system (skin, fascia, muscle, ligament, etc.). Tissue texture abnormalities are identified by observation and a number of different palpatory tests. Some authors add one of two other letters to this mnemonic, "P" or a second "T." "P" stands for pain associated with other findings, and "T" stands for tenderness on palpation of the area. Tenderness is particularly diagnostic if localized to a ligament. A normal ligament is not tender. A tender ligament is always abnormal. However, both pain and tenderness are subjective findings instead of the objective findings of asymmetry, altered range of motion, and tissue texture abnormality. By the use of these criteria, one attempts to identify the presence of somatic dysfunctions, their location, whether they are acute or chronic, and particularly whether they are significant for the state of the patient's wellness or illness at that moment in time. In addition to the diagnostic value, changes in these criteria can be of prognostic value in monitoring the response of the patient, not only to manipulative treatment directed toward the somatic dysfunction, but also to other therapeutic interventions.

SUGGESTED READINGS

Buerger AA, Greenman PE, eds. *Empirical approaches to the validation of spinal manipulation.* Springfield, IL: Charles C. Thomas Publisher, 1985.

Buerger AA, Tobis JS. *Approaches to the validation of manipulative therapy.* Springfield, IL: Charles C. Thomas Publisher, 1977.

Buzzell KA. The cost of human posture and locomotion. In: Northup GW, Korr IM, Buzzell KA, et al., eds. *The physiological basis of osteopathic medicine.* New York: Postgraduate Institute of Osteopathic Medicine and Surgery, 1970; (63–72).

Cyriax J. *Textbook of orthopedic medicine,* 7th ed. Vol. 1. East Sussex, England: Bailliere-Tindall, 1978.

DiGiovanna EL, Schiowitz S. *An osteopathic approach to diagnosis and treatment.* Philadelphia: JB Lippincott Co., 1991.

Gevitz N. *The D.O.'s: osteopathic medicine in America.* Baltimore, MD: Johns Hopkins University Press, 1982.

Greenman PE. The osteopathic concept in the second century: is it still germane to specialty practice? *J Am Osteopath Assoc* 1976; 75:589–595.

Greenman PE, ed. *Concepts and mechanisms of neuromuscular functions.* Berlin: Springer-Verlag, 1984.

Greenman PE. *Models and mechanisms of osteopathic manipulative medicine.* Osteopathic Medical News 4(5) 1–20, 1987.

Grieve GP. *Common vertebral joint problems.* Edinburgh: Churchill Livingstone, 1981.

Haldeman S. *Modern developments in the principles and practice of chiropractic.* East Norwalk, CT: Appleton-Century-Crofts, 1980.

Hildreth AG. *The lengthening shadow of Dr. Andrew Taylor Still.* Macon, MO: Hildreth, 1938.

Hoag JM, Cole WV, Bradford SG. *Osteopathic medicine.* New York: McGraw-Hill, 1969.

Hood W: On so-called "bone setting" its nature and results. *Lancet* 1871;Apr 1:336–338, 373–374, 441–443, 499–501.

Hospital adaptation of the international classification of disease, 2nd ed. Ann Arbor, MI: Commission on Professional and Hospital Activities, 1973.

Korr IM, ed. *The neurobiologic mechanisms in manipulative therapy.* New York: Plenum Publishing, 1978.

Lamax E. Manipulative therapy: a historical perspective from ancient times to the modern era. In: Goldstein M, ed. *The research status of spinal manipulative therapy.* National Institute of Neurological and Communicative Disorders and Stroke, Monograph No. 15. 1975;11–17.

Lewit K. *Manipulative therapy in rehabilitation of the locomotor system,* 2nd ed. Oxford: Butterworth-Heinemann, 1991.

Maigne R. *Orthopedic medicine.* Springfield, IL: Charles C. Thomas Publisher, 1972.

Maitland GD: *Vertebral Manipulation,* 4th ed. Stoneham, MA: Butterworths, 1980.

Mennell JM. *Back pain.* Boston: Little, Brown and Company, 1960.

Mennell JM. *Joint pain.* Boston: Little, Brown and Company, 1964.

Northup GW, ed. *Osteopathic research: growth and development.* Chicago, IL: American Osteopathic Association, 1987.

Northup GW. *Osteopathic medicine: an American reformation,* 2nd ed. Chicago, IL: American Osteopathic Association, 1979.

Northup GW, Korr IM, Buzzell KA, et al. *The physiological basis of osteopathic medicine.* New York: Postgraduate Institute of Osteopathic Medicine and Surgery, 1970.

Page LE. *The principles of osteopathy.* Kansas City, MO: American Academy of Osteopathy, 1952.

Paris SA. Spinal manipulative therapy. *Clin Orthop* 1983;179:55–61.

Schiotz EH. Manipulation treatment of the spinal column from the medical-historical viewpoint. *Tidsskr Nor Laegeforn* 1958;78:359–372, 429–438, 946–950, 1003 [NIH Library Translation NIH 75-22C, 23C, 24C, 25C].

Schiotz EH, Cyriax J. *Manipulation past and present.* London: William Heinemann Medical Books, 1975.

Schneider W, Dvorak J, Dvorak V, et al. *Manual medicine: therapy.* New York: Thieme Medical Publishers, 1988.

Stoddard A. *Manual of osteopathic technique.* London: Hutchinson Medical Publications, 1959.

Stoddard A. *Manual of osteopathic practice.* New York: Harper & Row, 1969.

Ward RC, ed. *Foundations for osteopathic medicine.* Baltimore: Williams & Wilkins, 1997.

Zink JG. Respiratory and circulatory care: the conceptual model. *Osteopath Annals* 1977;5:108–124.

2

PRINCIPLES OF STRUCTURAL DIAGNOSIS

Structural diagnosis in manual medicine is directed toward evaluation of the musculoskeletal system with the goal of identification of the presence and significance of somatic dysfunction(s). It is a component part of the physical examination of the total patient. Most of the evaluation of the internal viscera takes place by evaluation of these structures through the musculoskeletal system. Therefore, it is easy to examine the musculoskeletal system while evaluating the internal viscera of the neck, chest, abdomen, and pelvic regions. Structural diagnosis uses the traditional physical diagnostic methods of observation, palpation, percussion, and auscultation. Of these, observation and palpation are the most useful. Structural diagnosis of the musculoskeletal system should never be done in isolation and should always be done within the context of a total history and physical evaluation of the patient. It has been said that 90% of a physician's decision making is from the history and physical examination.

The diagnostic entity sought by structural diagnosis is somatic dysfunction. It is defined as follows:

Somatic dysfunction: impaired or altered function of related components of the somatic (body framework) system; skeletal, arthrodial, and myofascial structures; and related vascular, lymphatic, and neural elements.

The three classical diagnostic criteria for somatic dysfunction can be identified with the mnemonic **ART** as follows:

A for asymmetry: asymmetry of related parts of the musculoskeletal system either structural or functional. Examples might be the height of each shoulder by observation, height of iliac crest by palpation, and contour and function of the thoracic cage by observation and palpation. Asymmetry is usually discerned by observation and palpation.

R for range-of-motion abnormality: Alteration in range of motion of a joint, several joints, or region of the musculoskeletal system is sought. The alter-

ation may be either restricted or increased mobility. Restricted motion is the most common component of somatic dysfunction. Range-of-motion abnormality is determined by observation and palpation, using both active and passive patient cooperation.

T for tissue texture abnormality (TTA): Alteration in the characteristics of the soft tissues of the musculoskeletal system (skin, fascia, muscle, ligament) is ascertained by observation and palpation. Percussion is also used in identifying areas of altered tissue texture. A large number of descriptors are used in the literature to express the quality of the abnormal feel of the tissue. There are two primary tissue abnormalities that account for palpable changes, namely muscle hypertonicity, secondary to increased alpha motor neuron stimulation, and altered activity of the "skin viscera," the pilomotor, vasomotor, and secretomotor functions that are under the control of the sympathetic division of the autonomic nervous system.

HAND-EYE COORDINATION

In structural diagnosis, it is important for the physician to maximize the coordinated use of the palpating hands and the observing eyes. When using vision for observation, it is important to know which eye is dominant so that it can be appropriately placed in relation to the patient for accuracy in visual discrimination. Since most structural diagnosis uses hand–eye coordination with the arms extended, it is best to test for the dominant eye at arm's-length distance (Fig. 2.1). The test is as follows:

1. Extend both arms and form a small circle with the thumb and index finger of each hand.
2. With both eyes open, sight through the circle formed by the thumbs and fingers at an object at the other end of the room. Make the circle as small as possible.
3. Close your left eye only. If the object is still seen through the circle, you are right-eye

Figure 2.1.
Test for dominant eye.

dominant. If the object is no longer seen through the circle, you are left-eye dominant.
4. Repeat the procedure closing the right eye and note the difference.

When looking for symmetry or asymmetry, it is important that the dominant eye be located midway between the two anatomic parts being observed and/or palpated. For example, when palpating each acromial process to identify the level of the shoulders, the dominant eye should be in the mid-sagittal plane of the patient, equidistant from each palpating hand. In other words, the dominant eye should be on the midline of the two anatomic parts being compared. With a patient supine on the examining table, a right-eye–dominant examiner should stand on the right side of the patient and a left-eye–dominant examiner should stand on the left side of the patient. Remember that the hands and eyes should be on the same reference plane when one is attempting to determine if paired anatomic parts are symmetrically placed. For example, when evaluating the height of the shoulders by palpating the two acromial processes and visualizing a level against the horizontal plane, the eyes should be on the same horizontal plane as the palpating hands. When palpating the two iliac crests to identify if they are level against the horizontal plane, the eyes should be at the level of the iliac crests in the same plane as the palpating hands. Whenever possible, the eyes should be in the plane against which anatomic landmarks are being compared for symmetry or asymmetry.

All physicians use palpation in physical examination of the abdomen for masses, normal organs for size and position, point of maximum impulse of the heart, tactile fremitus of the lungs, and pulsations of the peripheral vessels. Palpation is also used to identify masses, normal and abnormal lymph nodes, and other changes of the tissues. In structural diagnosis, palpation requires serious consideration and practice to develop high-level diagnostic skills. Palpatory skills affect the following:

1. The ability to detect Tissue Texture Abnormality
2. The ability to detect asymmetry of position, both visual and tactile
3. The ability to detect differences of movement in total range, quality of movement during the range, and quality of sensation at the end of the range of movement
4. The ability to sense position in space of both the patient and examiner
5. The ability to detect change in palpatory findings, both improvement and worsening, over time

It is important to develop coordinated and symmetric use of the hands so that they may be linked with the visual sense. In developing palpatory skills, one must be aware that different parts of the hands are valuable for different tests. For example, the palms of the hands are best suited for use in the stereognostic sense of contour; the dorsum of the hands are more sensitive to temperature variations; the finger pads are best for fine discrimination of textural differences, finite skin contour, and so forth; and the tips of the fingers, particularly the thumbs, are useful as pressure probes for the assessment of differences in depth.

Three stages in the development and perception of palpatory sense have been described: reception, transmission, and interpretation. The proprioceptors and mechanoreceptors of the hand receive stimulation from the tissues being palpated. This is the reception phase. These impulses are then transmitted through the peripheral and central nervous systems to the brain where they are analyzed and interpreted. During the palpation process, care must be exercised to ensure efficiency of reception, transmission, and interpretation. Care must be taken of the examiner's hands to protect these sensitive diagnostic instruments. Avoidance of injury abuse is essential, hands should be clean, and nails an appropriate length. During the palpation process, the operator should be relaxed and comfortable to avoid extraneous interference with the transmission of the palpatory impulse. To accurately assess and interpret the palpatory findings, the physician must concentrate on the act of palpation, the tissue being palpated, and the response of the palpating fingers and hands. Reduce all extraneous sensory stimuli as much as possible. Probably the most common mistake in palpation is the lack of concentration by the examiner.

Tissue palpation can be further divided into light touch and deep touch. In light touch the amount of pressure is very slight and the examiner attempts to assess tissue change both actively and passively. By simply laying hands on the tissue passively, the examiner is able to make tactile observation of the quality of the tissues under the palpating hand. By moving the lightly applied hand in an active fashion, scanning information of multiple areas of the body can be ascertained, both normal and apparently abnormal. Deep touch is the use of additional pressure to palpate deeper into the layers of the tissue of the musculoskeletal system. Compression is palpation through multiple layers of tissue and shear is a movement of tissue between layers. Combinations of active and passive palpation and light and deep touch are used throughout the palpatory diagnostic process.

It is useful to develop appropriate terms to describe the changes in the anatomy being palpated and evaluated. The use of paired descriptors such as superficial–deep, compressible–rigid, moist–dry, warm–cold, painful–nonpainful, circumscribed–diffuse, rough–smooth, among others, are most useful. It is best to define both normal and abnormal palpatory clues in anatomic and physiologic terms. Second, it is useful to define areas of altered palpatory sense by describing the state of the tissue change as acute, subacute, or chronic in nature. Third, it is useful to develop a scale to measure the severity of the altered tissue textures being palpated. Are the tissues normal or are there changes that could be identified as mild, moderate, or severe? A zero, 1+, 2+, and 3+

scale is useful in diagnosing the severity of the problem and in monitoring response to therapeutic intervention over time. Try to use descriptive language that a colleague can comprehend.

LAYER PALPATION

The following describes a practice session that is helpful in learning skill in layer palpation of the tissues of the musculoskeletal system. Two individuals sit across from each other with their arms placed on a narrow table (Fig. 2.2). Each individual's right hand is the examining instrument and the left forearm is the part for the partner to examine. Starting with the left palm on the table, each individual places the right hand (palms and fingers) over the forearm just distal to the elbow.

1. The right hand gently makes contact with the skin. No motion is introduced by the operator's right hand. The operator "thinks" skin. How thick or thin is it? How warm or cold is it? How rough or smooth is it? The left forearm is now supinated and the examiner's right hand is placed on the volar surface of the forearm in the same fashion. Again analysis of the skin is made and comparison made between the dorsal and volar aspects (Fig. 2.3). Which is the thickest? Which is the smoothest? Which is the warmest? It is interesting to note the ability to identify significant differences between skin of one area and another by concentration on skin alone.

2. With the right hand firmly in contact with the skin, slight movement of the skin is made, both longitudinally and horizontally, to evaluate the subcutaneous fascia. You now concentrate on the second layer, the subcutaneous

Figure 2.2.
Layer palpation dorsal forearm.

Figure 2.3.
Layer palpation volar forearm.

fascia. How thick is the layer? How loose is it? Note that with movement in one direction the tissues are more "loose" and in the other direction are more "tight." It is within this layer that many of the TTAs associated with somatic dysfunction are found.

3. Within the subcutaneous fascia layer are found the vessels, arteries, and veins. Palpate these structures for their identification and description.

4. Gently increase the pressure until you sense the deep fascia layer that envelops the underlying structures. Think deep fascia. It can be described as smooth, firm, and continuous. By palpating the deep fascia layer, and moving the hand gently horizontally across the forearm, you can identify areas of thickening that form fascial compartments between bundles of muscle. The ability to define these enveloping layers of deep fascia is helpful, not only in separating one muscle from another, but as a means of getting deeper into underlying structures between muscle.

5. Palpating through the deep fascia, you now concentrate on the underlying muscle and, through concentration, identify individual fibers and the direction in which the fibers run. Move your hands both transversely and longitudinally, sensing for smoothness or roughness. As you palpate across muscle fiber it seems rougher, but as you move in the direction of the muscle fiber it feels smoother. While palpating muscle, both individuals slowly open and close their left hands, energizing the muscles of the forearm. Your right hand is now palpating contracting and relaxing muscle. Next, squeeze

the left hand as hard as possible and palpate muscle during that activity. You are now palpating "hypertonic" muscle. This is the most common TTA feel at the muscle level in areas of somatic dysfunction.

6. While palpating at the muscle level, slowly course down the forearm until you first feel change in the tissue and the loss of ability to the discern muscle fiber. You have now contacted the musculotendinous junction, a point in muscle that is vulnerable to injury (Fig. 2.4).

7. Continue to course down toward the wrist, beyond the musculotendinous junction, and palpate a smooth, round, firm structure called a tendon. Note the transition from muscle through musculotendinous junction to tendon.

8. Follow the tendon distally until you palpate a structure that binds the tendons at the wrist. Palpate that structure (Fig. 2.5). It is the transverse carpal ligament. What are its characteristics? What direction do its fibers traverse? How thick is it? How firm is it? Ligaments throughout the body feel quite similar.

9. Now return your palpating right hand to the elbow with your middle finger overlying the dimple of the elbow in the dorsal side and your thumb opposite it on the ventral side to palpate the radial head (Fig. 2.6). Stay on bone, and think bone. How hard is it? Is there any "life" in it?

10. Now move just proximal with your palpating thumb and index finger until you fall into the joint space. Underlying your palpating fingers is a structure that you should not be able to feel, namely, the joint capsule. Palpable joint capsules are present in pathologic joints

Figure 2.4.
Palpation musculotendinous junction.

Figure 2.5.
Palpation transcarpal ligament.

Figure 2.6.
Palpation of radial head.

and are not usually found in somatic dysfunction. In fact, some individuals believe that a palpable joint capsule, with the limited exception of the knee joint, is a contraindication to direct-action manipulative treatment.

You have now palpated skin, subcutaneous fascia, blood vessels, deep fascia, muscle, musculotendinous junction, tendon, ligament, bone, and joint space. After using the forearm as the model, these same structures are palpable throughout the body. Practice and experience can enhance your capability as a structural diagnostician.

Development of high-level palpation skill requires considerable practice, which is accumulated over time if a concentrated effort is made. It is also important to avoid the three most common errors in palpation, namely lack of concentration, too much pressure, and too much movement. As stated previously, the most common error is the lack of concentration on the task. The beginner frequently attempts to gain information rapidly and presses much too hard. Remember, the harder you press, the more stimulation you provide to your own mechanoreceptors thus increasing the amount of sensory impulse being transmitted. The beginner is also prone to use too much movement in searching for anatomic landmarks and in identifying layers of tissue. This is referred to as the "jiggling hands syndrome." One must remember that the more motion exerted by the hands, the more stimulation there is in the afferent system to be transmitted and interpreted by the nervous system. Therefore, concentrate, do not push too hard, and do not move too much.

MOTION SENSE

In identifying areas of somatic dysfunction by defining alterations in the diagnostic triad of asymmetry, altered range of motion, and TTA, a combination of ob-

servation and palpation is used. In palpation, both static and dynamic dimensions are present. Statically, we look for levels of paired anatomic parts to identify asymmetry. By static and dynamic palpation, we look for alterations in TTA. In palpating tissues without movement, the examiner is interested in such things as skin temperature, smoothness, thickness, and other qualifiers of the state of the tissue. In dynamic palpation, one evaluates, by compression and shear movement within the tissue, the thickness of the tissue, the amount of normal tissue tone, and a sense of which tissues are abnormal. It is within the evaluation of the range of motion that the palpatory sense becomes highly refined. Because restoration of the maximal normal amount of motion possible in the tissue is the desired end point, it is essential that we be able to identify normal and abnormal ranges of motion within both soft tissue and arthrodial structures.

Motion sense is an essential component of the palpatory art in structural diagnosis. The examiner attempts to identify whether there is normal mobility, restricted movement (hypomobility), or too much movement (hypermobility). In motion testing, the examiner may put a region or part of the body through both active and passive movement to ascertain how that part complies with the motion demand placed on it. Information is sought as to whether the mobility is abnormal in a regional sense or confined to one segment. A wide variety of techniques can be used, both actively and passively, to test for motion.

The examiner must recognize that there is an inherent tissue motion that is continuous and palpable with practice. Return to the hand and forearm positions of Fig. 2.2 with very light contact. Close your eyes and concentrate on the behavior of the tissues under your palpating hand. With practice, you will note that the forearm is not static, but is inherently, dynamically moving. This inherent motion is thought to be a compilation of motions from transmission of the arterial pulse, effect of respiration, contraction and relaxation of muscle fibers during normal muscle tone, and the cranial rhythmic impulse.

It is essential that good contact be made with the examiner's hand(s) on the part(s) being palpated. As the part is taken through range of motion, either actively or passively, the examiner is interested in three elements, range of movement, quality of movement during the range, and "end feel." In determining range of movement, one is interested in the quantity of movement. Is it normal, restricted, or increased in range? Second, how does it feel during the movement throughout the range? Is it smooth? Is it "sticky" or "jerky" or "too loose"? There are a number of alterations in movement feel during the range that can be of assistance to the examiner in determining what factors might be altering the range of movement. Third, what is the feel at the end point of the range of movement? Is there symmetry to the range and does each extreme of the range of movement feel the same? If there is alteration in the end feel, what are the qualities of the end point? Is it hard? Is it soft? Is it spongy? Is it jerky? There are wide varieties of characteristic end feels that experience will teach the examiner. The quality of the end feel is most helpful in determining the cause of the restrictive movement and the type of manipulative therapy that might be most effective.

Hypermobility

Manual medicine procedures are used to overcome restrictions of movement. Techniques that increase mobility should not be used in the presence of hypermobility. Hypermobility is present when there is an increase in the range of movement, a loose feeling throughout the range of movement, and loss of normal tissue resiliency at the end feel. Hypermobility might be normal in certain highly trained athletes, such as gymnasts and acrobats, but in most individuals, it must be considered abnormal. In the vertebral complex, it is not uncommon to find relative hypermobility of one vertebral motion segment adjacent to a vertebral motion segment that is restricted. This has been described as "compensatory hypermobility" and has been explained as the body's attempt to maintain mobility of the total mechanism in the presence of restricted mobility of a part of the vertebral axis. It is common to find that hypermobile segments are the areas of symptomatology. As such, they gain a great deal of attention from the examiner. Care must be exercised not to provide manual medicine procedures that increase the relative hypermobility of these segments, rather than appropriately applying mobilizing techniques to the segment(s) with restricted mobility. Hypermobility can progress to the stage that can best be described as instability. Instability occurs when the integrity of the tissues supporting the joint structure cannot maintain appropriate functional apposition of the moving parts, thus, the relative stability of the motion unit is lost. The dividing line between hypermobility and instability is not always definite, and good objective measures to quantify instability are not available. Nonetheless, the skilled clinician must develop some sense of normal motion, hypomobility, hypermobility, and instability of anatomic structures within the musculoskeletal system. It is for this reason that the development of a motion sense is worth the effort.

One must also develop the skill of motion sense to identify change in the range of motion, quality of movement during a range, and the end feel after a manual medicine intervention. It is useful in prognosis as well as diagnosis. It should be possible to identify change in range of motion, and its quality, if a manual medicine intervention has been successful. Retesting the range of motion available is always the last step in any manual medicine therapeutic intervention.

Motion sense is an essential component of the palpatory art in structural diagnosis. As in any art form, practice is the major requirement for mastery.

SCREENING EXAMINATION

The screening examination evaluates the total musculoskeletal system as part of patient examination. It answers the question, "is there a problem within the musculoskeletal system that deserves additional evaluation?" There are numerous formats for a screening examination. The following 12-step procedure is comprehensive in scope and can be accomplished rapidly.

Step 1. Gait analysis in multiple directions
Step 2. Static posture and palpation of paired anatomic landmarks
Step 3. Dynamic trunk side bending
Step 4. Standing flexion test
Step 5. Stork test
Step 6. Seated flexion test
Step 7. Screening test of upper extremities
Step 8. Trunk rotation
Step 9. Trunk side bending
Step 10. Head and neck mobility
Step 11. Respiration of thoracic cage
Step 12. Lower extremity screening

Step 1. Gait Analysis

1. Observe gait with patient walking toward you (Fig. 2.7).

2. Observe patient walking away from you (Fig. 2.8).

3. Observe patient walking from the side (Figs. 2.9 and 2.10).

4. Observe length of stride, swing of arms, heel strike, toe off, tilting of the pelvis, and adaption of the shoulders.

5. One looks for the functional capacity of the gait, not the usual pathologic conditions. Of particular importance is the cross-patterning of the gait and symmetry of stride.

Figure 2.7.

Figure 2.9.

Figure 2.8.

Figure 2.10.

Step 2A. Static Analysis Posture

1. Observe from the front (Fig. 2.11), evaluating weight distribution, head carriage, shoulder level, and foot placement.

2. Observe from the back (Fig. 2.12), evaluating head carriage, shoulder height, level of pelvis, and weight distribution of the feet.

3. Observe from the side (Fig. 2.13), evaluating posture against the plumb line that drops from the external auditory meatus to the tip of the acromion through the femoral trochanter to just in front of the medial malleolus.

4. Observe from the opposite side (Fig. 2.14), again assess the plumb line and compare with the opposite side. Note head carriage, anteroposterior spinal curves, and extent of knee extension.

Figure 2.11.

Figure 2.12.

Figure 2.13.

Figure 2.14.

Step 2B. Static Posture Anatomic Levels

1. Combined palpation and observation is made of the levels of the acromion process (Fig. 2.15).

2. Palpation of the iliac crest (Fig. 2.16) is performed by pushing soft tissue out of the way from below and placing proximal phalanges of the index fingers on similar portions of the right and left hip bones.

3. Palpation and observation of the top of the greater trochanter require lateral-to-medial compression of the soft tissues of the lateral hip (Fig. 2.17).

4. Unleveling of the iliac crest and greater trochanter in the standing position is the first index of suspicion for a short-leg–pelvic-tilt syndrome.

5. Note that the eyes are on the same horizontal plane as the palpating fingers for better hand–eye coordination.

Figure 2.16.

Figure 2.15.

Figure 2.17.

Step 3. Trunk Sidebending

1. Observation is made from the back.

2. Patient is asked to sidebend left (Fig. 2.18) as far as possible without bending forward.

3. The patient repeats the sidebending to the right (Fig. 2.19), again without bending forward.

4. Observation is made of the symmetry of range right to left as a reflection of fingertip distance on the lateral leg.

5. Observation is made of the induced spinal curve, which should be a smooth symmetric C curve with fullness on the side of the induced convexity. Straightening of the segments of the induced curve and fullness on the side of the concavity are highly suggestive of significant vertebral motion segment dysfunction at that level.

6. Observation is made of the symmetry of the pelvic shift right to left during the side bending effort and whether the loading of the lower extremities appears symmetric.

Figure 2.18.

Figure 2.19.

Step 4. Standing Flexion Test

1. Patient stands with feet approximately 4 in. (10 cm) apart with weight under the hip joints (Fig. 2.20).

2. Operator palpates, with pads of the thumbs, the inferior slope of the posterior superior iliac spine.

3. Patient is instructed to bend forward as smoothly as possible, attempting to touch the floor (Fig. 2.21). Operator's thumbs follow the posterior superior iliac spines to see whether one appears to move more cephalward than the other.

4. The test is viewed as positive if one posterior superior iliac spine moves further cephalad or ventrally than the other does.

5. Observation is also made of the lower thoracic and lumbar spines for segmental rhythm and for the induction of side bending rotational curves.

6. This test is very sensitive to dysfunctions in the articulations of the bony pelvis and the fascias of the trunk and lower extremity. Its value is to lateralize dysfunction from one side to the other of the pelvis.

7. Repeating the standing flexion test beginning with the arms overhead (Fig. 2.22) and forward bending with the arms in that position (Fig. 2.23) alters the behavior of the pelvic girdle through loads from the fascias of the rib cage and upper extremity.

8. Different behavior of the posterior superior iliac spine in the two variations gives the examiner information as to whether major restrictors are above or below the pelvis.

Figure 2.20.

Figure 2.22.

Figure 2.21.

Figure 2.23.

Step 5. Stork Test

1. With the patient standing and the operator sitting behind, the operator's left thumb is placed over the most posterior portion of the left posterior superior iliac spine and the right thumb overlying the midline of the sacrum at the same level (Fig. 2.24).

2. Operator asks the patient to flex the left hip and knee to a minimum of 90 degrees of hip flexion (Fig. 2.25).

3. A negative test finds the left thumb on the posterior superior iliac spine moving caudad in relation to the right thumb on the sacrum.

4. The thumb placements are reversed, and the patient is asked to raise the right leg in similar fashion (Fig. 2.26).

5. A positive finding occurs when the thumb on the posterior superior iliac spine moves cephalad in relation to the thumb on the sacrum.

6. The findings of this test are correlated with those of the standing flexion test. The stork test is more specific for sacroiliac joint restriction.

7. If the patient has difficulty standing on one foot to perform the test, proprioceptive sensory motor balance deficit should be further evaluated.

Figure 2.25.

Figure 2.24.

Figure 2.26.

Step 6. Seated Flexion Test

1. Patient sitting on examining stool with knees apart and feet flat on the floor.

2. Operator's two thumbs contact the inferior slope of each posterior superior iliac spine (Fig. 2.27).

3. Patient is instructed to bend forward with the arms between the knees as far as possible (Fig. 2.28).

4. Operator monitors the movement of the two posterior superior iliac spines (Fig. 2.29). The one that moves the furthest in a cephalad or ventral direction is deemed positive, indicative of restricted mobility of that side of the pelvis.

5. Operator observes the behavior of the lower thoracic and lumbar spines for dysrhythmia and for the introduction of side bending and rotational curves.

6. Comparison of findings with those of a standing flexion test evaluates the behavior of the pelvic girdle and vertebral complex without the influence of the lower extremities as the patient is sitting on the ischial tuberosity.

7. Unleveling of the iliac crest when seated to perform this test is presumptive evidence of inequality in size of the right and left hip bones.

Figure 2.28.

Figure 2.27.

Figure 2.29.

Step 7. Upper Extremity Screen

1. Patient seated on examining stool or table.

2. Patient instructed to fully abduct both upper extremities in the coronal plane, reach to the ceiling, and turn the backs of the hands together (Fig. 2.30).

3. Observation is made from the front.

4. Observation is also made from behind (Fig. 2.31).

5. This maneuver requires mobility of the sternoclavicular, acromioclavicular, glenohumeral, elbow, and wrist joints.

6. Any asymmetry indicates the need for additional evaluation.

Figure 2.30.

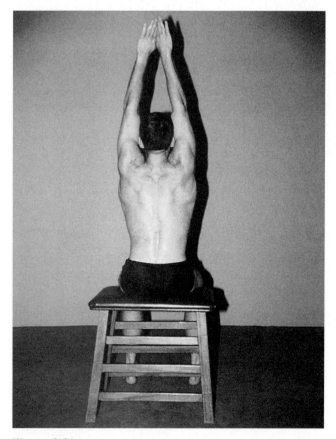

Figure 2.31.

Step 8. Trunk Rotation

1. Patient sitting on table with operator standing behind.

2. Operator grasps each shoulder (Fig. 2.32).

3. Operator introduces trunk rotation through the shoulders (Fig. 2.33) sensing for range, quality of movement, and end feel.

4. Operator rotates trunk to the left (Fig. 2.34) comparing range, quality of movement, and end feel with those of right rotation.

5. Asymmetry of right-to-left rotation indicates additional diagnostic procedures for the vertebral column and rib cage.

Figure 2.33.

Figure 2.32.

Figure 2.34.

Step 9. Trunk Side Bending

1. Patient sitting with operator behind.

2. Operator grasps each shoulder (Fig. 2.35).

3. Operator presses downward on right shoulder with the right hand, introducing right-side bending (Fig. 2.36) sensing for range, quality of movement, and end feel.

4. Operator pushes left shoulder inferiorly to introduce left-side bending (Fig. 2.37), sensing for range, quality of movement, and end feel.

5. Comparison is made of left- and right-side bending for symmetry or asymmetry. Asymmetry demonstrates need for additional diagnostic evaluation of the vertebral column and the rib cage.

Figure 2.36.

Figure 2.35.

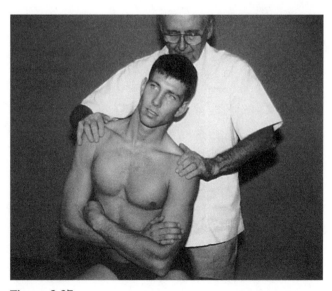

Figure 2.37.

Step 10. Mobility of the Head and Neck

1. Patient sitting on the table with the operator standing behind.

2. Operator grasps head between the two hands (Fig. 2.38).

3. Operator introduces backward bending (Fig. 2.39). Normal extension is 90 degrees.

4. Operator introduces forward bending (Fig. 2.40). Normal range is 45 degrees of flexion.

Figure 2.39.

Figure 2.38.

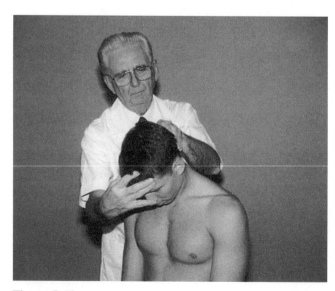

Figure 2.40.

5. Operator introduces right side bending (Fig. 2.41) and left side bending (Fig. 2.42). Normal range is 45 degrees to each side.

6. Operator introduces rotation to the left (Fig. 2.43) and to the right (Fig. 2.44). Normal range is 80 to 90 degrees on each side.

7. Operator evaluates range, quality of movement during the range, and end feel, looking for symmetry or asymmetry. If asymmetric, additional diagnostic evaluations of the cervical spine, upper thoracic spine, and rib cage are necessary.

Figure 2.41.

Figure 2.43.

Figure 2.42.

Figure 2.44.

Step 11. Respiratory Movement of Thoracic Cage

1. Patient supine on the table with operator standing at side with dominant eye over the midline of the patient.

2. Operator symmetrically places hands over the anterolateral aspect of the lower rib cage bilaterally (Fig. 2.45).

3. Patient is instructed to deeply inhale and exhale while operator follows lower thoracic cage movement during respiration, looking for symmetry or lack of it.

4. Operator places hands in intercostal spaces of the anterolateral aspect of the upper rib cage (Fig. 2.46) to evaluate bucket-handle movement of the upper ribs during inhalation and exhalation.

5. Operator's hand are placed vertically over anterior aspect of the upper rib cage with the longest finger in contact with the cartilage of the first rib under the medial end of the clavicle (Fig. 2.47) and assesses pump handle motion response of the upper ribs to inhalation and exhalation.

6. Asymmetry of movement of inhalation and exhalation effort calls for more definitive diagnosis of the thoracic spine and rib cage.

Figure 2.45.

Figure 2.46.

Figure 2.47.

Step 12. Lower Extremity Screen

1. Patient supine on table with operator standing at side.

2. Operator grasps left ankle, monitoring the right anterior superior iliac spine (Fig. 2.48).

3. Operator lifts left leg until first movement of the right anterior superior iliac spine is felt, indicative of length of the hamstring muscle group (Fig. 2.49).

4. Comparison is made with the opposite side for symmetry or asymmetry.

Figure 2.48.

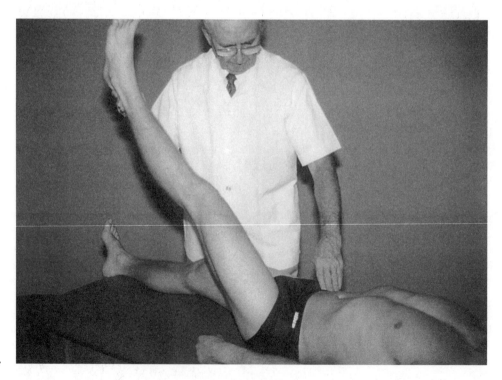

Figure 2.49.

5. Operator flexes, externally rotates, and abducts the patient's right hip (Fig. 2.50). Comparison is made with the opposite side for symmetry or asymmetry. Restricted motion suggests dysfunction and pathology of the right hip joint.

6. Patient is instructed to do a deep knee bend, maintaining the heels on the floor (Fig. 2.51). This squat test requires mobility of the foot, ankle, knee, and hip joints bilaterally. Inability to perform the squat test indicates additional diagnostic evaluation of the lower extremities.

Figure 2.50.

Figure 2.51.

SCANNING EXAMINATION

Once an area of the musculoskeletal system has been identified during the screening examination as being of sufficient abnormality for further investigation, a scanning procedure of that region is initiated. The scanning examination is designed to answer the following questions: What part of the region, and what tissues within the region, are significantly dysfunctional? The object is to locate the areas that might account for the abnormal finding. By using the analogy of a microscope, we have gone from low power (the screening examination) to high power (scanning examination). More definitive evaluation of soft tissue can be accomplished with active and passive light and deep touch. Thumbs or fingers can be used as a pressure probe searching for areas of tenderness or more specific signs of tissue texture change. Multiple variations of motion scanning can be introduced to look for alterations in symmetry of range, quality of movement, and sensations at end feel. Respiratory effort might be used to evaluate the response of the region to inhalation and exhalation efforts. Responses within the region to demands placed on it from more remote areas of the musculoskeletal system are frequently useful in better defining the area requiring specific attention.

SKIN ROLLING TEST

One valuable diagnostic test for scanning procedures is the skin-rolling test. In this examination, a fold of skin is grasped between the thumb and index finger and rolled as if one were rolling a cigarette (Fig. 2.52). Skin rolling can be accomplished symmetrically on each side of the body, testing for normal pain-free laxity of the skin and subcutaneous fascia. A positive finding is tenderness and pain provocation in certain dermatomal levels of skin, with tightness and loss of resiliency within the skin and subcutaneous fascia. Frequently, tender nodules will be palpated while accomplishing this test. They are interpreted to represent alteration in dermatomal innervation from dysfunctions within the vertebral axis. In the examination of the thoracic and lumbar regions of the spine, it is recommended that the skin be rolled in the midline overlying the spinous processes and, more laterally, coursing from below upward, comparing changes on one side to the other. Although defined as a scanning procedure, skin rolling can be quite specific in defining specific segmental dysfunction because of the clinically observable dermatomal relationship to altered vertebral motion segment function.

SEGMENTAL DEFINITION

The third element to the diagnostic process is segmental definition, used to identify the specific vertebral motion segment, or peripheral joint, that is dysfunctional. It is also used to determine the specific motion restriction that is involved. An attempt is made to identify the tissue(s) that are most involved in the dysfunctional segment.

One method of identifying the specific joint that is dysfunctional, and the motion that is lost, is to test for joint-play movements. Mennell has advocated this concept for many years. Joint-play movements are defined as being independent of the action of voluntary muscle and are found within synovial joints. The range of joint play is very small but very precise. Normal joint-play movement allows for easy, painless performance of voluntary movement. The amount of joint play is usually less than one eighth of an inch in any one plane within a synovial joint. Mennell defines joint dysfunction as the loss of joint-play movement that cannot be recovered by the action of voluntary muscles. Once the precise system for identifying joint play is learned, very similar maneuvers can be used therapeutically in restoring anatomic and physiologic function to the joint by reestablishing its normal joint play.

Numerous diagnostic procedures can specifically define, within the vertebral motion segment or the synovial extremity joint, the specific dysfunction that is present. Subsequent chapters will describe the methods most commonly used by this author. The primary goal is to determine which vertebral motion segment is dysfunctional, which joint within that vertebral motion segment is dysfunctional, the direction of altered motion(s), and some estimate of the tissue involved in the restricted motion. Primary emphasis is placed on motion loss and its characteristics. Many diagnostic systems depend upon localization of pain or provocation of

Figure 2.52.
Skin rolling.

pain by certain motion introductions. In the opinion of this author, motion loss and its characteristics are more valuable diagnostic criteria than the presence of pain and the provocation of pain by movement. Pain and its provocation can be of assistance in diagnosis, but they are not diagnostic in and of themselves.

These principles of structural diagnosis need to be studied extensively and mastered by the physician who wishes to be skilled in the field of manual medicine. An accurate and specific diagnosis is essential for successful results from manual medicine therapeutic interventions.

SUGGESTED READINGS

Dvorak J, Dvorak V. *Manual medicine, diagnostics.* New York: Thieme-Stratton, 1983.

Dvorak J, Dvorak V, Schneider W, eds. *Manual medicine 1984.* New York: Springer-Verlag, 1984.

Farfan HF. The scientific basis of manipulative procedures. *Clin Rheum Dis* 1980;6:159–178.

Fisk JW. *The painful neck and back.* Springfield, IL: Charles C Thomas Publisher, 1977.

Greenman PE. Layer palpation. *Mich Osteopath J* 1982;47:936–937.

Mennell J McM. *Joint Pain,* Boston: Little Brown & Co, 1964.

Ward RC, Sprafka S. Glossary of osteopathic terminology. *J Am Osteopath Assoc* 1981;80:552–567.

The Glossary Review Committee of the Educational Council on Osteopathic Principles in Allen TW ed. AOA yearbook and Directory of Osteopathic Physicians. Chicago, Illinois AOA, 1993.

3

BARRIER CONCEPTS IN STRUCTURAL DIAGNOSIS

Within the diagnostic triad of asymmetry, range of motion abnormality, and tissue texture abnormality, perhaps the most significant is alteration in the range of joint and tissue movement. Loss of normal motion within the tissues of the musculoskeletal system, or one of its component parts, responds most favorably to appropriate manual medicine therapeutic intervention. To achieve the goal of manual medicine intervention and restore maximal, pain-free movement to a musculoskeletal system in postural balance, we must be able to identify both normal and abnormal movements. In the presence of altered movement of the hypomobility type, an appropriate manual medicine intervention might be the treatment of choice. We must strive to improve mobility of all of the tissues of the musculoskeletal system, bone, joint, muscle, ligament, fascia, and fluid, with the anticipated outcome of restoring normal physiologic movement and maximum functional physiology as well.

In the musculoskeletal system, there are inherent movements, voluntary movements, and involuntary movements. The inherent movement has been described by some authors as relating to the recurrent coiling and uncoiling of the brain and longitudinal movement of the spinal cord, together with a fluctuation of the cerebral spinal fluid. Inherent motion is also the movement of the musculoskeletal system in relation to respiration. It has been observed that during inhalation the curves within the vertebral column straighten and with exhalation the curves are increased. With inhalation the extremities rotate externally, and with exhalation, internally. The voluntary movements of the musculoskeletal system are active movements resulting from contraction of muscle from voluntary conscious control. The involuntary movements of the musculoskeletal system are described as passive movements. An external force moving a part of the musculoskeletal system through an arc of motion induces passive movement. The joint-play movements described by Mennell are also involuntary movements. They are not a component of the normal active or passive range of movement but are essential for the accomplishment of normal active and passive movement.

In structural diagnosis, we speak of normal and abnormal barriers to joint and tissue motion. The examiner must be able to identify and characterize normal and abnormal range of movement and normal and abnormal barrier to movement in order to make an accurate diagnosis. Most joints have motion in multiple planes, but for descriptive purposes we describe barriers to movement within one plane of motion for one joint. The total range of motion (Fig. 3.1) from one extreme to the other is limited by the anatomic integrity of the joint and its supporting ligaments, muscles, and fascia. Exceeding the anatomic barrier causes fracture, dislocation, or violation of tissue such as ligamentous tear. Somewhere within the total range of movement is found a midline neutral point.

Within the total range of motion there is a range of passive movement available that the examiner can extraneously introduce (Fig. 3.2). The limit of this passive range of motion has been described as the elastic barrier. At this point, all tension has been taken within the joint and its surrounding tissues. There is a small amount of potential space between the elastic barrier and the anatomic barrier described by Sandoz as the paraphysiologic space. It is within this area that the high-velocity, low-amplitude thrust appears to generate the popping sound that results from the maneuver.

The range of active movement (Fig. 3.3) is somewhat less than that available with passive movement, and the end point of the range is called the "physiologic barrier." The normal end feel is due to resilience and tension within the muscle and fascial elements.

Frequently there is reduction in available active motion due primarily to myofascial shortening (Fig. 3.4). This is often seen with aging but it can occur at all ages. It is the stretching of this myofascial shortening that all individuals, particularly athletes, should do as part of physical exercise. Stretching exercise to the muscles and fascia enhances the active motion range available and the efficiency of myofascial function.

When motion is lost within the range it can be described as major (Fig. 3.5) or minimal (Fig. 3.6). The barrier that prevents movement in the direction of

Figure 3.1.
Total range of motion.

Figure 3.2.
Range of passive movement.

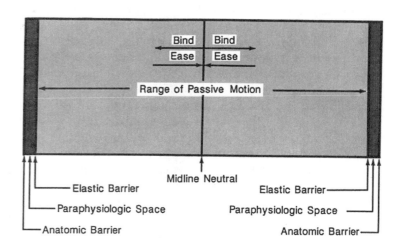

Figure 3.3.
Range of active movement.

motion loss is defined as the restrictive barrier. The amount of active motion available is limited on one side by the normal physiologic barrier and on the opposite side by the restrictive barrier. The goal of a manual medicine intervention is to move the restrictive barrier as far into the direction of motion loss as possible. Another clinically describable phenomenon associated with motion loss is the shifting of the neutral point from midline to the middle of the available

active range. This is described as the "pathologic" neutral and is usually, but not always, in the midrange of active motion available.

Each of the barriers described have palpable findings that can be described as either normal or abnormal end feel. Within a normal range of passive movement, the elastic barrier will have a normal sensation at the end point as a result of the passively induced tension within the joint and its surrounding struc-

Figure 3.4.
Reduced range from myofascial shortening.

Figure 3.5.
Major motion loss.

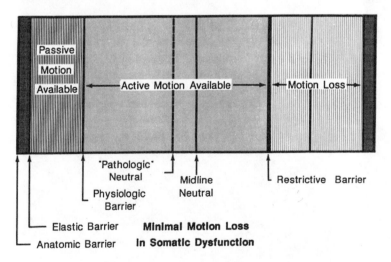

Figure 3.6.
Minimal motion loss.

tures. At the end of the range of active movement, the physiologic barrier likewise has a characteristic feel that results from the voluntary increase in resistance due to the apposition of the joints and the myofascial tension developed during voluntary muscular activity.

Let us return to the layer palpation exercise (see Chapter 2) and begin at the point where one exam-

iner was evaluating the joint space at the proximal radiohumeral joint (Fig. 3.7). While palpating this joint with the thumb placed anteriorly and the index finger placed posteriorly, have the subject actively introduce pronation and supination (Fig. 3.8). You will note that the range is not symmetric in pronation and supination and that the end feel is not the same at the terminal range of pronation and supination. Which range is greater? Which end feel seems tighter? Now grasp the subject's hand and wrist and passively introduce pronation and supination while monitoring at the proximal radiohumeral joint (Fig. 3.9). Note that you are now receiving proprioceptive impulse from your palpating hand at the radiohumeral joint, as well as from your hand as it passively introduces, through the subject's hand and wrist, the pronation and supination effort (Fig. 3.10). Again, look for total range of movement, the quality of movement during the range, and the end feel. In supination and pronation, which has the greatest range? Which has the tighter or looser end feel? How does this compare with the active movement? Now let us take it one step further. While passively introducing pronation and supination you should notice that tension increases

the closer you get to the end points of the range. As you move in the opposite direction, it appears to be easier or freer. See if you can, by decreasing increments of pronation and supination, find the point between the two extremes of movement wherein the joint feel is the freest. Even though pronation and supination are not a symmetric range of movement at this joint, it is possible to find a point within the range that is the freest and could be described as the physiologic neutral point.

We now have another concept of joint motion, the concept of "ease" and "bind" (Fig. 3.11). The more one moves in the direction of the neutral point, whether a midline neutral point in a normal range of motion or a "pathologic" neutral point somewhere within the range of altered motion, it becomes more free, or there is more "ease." Conversely, as one moves

Figure 3.7.
Palpate radiohumeral joint.

Figure 3.9.
Passive pronation–supination.

Figure 3.8.
Active pronation–supination.

Figure 3.10.
Sensing hand of pronation–supination.

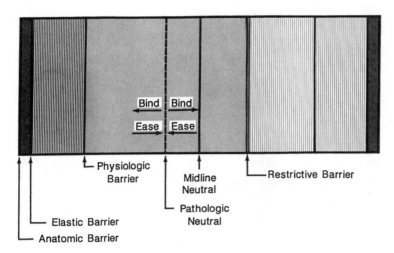

Physiologic
Barrier

Midline
Neutral

Restrictive Barrier

Pathologic
Neutral

Elastic Barrier

Anatomic Barrier

Figure 3.11.
Neutral ease–bind point.

away from the neutral "free" point, one begins to sense a certain amount of "bind," or increase in resistance to the induced movement. Understanding this concept of ease and bind, and the ability to sense this phenomenon, is essential to mastering the functional (indirect) techniques (see Chapter 10). In the elbow exercise that you just accomplished, the hand palpating over the proximal radiohumeral joint was the "sensing hand," and your other hand that introduced passive supination and pronation at the subject's hand was the "motor hand."

RESTRICTIVE BARRIERS

The restrictive barriers limit movement within the normal range of motion and have palpatory characteristics different from the normal physiologic, elastic, and anatomic barriers. The restrictive barrier can be within the following tissues:

> Skin
> Fascia
> Muscle, long and short
> Ligament
> Joint capsule and surfaces

Restrictive barriers can be found within one or more of these tissues and the number and type contribute to the palpable characteristics at the restrictive barrier. Different pathologic changes within these tissues can give quite different end feel sensations. For example, congestion and edema within the tissues will give a diffuse, boggy sensation quite like a sponge filled with water. Chronic fibrosis within these tissues will give a harder, more unyielding, rapidly ascending end feel when compared to the more boggy, edematous sensation. A restrictive barrier due to altered muscle physiology, whether it be spasm, hypertonus, or contracture, will give a more jerky and tightening type of end feel than one due to edema or fibrosis. Do not forget that pain can be a restrictive barrier as well. If a movement is

painful, it will result in restriction as the body attempts to compensate for relief of pain by reduction of movement. When examining ranges of movement, and particularly when looking for normal and abnormal barriers to movement, one should constantly keep in mind the potential for hypermobility. The classic feel of a hypermobile range of motion is one of looseness for a greater extent of the range than would be anticipated, and with a rapidly escalating, hard end feel when one approaches the elastic and anatomic barriers.

Restrictive barriers may be long or short. They may involve a single joint or spinal segment, or cross over more than one joint or series of spinal segments. It is important to identify the tissue or tissues involved in the restrictive barrier, their extent, and the functional pathology found within the tissues. Some types of manual medicine intervention are more appropriate for certain restrictive barriers than others.

In structural diagnosis, alteration of range of movement is an essential criterion for a diagnosis of somatic dysfunction. It is necessary to evaluate the total range of movement, the quality of movement available during the range, and the feel at the end point of movement in order to make an accurate diagnosis of the restrictive barrier. Therapeutic intervention by manipulative means can be described as an approach to these pathologic barriers. Multiple methods are available and different activating forces can be used toward the goal of restoring maximal physiologic movement available within the anatomy of the joint(s) and tissue(s).

DEFINITIONS

1. *Active motion:* Movement of an articulation between the physiologic barriers limited to the range produced voluntarily by the patient.
2. *Anatomic barrier:* The bone contour and/or soft tissues, especially ligaments, which serve as the final limit to motion in an articulation beyond which tissue damage occurs.

3. *Barrier.* An obstruction; a factor that tends to restrict free movement.
4. *Elastic barrier.* The resistance felt at the end of passive range of motion when the slack has been taken out.
5. *Motion:* Movement, act, process, or instance of changing places.
6. *Paraphysiologic space.* The sensation of a sudden "give" beyond the elastic barrier of resistance, usually accompanied by a "cracking" sound with a slight amount of movement beyond the usual physiologic limit but within the anatomic barrier.
7. *Passive motion:* Movement induced in an articulation by the operator. This includes the range of active motion as well as the movement between the physiologic and anatomic barriers permitted by soft-tissue resiliency that the patient cannot do voluntarily.

8. *Physiologic barrier.* The soft-tissue tension accumulation that limits the voluntary motion of an articulation. Further motion toward the anatomic barrier can be induced passively.
9. *Restrictive barrier.* An impediment or obstacle to movement within the physiologic limits of an articulation that reduces the active motion range.

SUGGESTED READINGS

Beal MC. Motion sense. *J Am Osteopath Assoc* 1953;53:151–153.

Good AB. Spinal joint blocking. *J Manipulative Physio Therapy* 1985;8:1–8.

Sandoz, R. Some Physical Mechanisms and effects of Spinal Adjustments. *Ann Swiss Chiro Assoc.* 6:91–141, 1976.

4

THE MANIPULATIVE PRESCRIPTION

In the practice of medicine, it is essential that an accurate diagnosis be made before the institution of either curative or palliative therapy. When a therapeutic intervention is indicated, particularly when using pharmacotherapeutic agents, a specific and accurate prescription must be written. No self-respecting physician would make a diagnosis of throat infection and write a prescription for an antibiotic.

Diagnosis (DX)—Throat infection
Prescription (RX)—Antibiotic

The physician would seek to identify the infectious agent, either bacterial or viral, causing the throat infection. When a specific infectious agent responsive to antibiotic therapy was identified, a specific prescription would be written for the antibiotic agent. A prescription would identify the antibiotic to be used, the strength of each dose, the number of doses per day, and the duration of therapy.

In manual medicine it is common for practitioners to be lax in their specificity for the structural diagnosis and prescription of the manual medicine intervention to be applied. Too often, a diagnosis is made of somatic dysfunction and manual medicine is the prescription, such as:

DX—Somatic dysfunction
RX—Manipulative treatment

In manual medicine, it is just as important to know the location, nature, and type of somatic dysfunction before a specific manual medicine therapeutic intervention is prescribed. The same elements are needed for a manual medicine prescription as for a pharmaceutical agent. One wants to be specific about the type of manual medicine, the intensity, the frequency, and the total length of the treatment plan. Therefore, the manipulative prescription requires an accurate diagnosis of the somatic dysfunction to be treated and a specific description of the type of manipulative procedure, the intensity, and the frequency.

Manipulative therapeutic procedures are indicated for the diagnostic entity somatic dysfunction or the manipulable lesion.

SOMATIC DYSFUNCTION

Somatic dysfunction is impaired or altered function of related components of the somatic (body framework) system: skeletal, arthrodial, and myofascial structures, and the related vascular, lymphatic, and neural elements.

MANIPULABLE LESION SYNONYMS

- Joint blockage
- Joint lock
- Chiropractic subluxation
- Osteopathic lesion
- Loss of joint play
- Minor intervertebral derangements

DIAGNOSTIC TRIAD

In defining somatic dysfunction, one uses three elements:

A for asymmetry of form or function of related parts of the musculoskeletal system.
R for range of motion, primarily alteration of motion, looking at range, quality of motion during the range, and the "end feel" at the limit of movement.
T for tissue texture abnormality with alteration in the feel of the soft tissues, mainly muscle hypertonicity, and in skin and connective tissues, described as hot/cold, soft/hard, boggy, doughy, and so forth. Most of the tissue texture abnormalities result from altered nervous system function with increased alpha motor neuron activity maintaining muscle hypertonicity and altered sympathetic autonomic nervous system function to the skin viscera, vasomotor, pseudomotor, and pilomotor activity.

CLINICAL GOALS FOR MANIPULATIVE TREATMENT

As previously stated, the goal of manipulation is the use of the hands in a patient-management process using instructions and maneuvers to achieve maximal, painless, movement of the musculoskeletal (motor) system in postural balance. In achieving this goal, different types of therapeutic effects upon the patient can be sought. They can be classified as follows:

1. Circulatory effects
   A. Move body fluids
   B. Provide tonic effect
2. Neurologic effect—modify reflexes
   A. Somato-somatic
   B. Somato-visceral
   C. Viscero-somatic
   D. Viscero-visceral
   E. Viscero-somato-visceral
   F. Somato-viscero-somatic
3. Maintenance therapy for irreversible conditions

Depending on the desired outcome, the therapeutic application will use different models of manual medicine.

MODELS AND MECHANISMS OF MANUAL MEDICINE INTERVENTION

Several different conceptual models can be used in determining the manual medicine approach to a patient. Five such models will be described, but it should be evident that when a manual medicine procedure is provided, it has multiple effects and is mediated through a number of different mechanisms.

Postural Structural or Biomechanical Model

The postural structural model is probably the one most familiar to practitioners of manual medicine. In this model, the patient is approached from a biomechanical orientation toward the musculoskeletal system. The osseous skeleton is viewed as a series of building blocks piled one on top of the other, starting with the bones of the foot and ending with the skull. The ligamentous and fascial structures are the tissues that connect the osseous framework, and the muscles are the prime movers of the bones of the skeleton, working across single and multiple joint structures. Alteration of the patient's musculoskeletal system is viewed from the alignment of the bones and joints, the balance of muscles as movers and stabilizers of the skeleton, the symmetry of tone of the ligaments, and the integrity of the continuous bands of fascia throughout. Alteration in joint apposition, alteration in muscle function due to hypertonicity or weakness, tightness or laxity of ligament(s), and shortening or lengthening of fascia are all considered when approaching a patient from this perspective. The manual medicine treatment would be directed toward restoring maximal motion to all joints, symmetry of length and strength to all muscles and ligaments, and symmetry of tension within fascial elements throughout the body. The goal is to restore maximal function

of this musculoskeletal system in postural balance. The patient can be approached starting at the feet and ending with the head, or vice versa, starting from the top and ending at the feet.

The most important element of the postural structural model in this author's experience has been the restoration of maximum pelvic mechanics in the walking cycle. The pelvis becomes the cornerstone of the postural structural model. Influences from below or above must be considered to achieve symmetric movement of the osseous pelvis during walking.

This model is most useful in approaching patients with pain resulting from either single instances of trauma or microtrauma over time due to postural imbalance from such entities as anatomic shortening of one leg, unilateral fallen arch, and so forth. This conceptual model includes much of the current biomechanical engineering research in the areas of joint mechanics; properties of ligaments, tendons, and fascia; and kinetics and kinematics.

Neurologic Model

The neurologic model concerns influencing neural mechanisms through manual medicine intervention. One mechanism of action is through the autonomic nervous system. There is a large body of basic research regarding the influence of the somatic (motor) system on the function of the autonomic nervous system, primarily the sympathetic division. This basic research is consistent with clinical observations, but additional clinical research is needed into the influence of alteration in function of the musculoskeletal system on total body function mediated through the sympathetic division of the autonomic nervous system.

Autonomic Nervous System Model The concept is based on the organization of the sympathetic nervous system. The preganglionic fibers take their origin from the spinal cord from T-1 to L-3. The lateral chain ganglia are paired and overlie the posterior thoracic and abdominal walls, where synaptic junction occurs with postganglionic fibers. The lateral chain ganglia in the thoracic region are tightly bound by the fascia to the posterior chest wall and overlie the heads of the ribs. It is hypothesized that altered mechanics of the costovertebral articulations could mechanically influence the lateral chain ganglia. There are peripheral ganglia through which the sympathetic nervous system synapses with postganglionic fibers that are relatively adjacent to the organs being innervated.

The sympathetic nervous system is the sole source of autonomic nervous system activity to the musculoskeletal system. There is no parasympathetic innervation to the somatic tissues. The sympathetic nervous system has wide influence on visceral function, endocrine organs, reticuloendothelial system, circulatory system, peripheral nervous system, central nervous system, and muscle. Korr has worked extensively on the function of the sympathetic nervous system and points out the wide diversity of influence that sympathetic hyperactivity has on target end organs. Many factors can affect sympathetic hypertonia, one of which is afferent impulses from segmentally related areas of soma. It would seem reasonable, therefore, to attempt to reduce aberrant afferent stimulus to hyperirritable sections of the sympathetic nervous system to reduce the hyperactivity on target end organs.

Because the sympathetic nervous system is organized segmentally, it can be used in a maplike fashion to look for both alterations of afferent stimulus, and areas that might be influenced through manual medicine intervention. All of the viscera and soma above the diaphragm receive their preganglionic sympathetic nervous system fibers from above cord level T-4. All visceral and soma below the diaphragm receive preganglionic sympathetic nervous system fibers from T-5 and below. Understanding this anatomy helps in relating identified somatic dysfunction to the patient's problem and can lead the physician to give appropriate manual medicine treatment to those areas of somatic dysfunction thought to contribute increased somatic afferent stimuli to cord levels with manifestations of increased sympathetic nervous system activity.

The parasympathetic nervous system takes its origin from the brain, brainstem, and sacral segments of the cord. Its organization differs from the segmental aspects of the sympathetic division, but its segmentation relates to the origin of the cranial nerves in the brainstem and the segmentation of the sacral cord. The cranial nerves, including those with parasympathetic activity, exit from the skull through numerous foramina and penetrate the dura. These nerves are at risk for entrapment with alteration of cranial mechanics and dural tension. Often, the clinical goal of craniosacral technique is to improve the function of cranial nerves as they exit the skull and sacrum. The autonomic nervous system neurologic model leads the therapist toward a patient approach based on the anatomy/physiology of the two divisions of the autonomic nervous system and how best to affect them through manual medicine means.

Pain Model A second neurologic model focuses more on the interrelationships of the peripheral and central nervous systems, their reflex patterns, and their multiple pathways. This model is particularly useful in managing patients with pain syndromes, such as back pain. Although controversy remains about the origin of back pain, much is known about the location and type of nociceptors and mechanoreceptors within the musculoskeletal system. The pain stimulus can originate in a number of tissues and be transmitted by peripheral afferent neurons to the spinal cord for integration and organization. Different neurons end in different laminae of the dorsal horn and synapse with interneurons that transmit information up and down the spinal cord, thus affecting other neuronal pools through propriospinal pathways. Transmission up the cord to higher centers can be through the fast or slow pain pathways. Pain is perceived in the brain and stimulatory or inhibitory activities can enhance or reduce the pain perception. These processes are programmed through the brainstem and back down the cord to modulate activity at cord segmental level.

An understanding of the anatomy and physiology of the musculoskeletal system and nervous systems, particularly the spine and paraspinal tissues, is necessary to develop a therapeutic plan to manage the patient's pain syndrome. A clear distinction must be made between acute pain and chronic pain. Acute pain is that which is best known to the clinician. It results from tissue damage, is well localized, has clear objective evidence of injury, and has a sharp pricking quality. There may be some lingering burning and aching. Acute pain responds well to treatment and abates when the tissue damage has resolved. Chronic pain persists despite the lack of ongoing tissue damage. It is poorly localized with no objective evidence present. It has a burning aching quality with a strong associated affective component. Changes have occurred in the central pathways and central endogenous control. It is unclear as to when chronic pain begins, but it is generally accepted that ongoing pain beyond three months results in central pathway changes. Acute and chronic pains respond differently to therapeutic interventions. Manual medicine has a role in the treatment of both acute and chronic musculoskeletal pain syndromes. In the acute condition, manual medicine attempts to reduce the ongoing afferent stimulation of the nociceptive process. If it is determined that muscle contraction and hypertonicity are primary factors, muscle energy procedures might be most beneficial. If it is believed that altered mechanoreceptive behavior in the articular and periarticular structure of the zygapophyseal joint is the primary factor, a mobilizing procedure with or without impulse might be more appropriate. The goal of manual medicine in the patient with chronic pain is to restore the maximum functional capacity of the musculoskeletal system so that exercises and increased activities of daily living can occur. It is difficult for a patient with chronic pain to undergo exercise therapy and reconditioning rehabilitative processes in the presence of restricted mobility of the musculoskeletal system.

Neuroendocrine Model The third concept within the neurologic model is that of neuroendocrine control. Since the late 1970s, there has been a rapidly expanding body of knowledge about the role of endorphins, enkephalins, and other neural peptides. These substances are not only active in the nervous system but also profoundly affect the immune system. There appears to be ample evidence that alteration in musculoskeletal activity influences their liberation and activity. It has been hypothesized that some of the beneficial effects of manipulative treatment might result from the release of endorphins and enkephalins with subsequent reduction in the perception of pain. Because of the influence of the substances in areas other than the central nervous system, other systemic effects may result from manual medicine procedures. This neuroendocrine mechanism might explain some of the general body tonic effects of manual medicine interventions.

All of these neurologic mechanisms are highly complex and have been only superficially dealt with here. They can be used, however, as conceptual models to approach a patient with a myriad of problems.

Respiratory Circulatory Model

The respiratory circulatory model looks at a different dimension of musculoskeletal system activity. In this model, the patient is viewed from the perspective of blood and lymph flow. Skeletal muscles and the diaphragm are the pumps of the venous and lymphatic systems. The goal is restoring the functional capacity of the musculoskeletal system to assist return circulation and the work of respiration. The function of the diaphragm to modify the relative negative intrathoracic pressure to assist in inhalation and exhalation requires that the torso, including the thoracic cage and the abdomen, have the capacity to respond to these pressure gradient changes. Thus the thoracic spine and the rib cage must be functionally flexible, particularly the lower six ribs where the diaphragm attaches. The lumbar spine must be flexible enough to change its anterior curvature for breathing. The abdominal musculature should have symmetric tone and length and the pelvic diaphragm should be balanced and nonrestrictive.

The respiratory circulatory model looks at somatic dysfunction(s) and its influence on fluid movement and ease of respiration, rather than neural entrapment or biomechanical alteration. Thus, some of the techniques applied are less segmentally specific and are more concerned with tissue tension that might impede fluid flow. The guiding principle of this model is the progression from central to distal. The beginning point is usually in the thoracic cage, primarily at the thoracic inlet, so that the tissues of the thoracic cage are able to respond to respiratory effort and the pumping action of the diaphragm to receive the fluids trapped in the peripheral tissues. Attention to the thoracic inlet also aids in the drainage of fluid from the head, neck, and upper extremities. Recall that all of the lymph ultimately drains into the venous system at the thoracic inlet behind the anterior extremity of the

first rib and the medial end of the clavicle. When the thoracic cage is functioning at maximal capacity, one progresses to the lumbar spine, pelvis, and lower extremities attempting to remove any potential obstruction to fluid flow that occurs in these tissues. The therapeutic goals of the respiratory–circulatory model are to reduce the work of breathing and to enhance the pumping action of the diaphragm and the extremity muscles to assist lymphatic and venous flow.

Bioenergy Model

The bioenergy model is somewhat more ethereal than the preceding and focuses on the inherent energy flow within the body. Some clinicians are skilled at both observing and feeling energy transmission, and the absence of it, from patients. We are all familiar with the phenomena of Kirlian photography that enables us to visualize radiant energy outside the anatomic limits of the body. This may be but one example of perceptible energy that emanates from the human organism. The bioenergy model focuses on the maximization of normal energy flow within the human body and its response to its environment. Many clinicians have reported sensations of release of energy that appear to emanate from the patient during manual medicine procedures.

There is also the element of the transfer of energy from the therapeutic touch of the physician. Many of the ancient, oriental forms of healing have focused on elements of "life force," "energy field," and so forth, and it is within this domain that a manual medicine practitioner can apply this conceptual model. The craniosacral manual medicine approach is one in which one of the major goals of treatment are to restore the normal inherent force of the central nervous system, including the brain, spinal cord, meninges, and cerebral spinal fluid, to maximize a symmetric, smooth, normal rhythmic CRI (cranial rhythmic impulse).

Psychobehavioral Model

The psychobehavioral model views the patient from the perspective of enhancing the capacity to relate to both the internal and external environments. There are many racial, social, and economic factors that influence the patient's perception of such things as pain, health, illness, disease, disability, and death. The patient's ability or inability to cope with all the stresses of life may manifest itself in a wide variety of symptoms and physical signs. The physician's ability to understand the patient's response to stress and coping mechanisms, and methods to assist the patient with this process, are important components of this conceptual model. "Therapeutic touch" is an integral part of the doctor–patient interaction in this model. The influence of manual medicine may be less a biomechanical, neurologic, or circulatory effect than just an important caring function. Awareness of this model is also important in understanding the difficulty in clinical research within manual medicine because of the "placebo" effect of the "laying on of hands."

It is beyond the scope of this volume to do anything but highlight the various models that are available for consideration when using a manual medicine intervention. It should be obvious that more than one model can be operative at the same intervention. It is strongly recommended, however, that the physician use some conceptual model before a manual medicine intervention. I support the contention of F.L. Mitchell, Jr. (personal communication) that manual medicine therapy is more than "a search and destroy mission of somatic dysfunction."

MANUAL MEDICINE ARMAMENTARIUM

Manual medicine procedures can be classified and described below.

Soft-Tissue Procedures

The soft-tissue procedures use manual application of force directed toward influencing specific tissue(s) of the musculoskeletal system or, by peripheral stimulation, enhancing some form of reflex mechanism that alters biologic function. The direct procedures include massage, effleurage, kneading, stretching, friction rub, and so forth. These procedures can prepare the tissues for additional specific joint mobilization or can be a therapeutic end in themselves. The therapeutic goals are to overcome congestion, reduce muscle spasm, improve tissue mobility, enhance circulation, and "tonify" the tissue. These procedures are some of the first learned and practiced by manual medicine physicians and can be used effectively in a variety of patient conditions.

A number of reflex mechanisms have been described that stimulate the peripheral tissues of the musculoskeletal system. These include acupuncture, reflex therapy, Chapman reflexes, Travell trigger points, and so forth. In these procedures, a manual, mechanical, or electrical stimulus is applied to certain areas of the body to enhance a therapeutic response. Some of these systems have been postulated for neurologic models, lymphatic models, neuroendocrine models, and in some instances, without any explanation for the observable clinical phenomena. Suffice it to say, many of these peripheral stimulating therapeutic points are consistent across patients, observable by multiple examiners, and provide a predictable response.

Articulatory Procedures

The articulatory procedures (mobilization without impulse) are used extensively in physiotherapy. They consist primarily of putting the elements of the musculoskeletal system, particularly the articulations, through ranges of motion in some graded fashion, with the goal of enhancement of the quantity and quality of motion. These procedures are therapeutic extensions of the diagnostic process of evaluating range of motion. If there appears to be a restriction of motion in one direction, with some alteration in sense of ease of movement in that direction, a series of gentle, rhythmic, operator-directed efforts in the direction of motion restriction can be found to be therapeutically effective. These articulatory procedures are especially useful for their tonic and/or circulatory effect.

Specific Joint Mobilization

The specific joint mobilization procedures all have two common elements: method, which is the method of approaching the restricted barrier, and activating force that is the intrinsic or extrinsic forces(s) exerted.

Methods   The specific joint mobilization methods are as follows.

1. *Direct method*: All direct procedures engage the restrictive barrier and by application of some force attempt to move the restrictive barrier in the direction of motion loss.
2. *Exaggeration method*: This therapeutic effort applies a force against the normal physiologic barrier in the direction opposite that of the motion loss. The force is usually a high-velocity, low-amplitude thrust and has been quite successful. There are systems of manual medicine that only provide therapeutic force in the direction of pain-free movement, and it is within this exaggeration method that such therapy seems to be operative.
3. *Indirect method*: In these procedures, the operator moves the segment away from the restrictive barrier into the range of "freedom" or "ease" of movement to a point of balanced tension ("floating" of the segment(s)). The segment can then be held in that position for 5 to 90 seconds to relax the tension in the tissues around the articulations so that enhanced mobility occurs. Procedures using this method are termed "functional technique," "balance-and-hold technique," and "release-by-positioning technique."
4. *Combined method*: Sometimes it is useful to use combinations of direct, exaggeration, and indirect methods in sequence to assist in the ultimate therapeutic outcome. Frequently, a combined method series of procedures is more effective than multiple applications of the same method.
5. *Physiologic response method*: These procedures apply patient positioning and movement

direction to obtain a therapeutic result. A series of body positions may use nonneutral mechanics to restore neutral mechanics to the spinal complex of the musculoskeletal system. Another example of a physiologic method is the use of respiratory effort to affect mobility of vertebral segments within spinal curvatures. Inhalation effort enhances straightening of the curves and hence backward bending movement in the thoracic spine and forward bending in the cervical and lumbar spines; exhalation effort causes just the reverse.

Activating Forces   The activating forces can be categorized as extrinsic and intrinsic. The extrinsic forces are those that are applied from outside the patient's body directly to the patient. These can include

1. Operator effort, such as guiding, springing, and thrust;
2. Adjunctive, such as straps, pads, traction, and so on;
3. Gravity, which is the weight of the body part, and the patient position.

The intrinsic group includes those forces that occur from within the patient's body and are used for their therapeutic effectiveness. They are classified as

1. Inherent forces, or nature's tendency toward balance and homeostasis
2. Respiratory force
   a. Inhalation, which straightens curves in vertebral column and externally rotates extremities
   b. Exhalation, which enhances curves in vertebral column and internally rotates extremities
3. Muscle force of the patient
   a. Muscle cooperation
   b. Muscle energy, especially isometrics
4. Reflex activity
   a. Eye movement
   b. Muscle activation

Afferent Reduction Procedures

The afferent reduction procedures appear to work on a model of reducing aberrant afferent activity from the various mechanoreceptors found within the various tissues of the musculoskeletal system. The working hypothesis is that altered behavior of the musculoskeletal system provides aberrant stimulation to the central nervous system that alters the programming of musculoskeletal function. Identifying various positions and maneuvers that reduce the afferent bombardment to the spinal cord and central levels can provide an opportunity to restore more normal behavior. It is thought that many of the indirect approaches, including the dynamic functional techniques, balance and hold techniques, and release by positioning techniques, work through this mechanism.

MANIPULATION UNDER ANESTHESIA

Manipulation under anesthesia has had a long history in manual medicine. It is used for dysfunction within the spinal complex, particularly the lumbosacral and cervical regions, as well as peripheral joints. The procedures performed are mobilization with impulse (high-velocity, low-amplitude thrust technique) with the patient under general, regional, or local anesthesia. Its use requires skilled anesthesia and a high level of competence of the manipulating practitioner. The indications are acute or chronic vertebral dysfunctions that cannot be managed by nonoperative, conservative means. Muscle spasm and irritability may preclude a successful manual medicine procedure without anesthesia. In chronic myofibrositis, manipulation under anesthesia may enhance the response unobtainable by more conservative measures. The indications are not high. Morey reported that only 3% of patients hospitalized with musculoskeletal disorders in a 3-year period required manipulation under anesthesia. Complications are rare, but the procedure is contraindicated in patients who cannot tolerate the anesthetic and those in whom manual medicine is not viewed as appropriate.

It is possible to design multiple variations of method and activating force to achieve the desired clinical goal. All of the procedures in manual medicine can be viewed as having a common goal, which is to reprogram the behavior of the central nervous system. Using the analogy of the computer, manual medicine deals with the "hardware" of the musculoskeletal system and modulates the behavior of the "software" in the central nervous system. The more optimal the behavior of the central nervous system, the better the function of the musculoskeletal system. The anatomy (hardware) may be altered by developmental variant; trauma, both single and repetitive; and surgery. Despite the changes in the anatomy, the goal of manual medicine is to restore the maximum functional capacity that the anatomy will allow. The more skilled one becomes in using different methods and activating forces, the more successful one becomes as a manual medicine therapist.

FACTORS INFLUENCING TYPE OF MANIPULATIVE PROCEDURES

In addition to a wide variety of types and styles of manual medicine procedures available and a number of different clinical goals, other factors influence the type of manual medicine procedure instituted.

1. Age of patient
2. Acuteness or chronicity of problem
3. General physical condition of patient
4. Operator size and ability
5. Location (office, home, hospital, etc.)
6. Effectiveness of previous and/or present therapy

If one were prescribing a pharmaceutical agent, the dosage would be adjusted to the age of the patient. This is also the case in the use of manual medicine. Clearly, one approaches an infant differently from a young adult. In an elderly debilitated patient, one is much more careful and judicious in the use of some of the more forceful direct action types of technique. Osteoporosis in the female is not necessarily a contraindication to manual medicine, but indirect procedures with intrinsic activating forces would be more appropriate.

The type of manual medicine procedure is also modified by the acuteness or chronicity of the problem. In acute conditions, inflammatory swelling and acute muscle spasms are frequently encountered. The physician might use the respiratory–circulatory model to relieve the inflammatory congestion and perhaps some soft-tissue procedure to reduce the amount of acute muscle spasm. In more chronic conditions with long-standing fibrosis in the ligaments, muscles, and fascia, a more direct action myofascial release or direct action mobilization with impulse (high-velocity thrust) procedure might be more appropriate. In the acutely ill patient with reduced capacity to withstand aggressive, intensive therapy, a more conservative approach such as indirect technique might be more appropriate. Remember that manual medicine procedures, particularly those using intrinsic activating forces, result in energy expenditure by the patient. Keep the therapeutic application within the physical capacity of the acutely ill patient. In chronic conditions, do not expect to overcome all of the difficulty with a single manual medicine intervention.

The operator's size, strength, and technical ability will also influence the type of procedure used. Although strength is not necessarily the primary determinant of a successful procedure, the proper application of leverage usually is. Understanding of and ability in a number of manual medicine procedures makes a more effective clinician. With only one antibiotic available, the ability to treat infectious disease is clearly hampered. Likewise, with only one form of manual medicine treatment, one is clearly hampered as an effective manual medicine practitioner.

The physician should have the capacity to provide an effective manual medicine treatment regardless of the location of the patient. Although there are some procedures that are more effective in the office setting with specific therapeutic tables, stools and other equipment, one should be able to devise an effective procedure anywhere. In a hospital bed or at home on a soft mattress, the capacity to use a high-velocity, low-amplitude thrust is compromised. Muscle energy activating forces and other intrinsic force techniques are more appropriate in such locations.

Past therapy is also highly important in determining the type of procedure to be used. You must know if there has been a previous surgical intervention, manual medicine intervention, or pharmacotherapeutic treatment. If surgery has changed the anatomy, you might wish to modify the therapeutic procedure to meet the altered anatomy. Lack of response to previous manual medicine is not necessarily a reason not to use a different manual medicine treatment. Previous medication, particularly muscle relaxants, tranquilizers, and antiinflammatory agents, might modify the type of procedure to be used. With long-standing steroid therapy, be aware of the potential for laxity of ligaments and softening of cancellous bone.

These are but a few of the factors that affect the choice of a manual medicine procedure. In addition, there are three cardinal rules for any effective manual medicine procedure: control, balance, and localization.

Control includes the physician's control of body position in relationship to the patient, control of the patient in a comfortable position, control of intrinsic or extrinsic forces, and control of the type of therapeutic intervention being applied. Balance of patient and operator ensures adequate patient relaxation and the ability of the operator to engage the restrictive barrier in comfort. Localization refers to adequate engagement of a restrictive barrier in a direct action procedure, localization on the point of maximum ease in a balance-and-hold indirect procedure, and localization of the most pain-free position in a release by positioning procedure.

CONTRAINDICATION TO MANUAL MEDICINE PROCEDURES

Much has been written about absolute and relative contraindications to manual medicine procedures. This author holds the view that there are none, if—and it is a big if—there is an accurate diagnosis of somatic dysfunction that requires treatment to effect the overall management of the patient, and the manual medicine procedure is appropriate for that diagnosis and the physical condition of the patient. However, there are a number of conditions that require special precautions. Some of these are as follows:

1. The vertebral artery in the cervical spine
2. Primary joint disease (e.g., rheumatoid arthritis, infectious arthritis, etc.)

3. Metabolic bone disease (e.g., osteoporosis, etc.)
4. Primary or metastatic malignant bone disease
5. Genetic disorders (e.g., Down syndrome), particularly in the cervical spine
6. Hypermobility in the involved segments. This should clearly be avoided. One should look for restricted mobility elsewhere in the presence of hypermobility.

Following these principles, a specific and appropriate manual medicine therapeutic prescription can be written for a diagnosis, much as with traditional therapeutic interventions. Returning to our original example, the thinking physician identifies the infectious agent in a throat infection before deciding on a therapeutic intervention. If, for example, the throat infection was due to a streptococcus, the physician might select ampicillin as the antibiotic of choice. With the specific infectious agent identified and an appropriate antibiotic chosen, then adequate dosage on an appropriate schedule for a sufficient length of time would be ordered.

DX—Throat infection (streptococcal)
RX—Ampicillin 250 mg every 6 hours for 10 days

With an appropriate diagnosis of somatic dysfunction, an accurate manual medicine prescription can be written on the basis of the principles addressed above. One would choose the type of procedure, specify the method, activating force, dosage, length of treatment time, and frequency of treatments.

DX—Somatic dysfunction, T-6, extended, rotated, and side bent right (ERS_{right})
RX—Manual medicine, direct action muscle energy type to flexion, left rotation, and left-side bending. Reexamine in 48 hours.

The specific somatic dysfunction has been identified with its position and subsequent motion restriction. A direct procedure and an intrinsic activating force were chosen. It was anticipated that the effectiveness of the procedure would last 48 hours and therefore reexamination at that time was indicated.

COMPLICATIONS

It is difficult to have an accurate estimation of the incidence of complications from manual medicine procedures. Some authors have defined the rate at one to two per million procedures. A well-controlled study by Dvorak and Orelli identified symptom exaggeration as one in 40,000 and a significant complication as one in 400,000. Most of the complications involve vascular and neural structures. Obvious complications occur when a procedure is contraindicated. Many of the complications occur from manipulation in the cervical spine resulting in insult to the vertebrobasilar artery system. Fractures and dislocations have been identified as well as spinal cord injury. Complications of exaggeration of disc herniation with progressive radiculopathy after manipulation are controversial. Some authors view mobilization with impulse as contraindicated in the presence of disc herniation, whereas others believe that it is indicated in certain conditions if appropriately applied. Postmanipulation injury to the vertebral basilar artery system occurs in the 30- to 45-year-old age group with a slight preponderance in the female population. Death rates approach 22% and significant disability in 75% to 80%. Complete recovery is available to only a small number. The avoidance of complications requires the practitioner to be knowledgeable about the patient's diagnosis, have an appreciation of their own level of skill and experience, and have the ability to deal with complications if they occur. Although the incidence is low, they are to be avoided if possible.

As manual medicine practitioners, we should all prescribe our therapy as precisely as we prescribe any other therapeutic agent. It is hoped that these principles will assist in the appropriate use of manual medicine.

SUGGESTED READINGS

Dvorak J, Orelli F. How dangerous is manipulation to the cervical spine? *Manual Medicine*, 1985;2:1–4.

Greenman PE. Manipulation with the patient under anesthesia. *J Am Osteopath Assoc* 1992;92:1159–1170.

Kimberly PK. Formulating a prescription for osteopathic manipulative treatment. *J Am Osteopath Assoc* 1976;75:486–499.

Korr IM. The segmental nervous system as a mediator and organizer of disease processes. The physiological basis of osteopathic medicine. Postgraduate Institute of Osteopathic Medicine & Surgery, New York, 73–84, 1970.

Mitchell FL Jr. Personal communication, 1974.

Mitchell FL Sr. *Motion discordance.* Carmel, CA: Yearbook of the Academy of Applied Osteopathy, 1967:1–5.

Morey LW Jr. Osteopathic manipulation under general anesthesia. *J Am Osteopath Assoc* 1973;73:84–95.

Morey LW Jr. Manipulation under general anesthesia. *Osteopath Annals* 1976;4:127–135.

Romney IC. Manipulation of the spine and appendages under anesthesia. *J Am Osteopath Assoc* 1968;68:235–245.

5

NORMAL VERTEBRAL MOTION

The vertebral column consists of 26 segments. There are usually seven cervical segments, twelve thoracic segments, and five lumbar segments. Anomalous development occurs in the spine and is most common in the lumbar region where four or six segments are occasionally found. The lumbar region is also the site of the greatest number of anomalous developmental changes, particularly in the shape of the transverse processes and zygapophysial joints. The first and second cervical segments are uniquely atypical. The vertebral motion segment consists of two adjacent vertebrae and the intervening ligamentous structures (Fig. 5.1). The typical vertebra consists of two parts, the body and the posterior arch. The vertebral body articulates with the intervertebral disc above and below at the vertebral end plate. The posterior arch consists of the two pedicles, two superior and two inferior zygapophysial joints, two laminae, two transverse processes, and a single spinous process. Two adjacent vertebrae are connected ventrodorsad by the anterior longitudinal ligament, the intervertebral disc with its central nucleus and surrounding annulus, the posterior longitudinal ligament, the articular capsules of the zygapophysial joints, the ligamentum flavum, the interspinous ligament, and the supraspinous ligament.

CERVICAL REGION

Atlas

In the cervical region, we find the atypical atlas (C-1) and axis (C-2). The atlas (Fig. 5.2) does not have a ver-

tebral body and consists primarily of a bony ring with two lateral masses. On the posterior aspect of the anterior arch is a small joint structure for articulation with the anterior aspect of the odontoid process of the axis. Each lateral mass consists primarily of the articular pillars. The shape of the superior zygapophysial joints is concave ventrodorsad and laterally. The long axis of each superior zygapophysial joint projects from the lateral to medial dorsoventrad. This results in an anterior wedging of the long axis of these joints. They articulate with the condyles of the occiput, and their shape is a major determinant of the amount and type of motion available between the occiput and the atlas. The inferior zygapophysial joints are quite flat but when the articular cartilage is attached, they become convex ventrodorsad and laterally. These inferior zygapophysial joints articulate with the superior zygapophysial joints of the axis. The transverse processes are quite long and are easily palpable in the space between the tip of the mastoid process of the temporal bone and the angle of the mandible.

Axis

The axis (C-2) (Fig. 5.3) has atypical characteristics in its superior portion and more typical characteristics in its inferior portion. The vertebral body is surmounted by the odontoid process, developmentally the residuum of the body of the atlas. On the anterior aspect of the odontoid process is an articular facet for the posterior aspect of the anterior arch of the atlas; the posterior aspect has an articular facet for the transverse atlas ligament. The superior zygapophysial

Figure 5.1.
Vertebral motion segment.

Figure 5.2.
Atlas (C-1).

Figure 5.3.
Axis (C-2).

Figure 5.4.
Typical cervical vertebra.

Figure 5.5.
Thoracic vertebra.

joints are convex ventrodorsad and laterally. They are higher on the medial than lateral aspect and their contour resembles a pair of shoulders. The spinous process of C-2 is quite long and is one of the more easily palpable spinous processes in the cervical region.

Typical Cervical Vertebrae

The typical cervical vertebrae, from the inferior surface of C2 down to the cervical thoracic junction have the following characteristics (Fig. 5.4). The vertebral body is relatively small in relation to the posterior arch. The superior surface is convex ventrodorsad and concave laterally, whereas the inferior surface is concave ventrodorsad and convex laterally. When the intervertebral disc joins two typical vertebral bodies, the shape is similar to a universal joint. At the posterolateral corner of each vertebral body is a small synovial joint called the uncovertebral joint of Luschka. These joints are found only in the cervical region and are subject to degenerative changes that occasionally encroach on the intervertebral canal posteriorly. The pedicles are quite short and serve as the roof and floor of the related intervertebral canal. The articular pillars are relatively large and are easily palpable on the posterolateral aspect of the neck. The zygapophysial joints are relatively flat and face backward and upward at approximately a 45-degree angle. The shape and direction of the zygapophysial joints, and the universal joint characteristics between the vertebral bodies, largely determine the type of movement available in the typical cervical spinal segments. The laminae are flat and the spinous processes are usually bifid with the exception on C7. The transverse processes are unique in this region, having on each side the intertransverse foramen for the passage of the vertebral artery. The tips of the transverse processes are bifid and serve as attachments for the deep cervical muscles. They are quite tender to palpation and are not easily used in structural diagnosis of the cervical spine. The intervertebral canals on each side are ovoid in shape and are limited by the inferior margin of the pedicle above, the posterior aspect of the intervertebral disc

and Luschka joints in front, the superior aspect of the pedicle of the vertebral below, and the anterior aspect of the zygapophysial joints behind. The vertebral canal is relatively large and provides the space necessary for the large area of the spinal cord in the cervical region.

Thoracic Vertebrae

In the thoracic region (Fig. 5.5), the vertebral bodies become somewhat larger as they descend and have unique characteristics for articulation with the heads of the ribs. T1 has a unifacet found posterolaterally for the articulation of the head of rib one bilaterally. From the inferior surface of T1 down are found demifacets, which together with the intervertebral disc provide an articular fossa for the head of each rib. The zygapophysial joints are vertical in orientation and the superior facets project backward and laterally. Theoretically, this should provide a great deal of freedom of movement in multiple directions but the attachment of the ribs to the thoracic vertebra markedly restricts the available motion. The transverse processes have an articular facet on their anterior aspect for articulation with the tubercle of the rib. This forms the costotransverse articulation bilaterally. The transverse processes become progressively narrower in descent, with those at T1 being widest at their tips and those at T12, the narrowest. The laminae are shingled and continue to the spinous processes, which are also shingled from above downward. The spinous processes are quite long and overlap each other, particularly in the mid to lower region. The relation of the palpable tips of the spinous processes to the thoracic vertebral bodies is referred to as "the rule of 3's" (Fig. 5.6). The spinous processes of T4 to T6 project one-half vertebra below that to which they are attached. The spinous processes of T7 to T9 are located a full vertebra lower than the vertebra to which they are attached. The spinous processes of T10 through T12 return to being palpable at the same level as the vertebral body to which they are attached.

Lumbar Vertebrae

In the lumbar region, the vertebral bodies (Fig. 5.7) become even more massive and support a great deal of weight. The spinous processes project posteriorly in relation to the vertebral body to which they are attached and are broad, rounded, and easily palpable. The transverse processes project laterally, with those attached to L3 being the broadest in range. The zygapophysial joints have a concave/convex relationship between the superior and inferior zygapophysial joints of adjacent vertebra that greatly restricts the amount of side bending and rotation available. The plane of zygapophysial joints is usually considered a sagittal (*yz*) plane with the lumbosacral zygapophysial joints considered closer to the coronal (*xy*) plane. However, in the lumbar region, asymmetric facing of the zygapophysial joints is not uncommon.

Figure 5.6.
Thoracic spine rule of 3's.

Figure 5.7.
Lumbar vertebra.

Vertebral Column Muscles

The muscles overlying the vertebral column are many and layered. They can be described as follows:

> Layer one: the trapezius, latissimus dorsi, and lumbodorsal fascia
> Layer two: the levator scapulae and major and minor rhomboids
> Layer three: the erector spinae mass including the spinalis, semispinalis, longissimus, and iliocostalis
> Layer four: multifidi, rotatores, and intertransversarii

The anteroposterior curves of the vertebral column develop over time. The primary curve at birth is convex posteriorly. The first secondary curve to develop is in the cervical region, which becomes convex anteriorly when the infant begins to raise its head. The second curve develops in the lumbar region on assuming the biped stance. This curve is convex anteriorly. Appropriate alignment of the three curves of the vertebral axis is an essential component of good posture (Fig. 5.8).

LAYER PALPATION

The palpation of these structures is an essential component of structural diagnosis. The following exercise in palpation might be useful in gaining familiarity with some of them for further use both diagnostically and therapeutically.

1. Place the palms and palmer surfaces of the fingers over the shawl area of the cervicothoracic junction (Fig. 5.9). Palpate the skin for thickness, smoothness, and temperature.
2. Move the skin on the subcutaneous fascia overlying the deep structures in a synchronous and alternating fashion anteroposteriorly and from medial to lateral (Fig. 5.10). Note that in one direction it will be more free and in the other, somewhat tighter. This tight/loose characteristic is a sensation of

Figure 5.8.
Normal vertebral curves.

Figure 5.9.
Layer palpation of shawl area.

Figure 5.10.
Skin motion on subcutaneous fascia.

great significance when using myofascial release technique.

3. Using the thumb and index finger on each hand, pick up the skin and subcutaneous fascia and gently roll the skin over your thumbs by the action of your index fingers coming from below upward (Fig. 5.11). Repeat starting medially and going laterally. Perform this procedure symmetrically on each side looking for differences in thickness and pliability of the skin and ascertaining if this procedure produces pain for the patient. Skin rolling that identifies tightness and tenderness is a valuable tool in identifying levels of somatic dysfunction.

4. Place the palm ·of your hand over each acromion process with the long finger extending to the anterior aspect of the shoulder girdle and the finger pad palpating the tip of the coracoid process (Fig 5.12). Be gentle because this location is quite tender in all subjects. Palpate for the sensation of the resilience of bone. Move your finger pad slightly inferiorly to palpate the rounded, smooth, firm tendon of the short head of the biceps brachii. Return

to the tip of the coracoid process, proceed medially, and palpate the broader, but still smooth and firm tendon of the pectoralis minor muscle.

5. Place the palms of the fingers of both hands overlying the upper thoracic region medial to the spinous process of the scapula (Fig. 5.13). Palpate through skin and subcutaneous fascia to palpate the deeper fascia overlying the first layer muscle, the mid portion of the trapezius. Move your fingers from side to side as well as superiorly to inferiorly sensing for muscle fiber direction. This is somewhat easier by hav-

ing the patient retract the scapulae actively. Note that it appears smoother to move your hands from side to side and more rough when you move your hands from above to below. That smoothness-versus-roughness characteristic is typical of muscle fiber direction.

6. Place your left hand where your right hand was in the last example and grasp the elbow with your right hand (Fig. 5.14). Palpate through the tissues, including the horizontal portion of the trapezius, and concentrate on the next layer of muscle below, the rhomboids. The rhomboid can be more easily pal-

pable if you resist the patient's effort to push the elbow toward the table. Note that the muscle has a different fiber direction than the trapezius at the same level. It is oblique from medial to lateral and from above downward. The inferior margin is easily palpable to give you the fiber direction.

7. Palpate the midline overlying the spinous processes (Fig. 5.15). As you move from above downward, note that the skin is very tightly attached at the midline. As you course from above downward, you will note a bump-and-hollow characteristic. The bumps are

Figure 5.11.
Skin rolling.

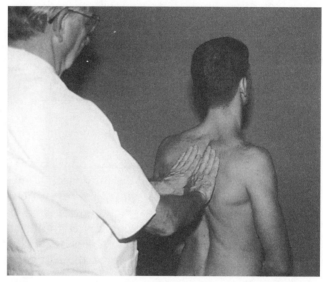

Figure 5.13.
Layer palpation of trapezius muscle.

Figure 5.12.
Palpation of shoulder girdle and coracoid process.

Figure 5.14.
Layer palpation of rhomboid muscle.

the bony spinous processes and the hollow is the interspinous space. Note the tension of the interspinous space reflecting the tension of the supraspinous and intraspinous ligaments.

8. Place three fingers in the interspinous spaces of the mid to upper thoracic spine. Introduce flexion through the head, sensing for opening of the interspinous spaces (Fig. 5.16). Reverse the process by taking the head and neck into extension and note that the interspinous spaces narrow (Fig. 5.17). Repeat this process several times noting how the interspinous spaces open and close. Attempt to move the head and neck so that you can localize the opening of the interspinous space beneath the middle finger during flexion, but not the finger below, and repeat the same process in extension so that you can close the interspinous space under the middle finger, but not the one below. This is an important exercise in identifying your capacity to localize to a single vertebral segment.

9. Place your index finger on one side of the spinous process and your middle finger on the other and palpate the fascial groove between the spinous process and the third layer of muscle, the erector spinae mass (Fig. 5.18). Actually, the fascial plane is between the spinalis muscle, which is intimately attached to the lateral aspect of the spinous processes, and the medial side of the longissimus, the easily pal-

pable "rope" of the erector spinae mass. As you move from cephalad to caudad in this groove, you should feel symmetry and no palpable structure. Should you palpate anything in this medial groove, it is a reflection of hypertonicity of the deeper fourth-layer muscle, primarily at the multifidus layer. Fourth-layer hypertonic muscle is rounded and tense and is

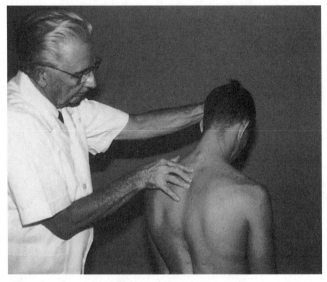

Figure 5.16.
Palpation of interspinous spaces during forward bending.

Figure 5.15.
Layer palpation of spinous processes.

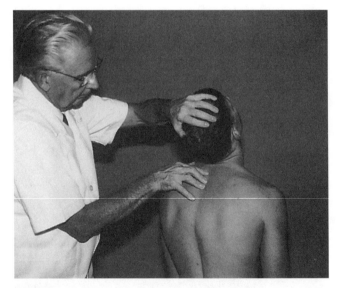

Figure 5.17.
Palpation of interspinous spaces during backward bending.

about the size of a Tootsie Roll candy. They are usually quite sensitive to the patient and found unilaterally. Occasionally, a bilateral fourth-layer muscle hypertonic area can be palpated in the presence of bilateral flexion or extension restrictions of a vertebral segment. Palpable fourth-layer hypertonic muscle (the "Tootsie Roll" sign) is one of the cardinal diagnostic findings in vertebral segmental somatic dysfunction.

10. Move laterally from the medial groove over the rounded mass of the longissimus muscle and note that there is a lateral deep fascial groove separating the lateral aspect of the longissimus from the medial aspect of the iliocostalis muscle. Place your thumbs on the lateral aspect of the longissimus in the lateral groove in a symmetric fashion (Fig. 5.19). Move your thumbs symmetrically in an anteromedial direction until you feel a deep resistance (Fig. 5.20). Note that there has been elevation of the belly of the longissimus. While maintaining your palpation at this deeper level, move your thumbs in a cephalic to caudad direction sensing for a bump and hollow contour similar to that identified over the spinous processes in the midline. At the level you are now palpating, you are overlying the transverse processes of the thoracic vertebrae, which are the bumps. The intertransverse space is the hollow. Try to palpate one pair of transverse processes in a symmetric fashion and ask the patient to actively flex

and extend his or her head and neck while you attempt to maintain contact with the transverse processes. Note that it is easier to feel the transverse process during the extension movement than during flexion. Acquisition of the skill of following transverse processes in three-dimensional space is most valuable in making a diagnosis of vertebral somatic dysfunction.

11. Move your hands more laterally overlying the most posterior aspect of the thoracic cage

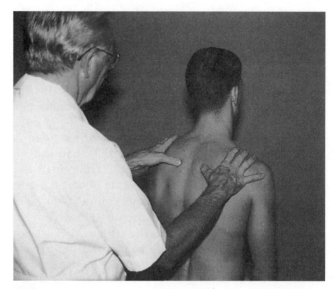
Figure 5.19.
Palpation of lateral groove erector spinae muscles

Figure 5.18.
Palpation of medial groove erector spinae muscles.

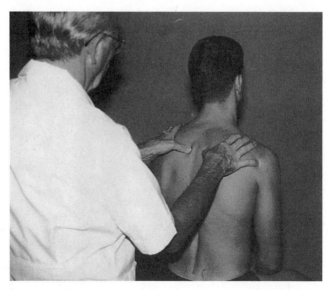
Figure 5.20.
Palpation of transverse processes.

(Fig. 5.21). You are palpating over the rib angles and the associated attachment of the iliocostalis muscle. Move from cephalad to caudad and note that the rib angles diverge from medial to lateral. Each rib angle should participate in the posterior convexity of the thoracic cage. The finding of one rib angle that is more or less prominent that its fellows above and below is significant in the diagnosis of rib somatic dysfunction. Any palpable hypertonicity of muscle at the rib angle is indicative of hypertonic iliocostalis, which is only found in the presence of rib dysfunction. Again, hypertonic iliocostalis at a rib angle is frequently tender to the patient.

12. Place your thumb overlying the rib angle of the most posterior aspect of the thoracic cage, usually the seventh rib (Fig. 5.22). Move your thumb over the rib shaft at the angle, noting the posterior convexity. Move to the superior and inferior aspect of the rib noting the rib edge. Most commonly, the inferior edge is somewhat more easily palpable than the superior. Of importance is the contour of the rib in comparison to the one above, the one below, and those on the contralateral side. Prominence of the superior or inferior rib edge is significant in the diagnosis of rib somatic dysfunction. Palpate the interspace above and below the rib and compare it with the opposite side. Is one narrower or wider than the other? Palpate the intercostal muscle to see if it is hypertonic and tender. Abnormal width above and below a rib and intercostal

hypertonicity are significant findings in certain rib somatic dysfunctions.

13. From the rib angle, continue to monitor rib shaft and move medially with the palm of your thumb on the rib shaft until the tip of your thumb runs into an obstruction (Fig. 5.23). The tip of your thumb has now struck the lateral aspect of the transverse process. The portion of bone from the rib angle to the tip of the transverse process is an important component of the rib that is used in some of the subsequently described tech-

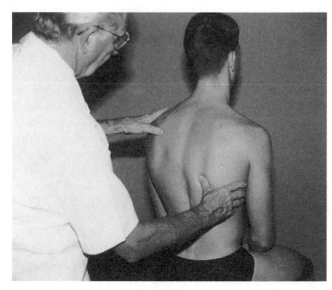

Figure 5.22.
Palpation of rib angle contour.

Figure 5.21.
Palpation of rib angles and iliocostalis muscle.

Figure 5.23.
Palpation of rib shaft to tip of transverse process.

niques for rib somatic dysfunction. Again note that the longissimus muscle becomes more prominent as you have moved from lateral to medial along the rib shaft.

This layer palpation exercise of the back will provide you with the ability to palpate anatomic structures necessary for the accurate diagnosis of vertebral axis and costal cage somatic dysfunction. Particularly important is the ability to follow paired transverse processes through a range of motion and the ability to identify tender, tense hypertonic muscle of the fourth layer. Practice this exercise on a regular basis until it becomes habitual.

VERTEBRAL MOTION

Certain conventions are used in describing all vertebral motion. The vertebral motion segment consists of the superior and inferior adjacent vertebrae and the intervening disc and ligamentous structures. By convention, motion of the superior vertebra is described in relation to the inferior. Motion is further defined as the movement of the superior or anterior surface of the vertebral body. In describing rotation, the anterior surface is used rather than the elements of the posterior arch. For example, in rotation of T3 to the right in relation to T4, the anterior surface of T3 turns to the right and the spinous process deviates to the left. Therefore, remember that descriptions relate to the anterior or superior surfaces of the vertebral body. In addition to describing characteristics of a vertebral motion segment, we also speak of movement of groups of vertebrae (three or more).

Vertebral motion is also described in relation to the anatomically oriented cardinal planes of the body using the right-handed orthogonal coordinate system. Most of the clinical literature relates to the anatomically described cardinal planes and axes, while the biomechanical research literature uses the coordinate system extensively. Motion can be described as rotation around an axis and translation along an axis with the body moving within one of the cardinal planes. By convention the horizontal axis is the x-axis, the vertical axis is the y-axis, and the anteroposterior axis is the z-axis. The coronal plane is the xy plane, the sagittal plane is the yz plane, and the horizontal plane is the xz plane. The ability to rotate around an axis and to translate along an axis results in 6 df for each vertebra. Vertebral motion can then be described as overturning moment (rotation around an axis) and translatory movement (translation along an axis).

TERMINOLOGY

At the present time, convention in clinical practice describes vertebral motion in the following terms: forward bending, backward bending, side bending right and left, and rotation right and left.

Forward Bending

A superior vertebra rotates anteriorly around the x-axis and translates somewhat forward along the z-axis. In forward bending (Fig. 5.24), the anterior longitudinal ligament becomes somewhat more lax, posterior pressure is placed upon the intervertebral disc, and the posterior longitudinal ligament becomes more tense as do the ligamentum flavum, the interspinous and supraspinous ligaments. The inferior zygapophysial facet of the superior vertebra moves superiorly in relation to the superior zygapophysial facet of the inferior vertebra. This has been described as "opening" or "flexing" of the facet.

Backward Bending

In backward bending, the vertebra rotates backward around the x-axis and moves posteriorly along the z-axis (Fig. 5.25). The anterior longitudinal ligament becomes more tense. There is less tension on the posterior longitudinal ligament, the ligamentum flavum, and the interspinous and supraspinous ligaments. The inferior zygapophysial facet of the superior segment slides inferiorly in relation to the superior zygapophysial facet of the inferior vertebra. The facets are spoken of as having "closed" or "extended." Forward bending and backward bending result in an accordion-type movement of the opening and closing of the zygapophysial joints. If something interferes with the capacity of a facet joint to open or close, restriction of motion of either forward bending or backward bending will result.

Figure 5.24.
Vertebral forward bending.

Figure 5.25.
Vertebral backward bending.

Side Bending

In side bending, there is rotation around the antero-posterior *z*-axis and translation along the horizontal *x*-axis. Side bending is seldom a pure movement and is usually coupled with rotation. In side bending to the right, the right zygapophysial joint "closes" and the left zygapophysial joint "opens." Interference with a facet's capacity to open or close can interfere with side bending and the coupled rotatory movement.

Rotation

Rotation of a vertebra is described as rotation around the *y*-axis with the translatory movement being dependent on the vertebral segment involved. Rotation is always coupled with side bending with the exception of the atlantoaxial joint.

COUPLED MOVEMENTS

Side bending and rotation are coupled movements and do not occur individually. In some instances, rotation is coupled in the same direction as side bending (e.g., side bending right, rotation right) and at other times at opposite directions (e.g., side bending right, rotation left). Coupled movements change in response to the anteroposterior curves of the vertebral axis.

Neutral Mechanics

Neutral mechanics, or its synonym Type I, results in coupled movement of side bending and rotation to opposite sides. Neutral mechanics occur when the patient is in the erect position with normal anteroposterior curves. For example, in the lumbar spine, with a normal lumbar lordosis present, side bending of the trunk to the left results in rotation of lumbar vertebrae to the right in three-dimensional space (Fig. 5.26). You

can demonstrate this on yourself by standing erect and placing four fingers of your hand over the posterior aspect of the transverse processes of the lumbar spine. Now side bend to the left and feel the tissues under your right hand become more full. This fullness is interpreted as posterior movement of the right transverse processes of the lumbar vertebrae as they rotate right in response to side bending left. If one looks at the behavior of each of the lumbar vertebra in relation to the segment below, they do not all side bend and rotate to opposite sides. In fact, in this example, the middle segment maximally side bends and rotates to the opposite side. The segments below the apex also side bend and rotate to opposite sides in a gradual fashion. The segments above the apex side bend and rotate to the same side and the curve gradually reduces. However, for descriptive purposes, the neutral group curve is described as being side bent and rotated to opposite sides in three-dimensional space.

Nonneutral Mechanics

A nonneutral mechanical coupling, or its synonym type II, results in side bending and rotation of vertebrae to the same side. This occurs when there is alteration in the anteroposterior curve into forward or backward bending. To demonstrate, stand and forward bend at the waist and place both fingers overlying the posterior aspect of the transverse processes of the lumbar spine. Introduce side bending to the right. You will feel fullness occur under the fingers of your right hand, interpreted as resulting from posterior orientation of the right transverse processes during a

Figure 5.26.
Neutral (type I) vertebral motion.

right rotational response to the right-side bending coupled movement (Fig. 5.27). Return to the midline before returning to the erect posture. Nonneutral mechanics occur in the lumbar spine when it is forward bent. In backward bending, the lumbar spine demonstrates neutral coupling.

In the thoracic spine, there is the capability for both neutral and nonneutral coupling. The type of coupling appears to be a function of where you are in the thoracic curve, above or below the apex, and whether you introduce side bending or rotation first. In general, if side bending is introduced first, rotation will occur to the opposite side. If rotation is introduced first, side bending couples to the same side.

Nonneutral (Type II) mechanics include the coupling of all three arcs of vertebral motion and all 6 degrees of freedom. Nonneutral coupling results in significant reduction in freedom of motion. It is for this reason that the vertebral column appears to be at risk for dysfunction when nonneutral mechanics are operative. Particularly in the lumbar region with the trunk forward bent, side bent, and rotated to the same side, any additional movement places the lumbar spine at risk for muscle strain, zygapophysial joint dysfunction, annular tear of the intervertebral disc, or posterolateral protrusion of nuclear material in a previously compromised disc annulus.

Type III Mechanics

Type III refers to the observation that when motion is introduced in the vertebral column in one direction, motion in all other directions is reduced. To demon-

Table 5.1.
Vertebral Motion

Segment	Type
C0-1 (occipitoatlantal)	I (neutral) (always)
C1-2 (atlantoaxial)	(rotation)
C2-7 (typical cervical)	II (nonneutral)
C7-L5 (typical thoracic and lumbar)	I (neutral) and II (nonneutral)

strate the phenomena have your patient sit erect on an examining couch and passively introduce rotation of the trunk to the right and left. Ascertain the range and quality of movement. Now have the patient slump on the table with a posterior thoracolumbar convexity and again introduce trunk rotation to the right and left. Note the reduction in range and the restricted quality of movement during the range with the patient in this slumped position. The phenomenon of type III vertebral motion is therapeutically applied during localization to dysfunctional segments. Introduction of motion above and below a dysfunctional vertebral segment can be accurately localized to a single vertebral motion segment that will then be treated by introduction of some activating force.

TYPES OF MOTION AVAILABLE

The type of coupled movement available in the vertebral column varies from region to region and from posture to posture. In the areas of the vertebral column that have both neutral and nonneutral movement capability, the vertebral segments can become dysfunctional with either type of motion characteristic (Table 5.1).

An understanding of the anatomy of the vertebral column, the ability to palpate the tissues therein, and an understanding of the concepts of vertebral motion are essential to understanding and diagnosing vertebral dysfunctions.

SUGGESTED READINGS

Fryette HH. *Principles of osteopathic technique.* Carmel CA: American Academy of Osteopathy, 1954.

Jirout J. Studies on the dynamics of the spine. *Excerpta Acta Radiol* 1955;46:55–59.

Kapandji IA. *The physiology of the joints.* Vol. 3. London: Churchill Livingstone, 1974.

Lovett RW. The mechanics of the lateral curvature of the spine. *Boston M S J* 1900;142:622–627.

Lovett RW. The study of the mechanics of the spine. *Am J Anat* 1902;2:457–462.

Pearcy MJ, Portek I, Shepherd J. Three dimensional x-ray analysis of normal movement of the lumbar spine. *Spine* 1984;9:294–297.

Pearcy MJ, Tibrewal SB. Axial rotation and lateral bending in the normal lumbar spine. *Spine* 1984;9:582–587.

Figure 5.27.
Nonneutral (type II) vertebral motion.

6

CONCEPTS OF VERTEBRAL MOTION DYSFUNCTION

In the application of manual medicine procedures to the vertebral column, it is essential to make appropriate, accurate diagnosis of vertebral somatic dysfunction.

Somatic dysfunction is defined as:

Impaired or altered function of related components of the somatic (body framework) system; skeletal, arthrodial, and myofascial structures; and related vascular, lymphatic, and neural elements.

This term is codable under current classification systems, *International Classification of Diseases, Ninth Revision, Clinical Modification*, (*ICD-9-CM*) codes 739.0 through 739.9. Somatic dysfunction replaces old terms such as "osteopathic lesion," "chiropractic subluxation," "joint blockage," "joint lock," "loss of joint play," or "minor vertebral derangement." Concern for the function of the musculoskeletal system requires a method of evaluating motion within the vertebral complex to determine if it is normal, increased, or decreased. The motion spectrum advances from ankylosis to hypomobility, to normal motion, to hypermobility, to instability. Manual medicine procedures are most appropriate for segments with hypomobility that retain the capacity to move.

THEORIES OF VERTEBRAL MOTION DYSFUNCTION

Many theories have been proposed to explain the clinically observed phenomena of hypomobility. One theory proposes that there is entrapment of synovial material or a synovial meniscoid between the two opposing joint surfaces. There is some anatomic evidence that meniscoids do occur but whether they actually cause joint restriction has not been demonstrated. The joint meniscoid has innervation by C-fibers that suggest nociception function.

A second theory suggests that there is lack of congruence in the point-to-point contact of the opposing joint surfaces. This theory postulates alteration in the normal tracking mechanism between the joint surfaces and that the role of manual medicine is to restore the joint to the "right track."

A third theory suggests an alteration in the physical and chemical properties of the synovial fluid and synovial surfaces. In essence, the smooth gliding capacity has been lost because the opposing surfaces have become "sticky." Following a mobilization with impulse (high-velocity, low-amplitude thrust) procedure, in both vertebral and extremity joints in which separation of the joint surfaces has occurred, the "cavitation" phenomenon has been demonstrated. In addition to the audible popping sound, there has been the observation of a negative density within the joint on x-ray. This "vacuum phenomenon" appears to have the density of nitrogen and this gaseous shadow is present for a variable period before it is no longer observable. This observation suggests a change from liquid to gaseous state as a result of the thrusting procedure.

A fourth theory regards the restriction of motion as a result of altered length and tone of muscle. Some muscles can become hypertonic and shortened in position, whereas others become lengthened and weaker. Of greatest significance is the loss of muscle control. Physiologic control of muscle is highly complex and includes the behavior of mechanoreceptors in joints and related soft tissue, muscle spindle and Golgi tendon apparatus, cord level and propriospinal pathway reflexes, pathways to the motor cortex, corticobulbar and corticospinal pathways modulated by the cerebellum, and the final common pathway of the alpha motor neuron to muscle fiber. Any alteration in afferent stimulus to this complex mechanism or alteration of function within the system can result in dysfunctional muscle activity and ultimately affect joint mechanics. Any alteration in muscle tone then restricts normal motion and serves as a perpetuating factor in altered joint movement. Whether the abnormal muscle activity is primary or secondary to the vertebral dysfunction is purely conjectural. However, altered muscle component of a vertebral dysfunction should always be dealt with in some fashion by the treatment provided. Using the analogy of a computer, the nervous system can be viewed as the software and the musculoskeletal system as the hardware. Altered function of the nervous system (the software) does not allow the musculoskeletal system (hardware) to function appropriately. Some manual medicine practitioners view the effectiveness of manual medicine treatment as being the reprogramming of the software through the alteration of mechanoreceptor behavior at the joint and soft tissue levels.

A fifth theory considers changes in the biomechanical and biochemical properties of the myofascial elements of the musculoskeletal system, the capsule, the ligamentous structures, and fasciae. When these structures are altered through traumatic, inflammatory, degenerative, or other changes, reduction of normal vertebral mobility can result.

Regardless of the theory to which one might subscribe, the clinical phenomenon of restricted vertebral motion can be viewed as the influence on the paired zygapophysial joints of the segment. We speak of the capacity of facets to open and close and refer primarily to the accordion-type movement, not separation-type movement. In forward bending, the facets should normally open and in backward bending, they should close. If something interferes with the capacity of both facets to open, forward-bending restriction will occur. Conversely, if something interferes with both facets' capacity to close, backward-bending restriction will occur. It is also possible for one facet to move normally and the other to become restricted. If, for example, the right facet does not open, but the left functions normally, right-side bending is possible, but left-side bending is restricted. Since side bending and rotation are coupled movements in the typical vertebral segments, rotation can also be affected by alteration in facet joint movement.

DIAGNOSIS OF VERTEBRAL MOTION DYSFUNCTION

Dysfunctions in the vertebral column can be described as single-segment dysfunctions involving one vertebral motion segment and group dysfunctions involving three or more vertebrae. After one completes a screening-and-scanning examination and fine-tunes the diagnostic process to segmental definition, one is particularly interested in the motion(s) lost by the vertebra(e) involved. There are many methods to accomplish the process. The most commonly used is palpating the same bony prominence of two or more vertebrae (e.g., spinous processes or transverse processes) and actively and/or passively putting the segment(s) through successive ranges of movement into forward bending, backward bending, side bending right, side bending left, rotation right, and rotation left, comparing the motion of one segment with another. These procedures are most frequently done passively and the operator attempts to define restriction and

quality of restriction of movement in one or more directions. Although this method is frequently effective, it does have two serious drawbacks. First, every time you introduce multiple-plane motion in a dysfunctional segment diagnostically, there is a therapeutic effect since you are accomplishing a mobilization without impulse (articulatory) procedure. This results in your finding being constantly under change. A second disadvantage is the difficulty in making an assessment following a treatment procedure, that is, knowing whether you have modified the amount of range present before the procedure. It is difficult to accurately remember all of the nuances of motion restriction that were present prior to the therapeutic intervention.

A second method, preferred by this author, is to follow a pair of transverse processes through an arc of forward bending and backward bending and interpret the findings on the basis of the phenomena of facets opening and closing. Regardless of the method used, one can describe vertebral motion from the perspective of the motion available, the position in which the segment is restricted, or the motion of the segment that is restricted.

In Table 6.1, a suffix is used in each term, either a static suffix representing the position of the segment, or a motion suffix, which describes the motion available or the motion lost. The current convention of describing vertebral dysfunction is either the position of the restricted segment or the motion that is lost in the restricted segment. Therefore, a segment that is backward bent (extended), right rotated, and right side bent has forward bending (flexion), left-side bending, and left rotation restrictions. A plea is made for the use of appropriate terminology either to describe position or motion restriction. One should learn to translate between the two systems of positional and motion restriction diagnosis but clearly a statement of terms is necessary for accurate communication between examiners.

DYSFUNCTIONS OF SINGLE VERTERAL MOTION SEGMENT

Single vertebral motion segment dysfunctions can be easily identified by the finding of hypertonicity of fourth-layer vertebral muscle in the medial grove ad-

Table 6.1.
Factors that Describe Vertebral Motion

	Position	Motion Restriction	Motion Available
T3 on flexed T4	Flexed	Extension	Flexion
	Left rotated	Right rotation	Left rotation
	Left side bent	Right side bending	Left side bending
	Extended	Flexion	Extension
	Right rotated	Left rotation	Right rotation
	Right side bent	Left side bending	Right side bending

Figure 6.1.
Single segment right prominent transverse process.

jacent to the spinous processes. Palpable fourth-layer muscle hypertonicity is not present in normal vertebral motion segments. When palpable at a vertebral level, the practitioner should identify the motion characteristics of that vertebra in relation to the one above and the one below. A second clue to the possibility of a single vertebral motion segment dysfunction is the scanning examination finding of prominence overlying one transverse process suggesting the possibility of rotation of the vertebra to that side (Fig. 6.1). The segmental definition diagnostic process is performed by placing the thumbs over the posterior aspect of the transverse process of a segment that is suspected of being dysfunctional. The patient then is put through a forward-to-backward bending movement arc either actively or passively. In the upper thoracic spine, the active movement of the head on the trunk is frequently used, whereas in the lower thoracic and lumbar regions, the patient is examined in three different positions: prone neutral on the table, fully backward bent (prone prop position), and fully forward bent

(Figs. 6.2, 6.3, and 6.4). One assesses the behavior of the superior segment in relation to the inferior segment that is level against the coronal plane. For the purpose of description, assume that something interferes with opening of the right zygapophysial joint. In the neutral position, the right transverse process appears to be more posterior than the left. As the patient increases the amount of forward bending, the right transverse process becomes more prominent compared with that of the left. The restricted right zygapophysial joint holds the right half of the posterior arch of that vertebra in a posterior position. The free-moving zygapophysial joint on the left side allows the left half of the posterior arch to move forward and superior with the left transverse process, seeming to become less prominent. In backward bending, both transverse processes appear to become more symmetric because the right transverse process is already held posterior by the restricted right zygapophysial joint, whereas the left zygapophysial joint closes in backward bending, thus allowing the left transverse process to move posteriorly and inferiorly, becoming more symmetric in appearance.

Now let us assume that something interferes with the left zygapophysial joint's ability to close. In this instance, we usually find the right transverse process a little more prominent in the neutral position. In asking the patient to move into backward bending, the right transverse process appears to become more prominent. This is the result of normal closure of the right zygapophysial joint allowing the transverse process to move posteriorly, while the left zygapophysial joint is restricted in its capacity to close and holds the left transverse process in a more anterior position. Upon forward bending, both trans-

Figure 6.2.
Vertebral motion testing prone neutral.

Figure 6.3.
Vertebral motion testing, backward bent.

Figure 6.4.
Vertebral motion testing, forward bent.

verse processes become more symmetric. The left transverse process is already held in an anterior position by the restricted left zygapophysial joint, and the motion of the right zygapophysial moving into an open position carries the right transverse process more anteriorly.

These single vertebral motor unit dysfunctions are also described as nonneutral dysfunctions because the restricted coupled movement is side bending with rotation to the same side. Historically, they have been described as type II dysfunctions. The characteristics are as follows:

1. Single vertebral motion unit involved
2. Includes either flexion or extension restriction component

3. Motion restriction of side bending and rotation to the same side

We have described the phenomenon that occurs if one or the other zygapophysial joint loses the capacity to open or close. If there is a single vertebral motion segment involved in which both zygapophysial joints are restricted, the transverse processes remain in the same relative position throughout forward- and backward-bending movement. One can determine the case of bilateral zygapophysial joints being closed or bilaterally being open by monitoring the interspace between the spinous process during forward and backward bending. If the z-joints are able to open, the interspinous distance will increase during forward bending. If the z-joints are able to close in a bilaterally symmetric fashion, the interspinous distance becomes smaller during backward bending.

There are several reasons why this method of vertebral motion testing is recommended. First, this method remains consistent and reproducible over time. The challenge to the motion segment is in only one plane of movement. No multiaxial changes in movement characteristics are introduced, as in the procedure described earlier. This method does not put the segment through an articulatory procedure and thus is not changing the vertebral mechanics to any appreciable amount. This makes it possible for the examiner to be more confident in the posttreatment evaluation of a segment to be sure that, in fact, some change has occurred in the motion present before and after treatment.

Second, this procedure is easier for multiple examiners to apply because of the nontreatment aspect of the method. This allows more consistent student teaching and evaluation of vertebral diagnostic procedures. If five separate examiners tested a given segment by putting it through multiple ranges of movement, by the time the fifth examiner described the findings, the first examiner would think it was a different patient. Using this single-plane movement challenge, the findings remain much more consistent across examiners and across time.

A third reason to recommend this process is the examiner's capacity to differentiate between structural and functional asymmetry of a vertebral segment. Structural asymmetries occur frequently, and palpation of a posterior transverse process cannot distinguish asymmetric development from actual dysfunction of a rotational nature. If the prominent transverse process is due to nonneutral (type II) single vertebral motion segment dysfunction, the prominence of the transverse process will change during a forward- and backward-bending arc. In one position, it will become worse, and in the other position, it will become more symmetric. If the transverse process is prominent because of asymmetric development and the segment is functional, the transverse process will retain the same amount of prominence throughout the forward to backward-bending movement arc. There is a third possibility for the finding of a transverse process being more prominent on one side than the other. This can occur when one zygapophysial joint does not open and the other does not close. This bilateral restriction retains the same amount of prominence of the posterior transverse process throughout the movement arc. One can distinguish this bilateral restriction from a structural asymmetry by evaluating the forward- to backward-bending capacity while monitoring at the interspinous space.

Figure 6.5 shows an example of the findings in the presence of nonneutral dysfunctions identified within

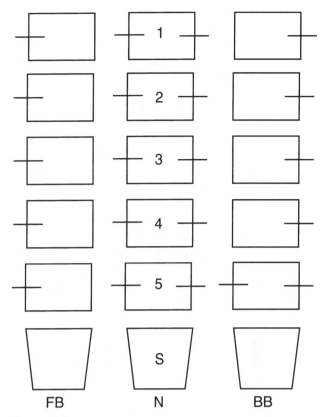

Figure 6.5.
Single-segment nonneutral vertebral dysfunction example.

the lumbar spine. A fundamental principle of the use of the diagnostic process is the importance of relating the behavior of the superior vertebra on the one below. The inferior segment is the plane of orientation against which the superior segment is related. The base reference plane is the coronal plane. If the inferior segment is rotated to the left, and the superior is level against the coronal plane, the superior vertebra in relation to the inferior segment is rotated to the right. Remember, always relate the behavior of the superior segment to that of the inferior. In this example, the sacrum is level against the coronal plane in all three positions of forward bending, neutral, and backward bending. At L5, the left transverse process becomes more prominent during forward bending whereas it is symmetric against the coronal plane in neutral and backward bending. This finding results from something interfering with the capacity of the left zygapophysial joint to open during forward bending. In both neutral and backward bending, the transverse processes are symmetric, indicating the capacity of the zygapophysial joints to close symmetrically in backward bending. The amount of restriction is not great because it is not evident by rotation to the left in neutral. The diagnosis would be the following: L5 is extended, rotated, and side bent left (ER-S_{left}), with motion restriction of forward bending, right-side bending, and right rotation. Also, note that in forward bending, the left transverse processes of L1, L2, L3, and L4 are also more prominent on the left. This finding is a result of the fact that L5 has rotated left during forward bending and the other four lumbar vertebrae have followed in a normal fashion with symmetric opening of their zygapophysial joints during forward bending. At L4, we have a different observation. At this level in backward bending, the right transverse process becomes more prominent in relation to the symmetric transverse processes at L5. In both neutral and forward bending, L4 follows the behavior of L5. In backward bending, it does not. In backward bending something has interfered with the capacity of the left zygapophysial joint to close. During backward bending, the normal closure of the right zygapophysial joint carries the vertebra into right rotation, right side bending, and backward bending on the right side. In this case, the diagnosis is as follows: L4 is Flexed, right rotated and right sidebent FRS$_{right}$ with motion restriction of backward bending, left-side bending, and left rotation. Again, note that the transverse processes of L1, L2, and L3 are also posterior on the right in backward bending. This is a normal finding because they follow the right rotation of L4. Their zygapophysial joints have the capacity to close symmetrically and follow the right rotation at L4.

NEUTRAL (GROUP) DYSFUNCTION

The characteristics of a neutral group dysfunction are

1. A group of segments (three or more)
2. Minimal flexion or extension component of restriction
3. Restriction of the group to side bending in one direction and rotation in the opposite (Fig 6.6)
4. The segments never become symmetric, maybe a little better or worse, but not symmetric

With three or more vertebral segments involved in motion restriction, a lateral curvature results to one side. There is prominence on the side of convexity of the group of segments due to rotation of the vertebrae to that side. On palpatory examination, one finds a fullness overlying the transverse processes of three or more adjacent vertebrae. This finding is frequently misdiagnosed as muscle hypertonicity or spasm because the muscle overlying the posterior transverse processes is more prominent and the impression is that the muscle is spastic, hypertonic, or tight. It is true that the muscle is more prominent, but it is the result of the rotation of the vertebrae that the transverse process is taking the muscle mass posteriorly.

During the diagnostic process of trunk, neutral, forward bending, and backward bending, the palpa-

Figure 6.6.
Neutral group vertebral dysfunction.

ble fullness over the transverse processes on one side is maintained. It may get a little better or a little worse in its deformity during the movement arc, but there is no position in which the transverse processes on each side become symmetric. The motion restriction found in this group of segments will be minimal forward- or backward-bending restriction, but with major restriction of side bending to the side of convexity and rotation to the side of concavity.

Neutral group dysfunctions are also called type I restrictions with a restricted coupled movement being side bending to one side and rotation to the opposite. These dysfunctions are present in compensatory scoliotic mechanisms and are frequently found above or below a single vertebral motion segment dysfunction. They are frequently secondary to change elsewhere, but because they involve a large number of vertebral segments they receive a lot of diagnostic attention. Because these dysfunctions are secondary to other findings, their treatment should follow appropriate treatment for the cause of the dysfunction, either a nonneutral dysfunction or unleveling of the sacral base.

Figure 6.7 portrays the findings in a group dysfunction. Again note that L5 shows a non-neutral single segment dysfunction that is ERS$_{left}$ as in Fig. 6.5. In this example, the left transverse processes are prominent from L1 to L4 in both forward bending, neutral, and backward bending. No matter what position the patient assumes, there is rotation of L1 through L4 to the left. This dysfunction is a neutral group dysfunction of L1 through L4 with the positional diagnosis being neutral, side bent right, and rotated left. Another diagnostic de-

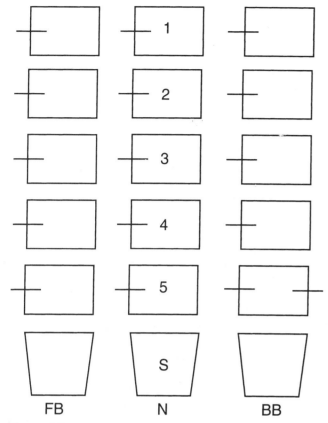

Figure 6.7.
Neutral group dysfunction example.

scription for this group dysfunction is L1 through L4 EN (easy normal) left (indicating left convexity).

In the therapeutic process, the practitioner identifies and treats all nonneutral dysfunctions first, and if any group dysfunctions remain, they are addressed separately.

Adaptation Versus Compensation

It is common to see an adaptive side bending to one side and rotation to the other in a group of vertebrae superior to a nonneutral dysfunction or an unleveled sacrum while the patient is in the neutral posture. This adaptation is the body's desire to remain in an upright position. The finding is reversible when the nonneutral dysfunction is corrected or the sacral base made level.

Compensation occurs over time with change in the anatomy and the curve remains despite correction of the underlying problem. It is not reversible.

HYPERMOBILITY

Manual medicine procedures are appropriate for restriction of articular structures (hypomobility), but if used on hypermobile segments they could be detrimental, enhancing the hypermobility. In structural diagnosis, we are concerned with three types of hypermobility: (a) hypermobility due to disease such as Ehlers–Danlos syndrome, Marfan syndrome, the mar-

fanoid hypermobility syndrome, and others even more rare; (b) physiologic hypermobility seen in certain body types (ectomorphic) and frequently observed in gymnasts, ballet dancers, and other athletes; and (c) compensatory hypermobility due to hypomobility elsewhere in the musculoskeletal system.

The pathologic hypermobilities are a group of conditions in which there is alteration in the histology and biochemistry of the connective tissues. In Ehlers–Danlos syndrome, there is articular hypermobility, dermal extensibility, and frequent cutaneous scarring. This condition has been noted in circus performers who are classified as "elastic people." The classic Marfan syndrome demonstrates long slender (Lincolnesque) limbs; ectopic lentis, dilatation of the ascending aorta, and mitral valve prolapse. While the severity of each of the components of the Marfan syndrome vary from patient to patient, all exhibit joint hypermobility. Following joint injury, the hypermobility is increased and it is very difficult to treat patients with this condition who have somatic dysfunction superimposed on their musculoskeletal anatomy. The marfanoid hypermobility syndrome has the same musculoskeletal system findings but seems not to demonstrate either the eye or the vascular changes.

The physiologic hypermobility group comprises hypermobility of fingers, thumbs, elbows, and knees and trunk forward bending. A 9-point scale has been devised for the paired fingers, thumbs, elbows, and knees, with one point assigned to trunk forward bending. Patients with this trait find it easy to become gymnasts and ballet dancers and increased mobility can result from training and exercise. In healthy individuals joint mobility reduces rapidly during childhood and then more slowly during adulthood. Patients with increased physiologic hypermobility are at risk for increased musculoskeletal system symptoms and diseases, particularly osteoarthritis.

It is in the secondary hypermobility states that the manual medicine practitioner becomes more involved. Compensatory hypermobility appears to develop in areas of the vertebral column as a secondary reaction to hypomobility within the complex. The segments of compensatory hypermobility can be adjacent to, or some distance from, the area(s) of major joint hypomobility. Clinically, there also appears to be relative hypermobility on the opposite side of a segment that is restricted. The major difficulty encountered with these areas of secondary compensatory hypermobility is that they are frequently the ones that are symptomatic. Because they attempt to compensate for restricted motion elsewhere, they receive excess stimulation from increased mobility and frequently become painful and tender. As the painful areas, they receive a great deal of attention from the manual medicine practitioner, who can become trapped into treating the hypermobile segment because it is symptomatic, not realizing that the symptom is secondary to restricted mobility elsewhere. In most instances of compensatory hypermobility, the condition requires little or no direct treatment but responds nicely to appropriate treatment of hypomobility elsewhere in the vertebral column. Many practitioners of musculoskeletal medicine use proliferent-type injection into the ligaments of a hypermobile segment as part of treatment. This system was used empirically for many years; however, recent findings from clinical and animal studies support the observation that proliferent therapy enhances joint stability and reduces nociception. In this author's experience most areas of secondary, compensatory hypermobility are self-correcting once the hypomobility areas are adequately treated and the total musculoskeletal system is restored to functional balance.

One cannot discuss hypermobility without referring to instability. Instability occurs when the damage is sufficient and the opposing joint structures lose their anatomic integrity. The dividing line between extensive hypermobility and instability is very hard to define. In actual instability, the appropriate treatment is either a stabilizing surgical procedure or a restraining orthopedic device.

Diagnosing Hypermobility

The diagnosis of hypermobility in the Ehlers–Danlos and Marfan syndrome group is not difficult as long as the index of suspicion is present and the other physical findings are identified. The 9-point scale mentioned in the previous section helps give an overall assessment of relative hypermobility. It is in the evaluation of local compensatory hypermobility that

the difficulty exists. The diagnostic procedures are variations on regional segmental motion testing. In these procedures, one attempts to hold one segment and move the other in relation to it, comparing it with the perceived normal of the segments above and below the segment suspected of hypermobility. Translatory motion challenges have been found to be the most effective. With the lumbar spine, the patient can be in the lateral recumbent position while the operator monitors each vertebral segment. By grasping two spinous processes with the thumb and index finger, a to-and-fro lateral translatory movement can be introduced and compared above and below (Fig. 6.8). Using the same lateral recumbent position with the knees and hips flexed, the operator can monitor a given segment holding the superior segment and introducing an anteroposterior translatory movement by movement of the operator's thigh against the patient's knees (Fig. 6.9). Combined side bending and rotation challenge can occur in the same position with the operator grasping the feet and ankles and lifting the extremities off the table (Fig. 6.10), and dropping them down below the table (Fig. 6.11), while monitoring the posterior elements of the lumbar vertebrae. Another hypermobility test builds on the fact that in backward bending, as the zygapophysial joints symmetrically close, there is reduction in available lateral translatory movement. With the patient in the prone prop, backward-bent position on the table (Fig. 6.12), the operator places thumbs on each side of the spinous process overlying the transverse processes of the vertebrae and translates from left to right (Fig. 6.13) and from right to left. Comparing the translatory mobility from segment to segment gives the operator an

Figure 6.8.
Hypermobility testing lateral translation.

Figure 6.9.
Hypermobility testing anteroposterior translation.

Figure 6.10.
Hypermobility testing, side-bending rotation.

Figure 6.12.
Hypermobility testing beginning with thumb contact of spinous and transverse processes while backward bent.

Figure 6.11.
Hypermobility testing, side-bending rotation.

Figure 6.13.
Hypermobility testing translation from left to right while backward bent.

impression of whether one is more mobile than the other. Testing for hypermobility requires a great deal of practice and the judgment is highly individualistic. If one suspects significant segmental hypermobility, stress x-ray procedures in the flexion–extension and right and left side-bending modes should be used to assist in the diagnosis.

CONCLUSION

While there is still a need for more research into the biomechanics of vertebral segmental motion and pathologies that might restrict vertebral motion, the concepts and methodologies described here will provide the

practicing manual medicine clinician with sufficient accurate diagnostic information for treatment purposes, for accurate records, and for communicating with a colleague. The hallmarks of structural diagnosis of restricted vertebral function are practice and experience.

SUGGESTED READING

Bogduk N, Jull G. The theoretic pathology of acute locked back: a basis for manipulative therapy. *Man Med* 1985;1:78–82.

International classification of diseases (ICD9cm) 9th Revision Commission on Professional and Hospital Activities. Ann Arbor, Mi, 1979 eg 637.

7

PRINCIPLES OF SOFT-TISSUE AND OTHER PERIPHERAL STIMULATING TECHNIQUES

Several techniques can be classified as peripheral stimulation therapies. They include soft-tissue technique procedures, Travell trigger points, Chapman reflexes, acupuncture, and others. The soft-tissue procedures to be described have had long acceptance and use in the field of manual medicine. Many of the procedures are the same as, or similar to, those found in traditional massage.

DEFINITION

Soft-tissue technique is defined as a procedure directed towards tissues other than the skeleton while monitoring response and motion changes using diagnostic palpation. It usually involves lateral stretching, linear stretching, deep pressure, traction, and/or separation of muscle origin and insertion (Glossary of Osteopathic Terminology, *J Am Osteopath Assoc* 1981;80:552–567).

PURPOSE OF SOFT-TISSUE TECHNIQUE

Soft-tissue procedures are widely used in a combined diagnostic and therapeutic mode. They are frequently a prelude to other more definitive manual medicine procedures to the underlying articular structures. They prepare the soft tissues for other technique procedures. They are also used as the only manual medicine intervention to achieve a specific therapeutic goal.

Mechanisms

These procedures have mechanical, circulatory, and neurologic effects and are useful in both acute and chronic conditions. Soft-tissue procedures can mechanically stretch the skin, fascia, and muscle tissues of the body to enhance their motion and pliability. These procedures are useful in encouraging circulation of fluid in and around the soft tissues of the musculoskeletal system, enhancing venous and lymphatic return, and decongesting parts of the body compromised by injury or a disease process. These same procedures can have a neurologic effect, particularly modifying muscle physiology to overcome hypertonicity and spasm. These neurologic effects can be stimulatory or inhibitory depending on how the procedure was applied. Another neurologic effect is the relief of musculoskeletal pain.

This may result from the release of endogenous opioids and other neurohumoral substances. Another possible mechanism is the modulation of spinal reflex pathways by the stimulation of mechanoreceptors, proprioceptors, and nociceptors in the soft tissues.

Tonic Effect

Soft-tissue procedures are also useful for their general "tonic" effect on patients, particularly those who have been bedridden for any period due to illness or injury. They seem to enhance general physical tone and level of well-being. Since many of these procedures seem general in application and result in various outcomes, the manual medicine practitioner must have a specific therapeutic goal in mind before instituting any soft-tissue procedure. Once the objective is clear, the procedure can be adapted to fit the patient's condition, patient's location, and operator's strength and ability.

TYPES OF SOFT-TISSUE PROCEDURES

Soft-tissue procedures are oriented toward the direction of a force being applied to the underlying muscle(s) (Fig. 7.1). A force at right angles to the long axis of the muscle is called lateral stretch. The force applied in the direction of the long axis of the muscle is called linear or longitudinal stretch. By applying a force in both directions along the long axis of a muscle, we achieve separation of origin and insertion. If steady deep pressure is applied to a muscle close to its attachment to the bone, the procedure is called deep pressure. Although these procedures are described in relation to muscle and its fiber direction, remember that application of external force to the muscle area also involves skin, subcutaneous fascia, and the deep fascia surrounding muscle. All of these tissues are affected by soft-tissue procedures.

THERAPEUTIC PRINCIPLES OF SOFT-TISSUE TECHNIQUE

As in all appropriate manual medicine procedures, the operator's body should be held in a posture that is comfortable and balanced to avoid undue strain or fa-

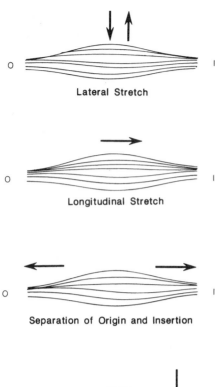

Figure 7.1.
Soft tissue procedures.

Figure 7.2.
Operator's stance.

tigue. The treatment table or bed should be at the appropriate height so that the operator need not bend forward unnecessarily (Fig. 7.2). The operator's stance should be relaxed with one foot slightly in front of the other so that the to-and-fro rocking of the operator's body mass provides the force, not operator muscle activity.

The patient should be in a comfortable and relaxed position. If the prone position is used, the head should be turned toward the operator so that lateral force does not put undue strain on the cervicothoracic junction. If a lateral recumbent position is used, an appropriate pillow height should maintain the head and neck in the long axis of the trunk. It is useful to have the patient's feet and knees together, with the knees and hips slightly flexed. This provides both comfort and stability for the patient. It is most important that the relationship of the patient and the operator be relaxed and synergistic.

The placement and use of the hands in soft-tissue procedures becomes most important. These procedures use mainly the finger pads, the thenar eminence of the hand, and the palmer aspect of the thumb. When the operator uses the finger pads to engage the tissues, the distal interphalangeal joint flexion that occurs is a function of the flexor digitorum profundus (Fig. 7.3). Beginners in manual medicine have to practice strengthening the profundus tendon flexor action in order to maintain appropriate application of force to soft tissues. The thenar eminence and palmer surface of the thumb can be laid along the long axis of muscle and used singly (Fig. 7.4), paired (Fig. 7.5), or with one hand reinforcing the other (Fig. 7.6). It is very important that the soft tissues be adequately and accurately engaged at the appropriate layer. In treating the erector spinae mass, there are two common errors to be avoided. The first is pressure toward the spinous processes instead of away from the spinous processes on the side being treated. This causes compression of the erector spinae mass against the lateral side of the spinous process, is painful to the patient, and is counterproductive. The second error is allowing the therapeutic hand to "snap over" an area of hypertonic muscle through failure of control at the muscle layer. Hand placement and control become most important.

Figure 7.3.
Soft-tissue, finger pad contact.

Figure 7.5.
Paired hand, soft-tissue contact.

Figure 7.4.
Single hand, soft-tissue contact.

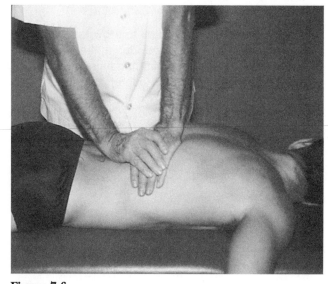

Figure 7.6.
Combined hand, soft-tissue contact.

The dosage of soft-tissue procedures is modified by the rate, rhythm, and length of time of application, and, most important, by the constant feedback of the tissues to the response obtained. Constant reassessment of the response is the hallmark of soft-tissue procedures. The operator should continue until the desired response is obtained or should stop as soon as it has been achieved. If the tissue response is not as anticipated, the procedure should be stopped and reassessment of the diagnosis and status of the patient should be made. Slow and steady soft-tissue procedures appear to have inhibitory effects on the tissues. More rapid and vigorous applications of force appear to be stimulatory. The goal to be achieved and the response of the tissues modify the application of force. The operator must also be aware of other reactions within the patient in addition to those of the tissue being treated. Sometimes patients become quite agitated and at other times, they become very relaxed and almost euphoric. It must be remembered that although these procedures are passive, they are still fatiguing, and the length of treatment might be modified by the response of the patient.

Soft-tissue Techniques

Cervical Spine

Procedure: Unilateral lateral stretch

1. Patient is supine on table with operator on side of the table facing the patient (example left side) (Fig. 7.7).
2. Operator's right hand stabilizes patient's forehead.
3. Operator's left hand grasps the patient's right cervical paravertebral musculature with fingertips medial to the muscle mass and just lateral to the spinous processes.
4. Lateral stretch is placed on the cervical musculature by the operator's left hand pulling laterally and somewhat anteriorly, with the operator's right hand maintaining the stability of the patient's head.
5. Lateral stretch is applied and released rhythmically throughout the cervical musculature with particular reference to areas of increased muscle tone and soft-tissue congestion.
6. The procedure can be varied to allow the patient's head to rotate toward the left during the application of force by the operator's left hand and a counterforce can be applied by the operator's right hand in a "push–pull" manner.
7. The procedure can be repeated on the opposite side by having the operator now stand on the patient's right.

Soft-tissue Techniques

Cervical Spine

Procedure: Bilateral–lateral stretch

1. Patient is supine on table with operator standing at head of table (Fig. 7.8).
2. Operator's finger pads contact the medial side of the cervical paravertebral musculature bilaterally.
3. The operator puts simultaneous lateral stretch on both sides of the cervical musculature, moving from above downward or below upward and focusing on side of greater tissue reaction and muscle hypertonicity.

Figure 7.7.
Soft-tissue, unilateral lateral stretch.

Figure 7.8.
Soft-tissue, bilateral lateral stretch.

Soft-Tissue Techniques

Cervical Spine

Procedure: Long axis longitudinal stretch

1. Patient is supine with operator standing or sitting at head of table.
2. Operator's one hand cradles the skull with the index finger and thumb in contact with the insertion of the cervical musculature into the occiput and the chin held by the other hand (Fig. 7.9).
3. By the use of body weight, the operator puts long-axis extension (traction) in a cephalic direction and then releases.
4. Repeat as necessary.

Caution: Too much traction is frequently counterproductive.

Soft-Tissue Techniques

Cervical Spine

Procedure: Suboccipital muscle deep pressure

1. Patient is supine with operator standing or sitting at head of table.
2. Operator's fingertips of each hand contact the bony attachment of the deep cervical musculature at the suboccipital region.
3. By flexing the distal interphalangeal joints, the operator puts sustained deep pressure over the muscular attachment to the occipital bone (Fig. 7.10).
4. Pressure is applied on each side to achieve balance in tension and tone.
5. Pressure is released when bilateral relaxation occurs.

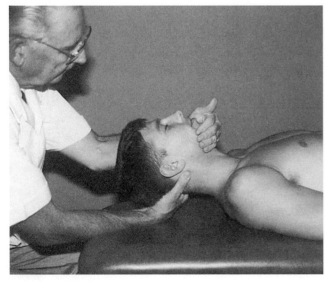

Figure 7.9.
Long axis, longitudinal stretch.

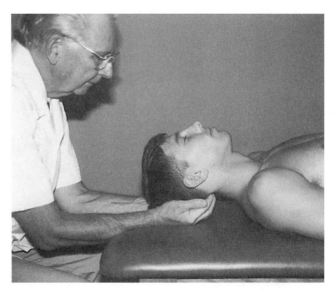

Figure 7.10.
Suboccipital muscle, deep pressure.

Soft-tissue Techniques

Cervical Spine

Procedure: Separation origin and insertion (example: right upper trapezius)

1. Patient is supine with operator standing at head of table.
2. Operator's left hand is placed over the patient's occiput and controls head and neck position.
3. Operator's right hand is placed over the patient's right acromion process (Fig. 7.11).
4. Operator's left hand side bends the head and neck to the left with some left rotation while right hand puts counterforce on the acromion process, separating the origin and insertion of the upper fibers of the trapezius.
5. By reversal of hand position, the opposite side can be treated with the goal of symmetry of length and tone of each trapezius.

Soft-tissue Techniques

Thoracic Spine

Procedure: Lateral stretch

1. Patient is in lateral recumbent position lying with involved side uppermost with operator standing and facing patient.
2. For upper thoracic region, patient's left arm is draped over operator's right arm and finger pads contact medial side of paravertebral musculature (Fig. 7.12).

3. Operator pulls thoracic paravertebral musculature laterally and releases in a rhythmic fashion.
4. A counterforce can be applied by the operator's left arm against the patient's left shoulder for additional leverage.
5. For rhomboid stretch, use the same body position as for upper thoracic spine but now finger pads are in contact with vertebral border of scapula (Fig. 7.13). The scapula is swept anterolaterally around the chest wall with stretch in the direction of the fibers of the rhomboid muscle.
6. Repeat as necessary.

Figure 7.12.
Lateral stretch, upper thoracic region.

Figure 7.11.
Separation of origin and insertion.

Figure 7.13.
Lateral stretch, rhomboid region.

Soft-tissue Techniques

Thoracolumbar Spine

Procedure: Lateral stretch

1. Patient lies in lateral recumbent position with involved side uppermost. Operator faces patient.

2. Operator's right hand grasps the thoracolumbar paravertebral muscle mass on the involved side with the left hand stabilizing the patient's left shoulder (Fig. 7.14).

3. An alternative hand position has the operator's left hand grasping the thoracolumbar paravertebral muscle mass and with the right hand stabilizing the patient's pelvis over the left ilium. (Fig. 7.15).

4. Operator's hand in contact with the paravertebral musculature stretches laterally against the counterforce applied at the pelvis or the shoulder girdle.

5. Repeat as necessary throughout the thoracolumbar muscle region.

6. Variation sometimes allows patient's left arm to be flexed at the elbow and the operator's left hand to be threaded through before application to paravertebral musculature.

Figure 7.14.
Lateral stretch, thoracolumbar region.

Figure 7.15.
Lateral stretch, thoracolumbar region.

Soft Tissue Techniques

Thoracolumbar Spine

Procedure: Lateral and longitudinal stretch

1. Patient in lateral recumbent position with involved side uppermost. Operator faces patient.
2. Operator's left forearm is threaded through the patient's left axilla and left hand in contact with the left paravertebral muscle mass.
3. Operator's right forearm is a superior aspect of the patient's left ilium with finger pads in contact with the left paravertebral musculature.
4. Finger-pad contact of both hands stretches paravertebral musculature laterally (Fig. 7.16).
5. Simultaneously with lateral stretch, the operator's forearms are separated with the right arm going caudally and the left cephalically applying a longitudinal stretch (Fig. 7.17).
6. Repeat as necessary throughout the lumbar and thoracic paravertebral musculature.

Soft Tissue Techniques

Thoracolumbar Spine

Procedure: Prone lateral stretch

1. Patient lies prone on table with arms at side and face turned toward operator.
2. Operator stands at side of table.
3. Operator's thumbs and thenar eminences are placed on medial side of involved paravertebral

musculature. Lateral stretch is applied rhythmically throughout the involved areas (Fig. 7.5).

4. A variation is applying lateral stretch using one hand on top of the other as reinforcement (Fig. 7.6).
5. Another variation is for the operator's right hand to grasp the patient's right anterior superior iliac spine while the left thumb and thenar eminence puts lateral stretch on paravertebral musculature (Fig. 7.18). Lifting the patient's right ilium provides a counterforce.
6. Repeat as necessary.

Figure 7.17.
Separation of origin and insertion.

Figure 7.16.
Lateral recumbent, lateral stretch with counterforce.

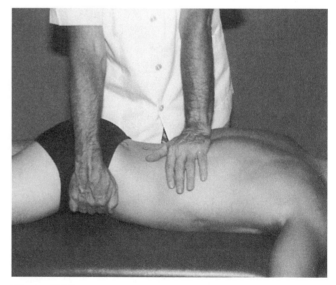

Figure 7.18.
Prone, lateral stretch with counterforce.

Soft-tissue Techniques

Thoracolumbar Spine

Procedure: Deep pressure

1. Patient is prone on table.
2. Operator places thumbs, or thumb reinforced by hand, over area of hypertonic muscle (Fig. 7.19). This is most effective in the medial groove between the spinous process and the longissimus, and overlying the hypertonic fourth-layer vertebral muscle.

3. Steady pressure is applied in a ventral direction and sustained until muscle release is felt.
4. A variation is the placement of the operator's olecranon process of the elbow overlying the hypertonic muscle. Body weight can be used to provide ventral compressive force against hypertonic muscle (Fig. 7.20).
5. Repeat as necessary.

Figure 7.19.
Deep inhibitory pressure with thumbs.

Figure 7.20.
Deep inhibitory pressure using elbow.

Soft-tissue Techniques

Gluteal Region

Procedure: Deep pressure

1. Patient is in prone or lateral recumbent position with involved side uppermost.

2. Operator can stand at the side or in front of the patient.

3. Reinforced thumbs are placed over hypertonic areas of gluteal musculature either near origin on the ilium, within the belly, or at insertion in greater trochanter (Fig. 7.21).

4. Deep pressure is maintained until relaxation is felt.

5. Variation can be the use of the olecranon process of the elbow as the contact point and body weight being applied against the hypertonic muscle (Fig. 7.22).

6. Repeat as necessary.

To this point, the soft-tissue techniques have been directed toward the skin, fascia, and muscle in a biomechanical or postural–structural model. Other soft tissues of the body respond well to appropriate soft-tissue technique using a different model, particularly the respiratory–circulatory model and the visceral model.

Lymphatic Pump Techniques

Lymphatic pump techniques are an application of the respiratory–circulatory model. The therapeutic goal is to enhance venous and lymphatic flow throughout the body and respiratory exchange. An underlying principle of the respiratory–circulatory model is to work from central to distal. Because all of the lymph flow of the body empties into the venous system through the subclavian veins at the thoracic inlet, the thoracic inlet is the place to start. The most effective thoracic inlet technique in this author's hand has been the necklace technique in the myofascial release technique system (see Chapter 11). The thoracoabdominal diaphragm is the most important "pump" of the venous and lymphatic systems. It is but one of several diaphragms in the body that must work synergistically for maximum total body efficiency. In addition to the thoracoabdominal diaphragm, there are three others from the functional perspective. One is in the cranium (see Chapter 12) and is the diaphragmatic function of the tentorium cerebelli. The aforementioned thoracic inlet also functions as a diaphragm exerting pumping action on the structures that pass through it. For the thoracic inlet to function effectively, there must be good biomechanics of T1 and the first ribs. The fourth is the pelvic diaphragm, which exerts a strong influence on the pelvic viscera in both males and females. The pelvic diaphragm is intimately related to the biomechanics of the pelvis, the sacrum, and the pubes. All four of these diaphragms need to function as a coordinated unit. Most of the lymph pump techniques focus on the chest wall and address primarily thoracoabdominal diaphragmatic function.

Figure 7.21.
Deep pressure gluteal region.

Figure 7.22.
Deep pressure using olecranon process.

Diaphramatic Techniques

Thoracic Inlet

See thoracic inlet (necklace technique) Chapter 11.

Pectoral Release

1. Patient supine with operator at head of table.
2. Operator's two hands, particularly the middle fingers, grasp patient's inferior border of the pectoral muscles (Fig. 7.23).
3. Operator applies bilateral cephalic traction on the inferior aspect of the pectoral muscles.
4. The response elicited is release of muscle tension.
5. Observe thorax and abdomen for change from thoracic to abdominal breathing.

Thoracoabdominal Diaphragm

Procedure: Diaphragmatic release patient supine

1. Patient supine on table with operator standing at side.
2. Operator's fingertips contact inferior surface of diaphragm below costal arch on each side. Operator's other hand stabilizes lower anterior rib cage (Fig. 7.24).

3. Operator maintains cephalic pressure on the inferior aspect of the diaphragm. Inhalation is resisted and exhalation encouraged. Fingertip compression is maintained until diaphragm is released.

Diaphragmatic Release Sitting Technique

1. Patient sits on table with operator behind.
2. Operator's fingertips bilaterally contact the inferior surface of the diaphragm below the costal arch (Fig. 7.25).

Figure 7.24.
Diaphragmatic release, supine.

Figure 7.23.
Pectoral release.

Figure 7.25.
Diaphragmatic release, sitting.

3. Patient slumps against the operator by forward bending the trunk (Fig. 7.26).

4. Operator maintains cephalic compression on the inferior aspect of the diaphragm during patient's inhalation effort.

5. Several applications may be necessary with fine-tuning of operator's fingers on specific areas of the diaphragmatic tension.

6. A variation finds the operator sitting in front of the patient with the thumbs in contact with the inferior surface of the diaphragm below the costal arch (Fig. 7.27). Patient slumps forward on operator's thumbs. Exhalation effort is followed by upward pressure by operator against points of diaphragmatic tension. Repeat until diaphragmatic release is obtained (Fig. 7.28).

Figure 7.27.
Diaphragmatic release, sitting.

Figure 7.26.
Diaphragmatic release, sitting.

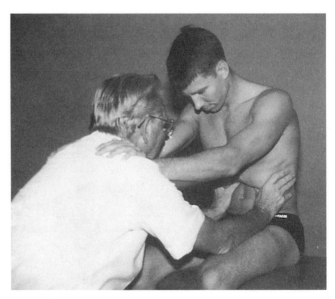

Figure 7.28.
Diaphragmatic release, sitting.

Pelvic Diaphragm

Procedure: Pelvic diaphragm release, lateral recumbent

1. Patient in lateral recumbent position with hips and knees flexed, involved side uppermost.
2. Operator stands in front of patient with extended fingers of right hand placed on medial side of left ischial tuberosity (Fig. 7.29).
3. Fingers move cephalad along ischium to the lateral side of the ischiorectal fossa until fingertips contact pelvic diaphragm.
4. During patient exhalation, operator's fingers move cephalad and hold against pelvic diaphragm as patient performs deep inhalation.
5. With release of diaphragmatic tension, the palpating fingers observe the diaphragm to move freely into fingers during inhalation and away during exhalation.
6. Repeat on both sides until symmetric balance is achieved.

Pelvic Diaphragm

Procedure: Pelvic diaphragm supine

1. Patient supine on table with hips and knees flexed.
2. Operator stands or sits at side of patient facing toward the head.
3. Operator's fingers contact medial side of right ischial tuberosity and move cephalad to contact the pelvic diaphragm at the superior aspect of the ischiorectal fossa (Fig. 7.30).
4. During patient inhalation the diaphragm should descend against operator's fingers and during exhalation should ascend away from fingers.
5. The most common dysfunction is the inability to fully ascend. Treatment consists of maintaining cephalic pressure on the diaphragm as the patient inhales. During exhalation, the operator follows the diaphragm cephalad as far as possible and repeats the respiratory action.
6. The procedure can be combined by having the operator's other hand contact the lower right costal cage to monitor the thoracoabdominal diaphragm to be sure the two diaphragms are working synchronously.

Figure 7.29.
Pelvic diaphragm, lateral recumbent.

Figure 7.30.
Pelvic diaphragm, supine.

Rib Raising Techniques

Rib raising techniques influence rib cage mechanics to enhance venous and lymphatic flow and respiratory exchange. They also have another benefit. The lateral chain ganglia of the sympathetic division of the autonomic nervous system lie on the posterior chest wall overlying the rib heads. Increased mobility of the rib heads appears to have a positive effect on the segmental function of the sympathetic nervous system. Rib raising in the upper thorax above T5 affects the intrathoracic viscera. Below T5, the effect is on the intraabdominal viscera. It is beneficial to maximize thoracic cage function before instituting lymph pump treatment.

Rib Raising Supine

1. Patient supine with operator standing or sitting at the side.

2. Operator's hands slide under the patient with finger contact medial to the rib angles and with forearms in contact with the table (Fig. 7.31).

3. Operator's fingers put lateral traction on the rib angles while lifting the rib cage by pushing down on the forearms. Do not try to lift the rib cage by wrist flexion.

4. Move up and down the rib cage on both sides. If a second operator is available, bilateral rib raising can be done.

Rib Raising Sitting

1. Patient sitting with operator standing in front.

2. Patient crosses forearms grasping the opposite elbow and places them on operator's chest. An alternate position places the patient's extended arms over the operator's shoulder.

3. Operator contacts medial to the rib angles bilaterally and pulls laterally while pulling the patient toward the operator (Fig. 7.32).

4. Operator moves from above downward or below upward while patient inhales when operator pulls patient forward and exhales on relaxation.

Figure 7.31.
Rib raising, supine.

Figure 7.32.
Rib raising, sitting.

Lymphatic Pump

Procedure: Thoracic lymphatic pump

1. Patient is supine on table with operator at head of table.
2. Operator has both hands in contact with anterior aspect of the thoracic cage with heel of hand just below the clavicle (Fig. 7.33).
3. Operator repetitively and rhythmically oscillates the chest at a rate of approximately 100 to 110 times per minute.
4. A preferred alternate technique has the patient inhale deeply and then exhale.
5. During exhalation phase, the operator puts oscillatory compression on chest cage.
6. At end of exhalation, patient is instructed to breathe in while operator holds chest wall in exhalation position for a momentary period.
7. Operator rapidly releases compression on chest during patient's inhalation effort.
8. Repeat steps 4 through 7 several times.

Lymphatic Pump

Procedure: Unilateral thoracic lymphatic pump

1. Patient is supine with operator at side of table.
2. Operator's left arm grasps the patient's right upper extremity.
3. Operator's right hand is in contact with right thoracic cage of patient (Fig. 7.34).
4. During patient's inhalation, operator puts traction on patient's right upper extremity.
5. During exhalation phase, traction on upper extremity is released, and operator puts oscillatory force against thoracic cage during exhalation.
6. Operator's right hand maintains compression on chest wall during initial phase of inhalation and gives rapid release, simultaneously cephalically lifting on patient's right upper extremity.

Figure 7.33.
Bilateral thoracic lymph pump, supine.

Figure 7.34.
Unilateral thoracic lymph pump.

7. Repeat steps 2 through 6 several times.

8. A lateral recumbent variation has the patient with the treated side being uppermost. The operator's left arm grasps the patient's right upper extremity while the operator's right hand is applied to the patient's right thoracic cage (Fig 7.35). Steps 2 through 6 are repeated several times.

Lymphatic Pump

Procedure: Lymphatic pump, lower extremity

1. Patient is supine with operator at end of table.

2. Operator grasps dorsum of both feet with each hand and introduces plantar flexion (Fig. 7.36).

3. Operator applies oscillatory movement in a caudad direction and notes oscillatory wave of lower extremities up to trunk.

4. Operator's grasps toes and ball of patient's foot and take foot into dorsi flexion (Fig. 7.37).

5. Cephalic oscillatory movement is applied to the dorsiflexed feet.

6. Repeat in the dorsiflexed and plantar-flexed directions several times.

Lymphatic Pump

Procedure: Lymphatic pump, upper extremity

1. Patient supine with operator at head of table.

2. Patient raises both hands above head and operator grasps each wrist (Fig. 7.38).

3. Operator applies intermittent cephalic oscillatory traction to patient's upper extremities noting response in the thoracic cage.

4. Repeat as necessary.

Figure 7.36.
Lymphatic pump, lower extremity.

Figure 7.35.
Unilateral thoracic lymph pump.

Figure 7.37.
Lymphatic pump, lower extremity.

Visceral Technique

The internal viscera are specialized soft tissues encased and suspended in specialized fasciae. As such they are subject to fascial drag, twisting, and compression. Visceral techniques are designed to enhance visceral mobility, reduce passive congestion, and increase drainage of hollow organs. In addition to direct approaches to the viscera it is important to recall the innervation to the viscera under treatment. All internal viscera receive parasympathetic and sympathetic innervation. The best approach to the parasympathetic division is through the craniosacral technique (see Chapter 12) giving particular attention to the cranial base and the jugular foramen. The vagus nerve has some connection with the C2 root. Therefore, good function of the cranial base and upper cervical spine seem to enhance good parasympathetic nerve function. The pelvic organs receive parasympathetic innervation from the sacral nerves. Normalization of sacral function from the craniosacral and biomechanical perspectives appears to have a beneficial effect on parasympathetic innervation to pelvic viscera. The sympathetic division innervation of the viscera is segmentally related with all of the viscera above the diaphragm having preganglionic origin in the spinal cord above T5, and all of the viscera below the diaphragm below T5. Rib raising described above is one way to positively influence sympathetic nervous system function. Visceral techniques need to be applied gently and with an appreciation of their structural anatomy. Visceral techniques found useful in this author's experience follow.

Visceral Technique

Procedure: Supine mesenteric release

1. Patient is supine on table with operator standing at side.

2. Operator places both hands on each side of the anterior abdomen (Fig. 7.39).

3. Operator applies clockwise and counterclockwise rotations to the anterior abdominal wall with some abdominal compression. The operator senses the mobility of the small and large intestines and follows their directions of motility.

4. Sensation of release of underlying abdominal contents is end point.

Figure 7.38.
Lymphatic pump, upper extremity.

Figure 7.39.
Supine mesenteric release.

Visceral Technique

Procedure: Mesenteric release prone position

1. Patient is prone on table in knee–chest position.

2. Operator stands at side or head of table.

3. Operator places both hands over lower abdomen just above pubic bones (Fig. 7.40).

4. Operator's hands lift abdominal contents out of pelvis in slow oscillatory fashion until release is felt.

5. Operator localizes lifting force in the right lower quadrant for the cecum, the left lower quadrant for the sigmoid colon, and the suprapubic area for the pelvic organs.

Visceral Technique

Procedure: Cecum and sigmoid lifts, lateral recumbent

1. Patient in right lateral recumbent position for the cecum.

2. Operator stands behind and reaches across abdomen to pick up the cecum and carry it cephalad and medially (Fig. 7.41).

3. Operator follows ascending colon to the hepatic flexure reducing restrictions.

4. Patient in left lateral recumbent position for the sigmoid colon.

5. Operator stands behind and reaches across abdomen to pick up sigmoid colon and carry it cephalad and medially (Fig. 7.42).

6. Operator follows descending colon to splenic flexure reducing restrictions.

Figure 7.41.
Lift of cecum.

Figure 7.40.
Prone mesenteric release

Figure 7.42.
Lift of sigmoid colon.

Visceral Technique

Procedure: Liver and gallbladder drainage

1. Operator begins by releasing tension around the liver and gallbladder area by modifying supine diaphragmatic release localizing to liver margin and gallbladder under right diaphragm (Fig. 7.24).

2. Patient supine and operator standing at right side.

3. Operator places one hand behind lower right rib cage and the other over the right costal arch (Fig. 7.43).

4. Operator alternately compresses and releases liver and gallbladder between two hands.

5. A variation has the patient in the left lateral recumbent position with the operator behind with hands in front and behind right costal arch and lower rib cage (Fig. 7.44).

6. Operator alternately compresses and relaxes pressure over liver and gallbladder.

7. A second variation is a repetitive percussive application of force through the forearm contact over the right costal arch (Fig. 7.45).

Figure 7.44.
Liver pump, lateral recumbent.

Figure 7.43.
Liver pump, supine.

Figure 7.45.
Liver percussion.

Visceral Technique

Procedure: Splenic drainage

1. Operator releases tension around spleen by modifying diaphragmatic release under left costal margin (Fig. 7.24).

2. Patient supine on table with operator standing at left side.

3. Operator places posterior hand over left lower rib cage and the anterior hand over left costal arch (Fig. 7.46).

4. Operator alternately compresses and releases over the spleen.

5. An alternative has the patient in the right lateral recumbent position and the operator behind and with hands in front and behind the spleen providing alternating pressure and relaxation (Fig. 7.47).

6. An alternative has the operator applying a percussive force over the left costal arch stimulating splenic drainage (Fig. 7.48).

Soft-tissue techniques can be quite helpful in treating a patient with any number of upper respiratory infections, otitis media, colds, flulike symptoms, and so forth. They are designed to assist in the drainage of the lymphatic channels from the head and neck. Again, the thoracic inlet should be examined and treated first to allow better drainage into the mediastinum.

Figure 7.47.
Splenic pump, lateral recumbent.

Figure 7.46.
Splenic pump, supine.

Figure 7.48.
Splenic percussion.

Soft Tissue Technique

Procedure: Mandibular drainage

1. Patient supine with operator standing opposite the side to be treated.
2. Operator places one hand over the frontal area to stabilize the head and the other hand grasps the ramus of the mandible as far as the angle (Fig. 7.49).
3. Patient relaxes the jaw and the operator puts rhythmic caudal and medial traction on the mandible stimulating drainage of the eustachian tube.
4. The procedure is applied bilaterally.

Soft Tissue Technique

Procedure: Hyoid mobilization

1. Patient supine on table with operator standing at the side.
2. Operator's one hand holds the frontal area stabilizing the head and the thumb and index finger of the other hand gently grasps the hyoid bone (Fig. 7.50).
3. Operator gently rocks the hyoid bone from side to side, relaxing tension in the supra- and infrahyoid muscles.

Figure 7.49.
Mandibular drainage.

Figure 7.50.
Hyoid mobilization.

Soft-tissue Technique

Procedure: Cervical lymphatic drainage

1. Patient supine on table with operator standing at side.

2. Operator stabilizes head with one hand on the frontal area with the other hand placed on the cervical lymphatic chain, first in front of (Fig. 7.51) then posterior to the sternocleidomastoid muscle (Fig. 7.52).

3. Operator gently and rhythmically "milks" the cervical lymphatic chain from above downward on each side, enhancing lymph drainage.

Figure 7.51.
Cervical lymphatic drainage.

Figure 7.52.
Cervical lymphatic drainage.

OTHER SOFT-TISSUE TECHNIQUES

There are a variety of peripheral stimulating techniques that have been described as beneficial. They include Chapman reflexes and Travell trigger points.

Chapman Reflexes

In the 1920s, Frank Chapman, D.O., originally described Chapman reflexes. The first definitive publication of the work was by Charles Owens, D.O., in cooperation with Chapman's widow, Ada Hinckley Chapman, D.O., and W. F. Link, D.O., in 1937. Chapman reflexes are found on the anterior and posterior surfaces of the body as small (2 to 3 mm), round, shotty, tender nodules in remarkably consistent locations usually near bony or cartilaginous structures. They have been correlated with disease or dysfunction of the internal organs. It has been postulated that they are related in some fashion to the lymphatic system and operate through the sympathetic nervous system. Attempts at histologic study of these reflexes have been disappointing, but many clinicians have corroborated the clinical observation of these reflex points. They have been deemed useful in the differential diagnosis of a patient with a difficult presentation and their inclusion in the physical examination can be helpful. The anterior points are used more for diagnosis and the posterior points for treatment. Most clinicians find them more useful diagnostically. Finding the reflex point in the appropriate area that is exquisitely tender while other reflex areas are silent makes the diagnosis. Treatment of both anterior and posterior reflexes is by rotary pressure for 10 to 30 seconds until the reflex point becomes less tender and appears to be less well localized. Addressing the Chapman reflexes as part of management may assist in treatment of the patient (Figs. 7.53 and 7.54).

Travell Trigger Points

Another system of soft-tissue peripheral stimulation technique was developed by Janet Travell, M.D. She observed the presence of tender "taut band" points in muscles that usually had specific referred pain patterns. Travell and her colleague, David Simons, M.D., have mapped out these localized areas of muscle irritability throughout the body. She originally treated these trigger points by the injection of local pro-caine. Subsequently, it was found that these trigger points responded to dry needling and localized cooling and stretching. These points are also similar to those subjected to sustained compression by "acupressure." Travell identified many of these trigger points as the cause of suspected visceral disease, particularly in the pectoral muscles simulating coronary heart disease. Autonomic nervous system effects have also been associated with the presence of trigger points. Identifying a trigger point in a muscle and observing its referral pattern on stimulation make the diagnosis. The exact mapping of the myriad of trigger points in the system is found in the two-volume text, *Myofascial Pain and Dysfunction.* Through experience, this author has found that there is relationship between the presence of myofascial trigger points and levels of vertebral segmental dysfunction. Many times, an identified trigger point will disappear when a manual medicine procedure has been applied to a vertebral dysfunction in a dermatomal relationship to the muscle trigger. Sometimes the trigger does not respond. Likewise, treating a trigger point, particularly with needling, will result in the resolution of the vertebral somatic dysfunction. There is currently no explanation for this observation. It is also interesting to note that myofascial trigger points are more commonly found in phasic muscles than in tonic muscles, with the exception of the levator scapulae and quadratus lumborum muscles. This author previously injected trigger points regularly but has recently experienced the need to only inject those that do not respond to treatment of the rest of the musculoskeletal system. The most common muscles still requiring injection are the levator scapulae and the quadratus lumborum. The reader is encouraged to study this system through the work of Travell and Simons. It will be found very worthwhile.

CONCLUSION

Soft-tissue procedures are useful in a wide variety of acute to chronic patient conditions. They are applicable to all regions of the body. They are useful as independent procedures or can be combined with other manual medicine procedures. Experience in palpating the tissue response to the soft tissue is necessary to properly use them for the appropriate diagnosis.

Figure 7.53.
Chapman reflexes: anterior points. (From Kuchera and Kuchera, *Osteopathic considerations in systemic dysfunction.* Kuchera ML and Kuchera WA, Columbus Ohio: Greyden Press, 1994, with permission.)

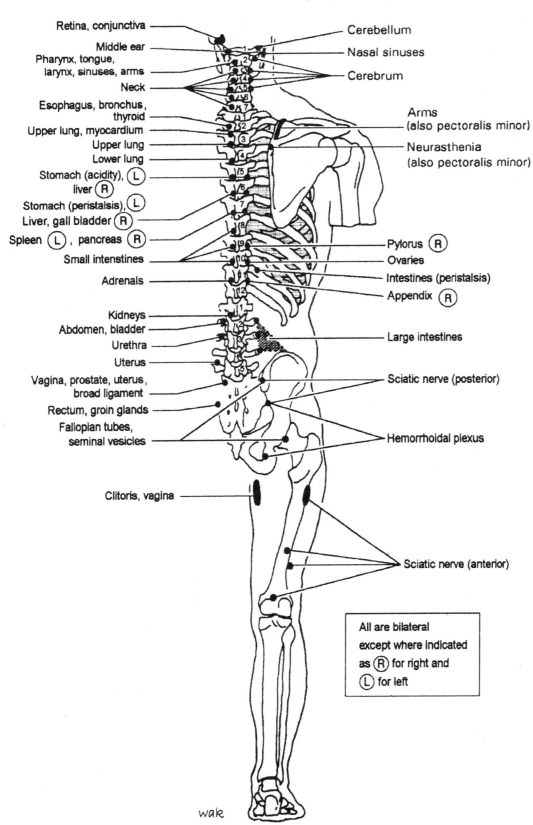

Figure 7.54.
Chapman reflexes: posterior points. (From Kuchera and Kuchera, *Osteopathic considerations in systemic dysfunction.* Greyden Press, 1994, with permission.)

SUGGESTED READING

Sandoz R. Some physical mechanisms and effects of spinal adjustments. *Ann Swiss Chiro Assoc* 1976;6: 91–141.

Travell J, Simons D. *Myofascial Pain and Dysfunction, the Trigger Point Manual.* Baltimore, Williams & Wilkins, 1983.

Tucker C, Deoora T. *Fundamental osteopathic techniques.* Melbourne: Research Publications, 1995.

Ward RL, Spraf Kas. Glossary of Osteopathic Terminology. *J Amer Osteopath Assn*, 1981 80: 552–567.

8

PRINCIPLES OF MUSCLE ENERGY TECHNIQUE

The heritage of the "bonesetters" gave all practitioners of manual medicine the aura of "putting a bone back in place." The muscle component of the musculoskeletal system did not receive as much attention. Early techniques did speak of muscle relaxation with soft-tissue procedures but specific manipulative approaches to muscle appear to be a 20th-century phenomena. In osteopathic medicine, Dr. T. J. Ruddy developed techniques that he described as resistive duction. The patient with a tempo approximating the pulse rate accomplished a series of muscle contractions against resistance. He used these techniques in the cervical spine and around the orbit in his practice as an ophthalmologist–otorhinolaryngologist.

Dr. Fred L. Mitchell, Sr., is acknowledged as the father of the system that we now call muscle energy technique. He took many of Ruddy's principles and incorporated them into a system of manual medicine procedures that could be applicable to any region of the body or any particular articulation. Mitchell was a great student of anatomy and a gifted osteopathic physician. He was influenced by the primary role of the pelvis in Chapman reflexes (see Chapter 7). He made a comprehensive study of the pelvis, its anatomy and biomechanics known at the time, and of the muscles action associated with pelvic function. He adapted muscle contraction to restore more normal motion to dysfunctional articulations in the extremities and the vertebral column. In the late 1950s and 1960s, he and Paul Kimberly, D.O., taught a 2½-day seminar under the aegis of the American Academy of Osteopathy entitled "The Pelvis and Its Environs." Despite the popularity of these offerings, the muscle energy techniques did not become integrated into common practice. In 1970, he taught an intensive weeklong tutorial in Ft. Dodge, Iowa for six students. Five members of this class became faculty in colleges of osteopathic medicine. He continued to teach in this tutorial fashion until his death in 1974. Upon his death, his tutorial students banded together to perpetuate and disseminate his work by developing three courses for the American Academy of Osteopathy. His son Fred Mitchell, Jr., with P.S. Moran and N.A. Pruzzo, first published the essence of the muscle energy system in 1973 entitled *An Evaluation and Treatment Manual of Osteopathic Manipulative Procedures*. Dr. Mitchell Jr. has recently published a three-volume work entitled *The Muscle Energy Manual*.

Dr. Mitchell, Sr., is given major credit for the muscle energy system, but his system could well be described as "Mitchell's biomechanical model of the pelvis." He believed that the pelvis is the key to the musculoskeletal system. Despite the great amount of research knowledge of the pelvis gained in the past 20 years, his concepts of pelvic function and dysfunction have stood the test of time and retain great clinical relevance.

Muscle energy technique has become incorporated into the practice of physical therapy; massage therapy, and manual medicine worldwide. The first use in Europe was the Geyman–Lewyt variation. Later, Lewyt and Bourdillon, the latter a British-trained orthopedic surgeon who became a student, practitioner, teacher and author in manual medicine, described it as postisometric technique. The Swiss neurologist and manual medicine practitioner, Jiri Dvorak, M.D., described it as NMT (neuromuscular therapy) and described three different muscle approaches.

WHAT IS MUSCLE ENERGY TECHNIQUE?

Muscle energy technique is a manual medicine treatment procedure that involves the voluntary contraction of patient muscle in a precisely controlled direction, at varying levels of intensity, against a distinctly executed counterforce applied by the operator. Muscle energy procedures have wide application and are classified as active techniques in which the patient contributes the corrective force. The activating force is classified as intrinsic. The patient is responsible for the dosage applied.

Muscle energy technique has many clinical uses. It can be used to lengthen a shortened, contractured, or spastic muscle; to strengthen a physiologically weakened muscle or group of muscles; to reduce localized edema and relieve passive congestion (the muscles are the pump of the lymphatic and venous systems); and to mobilize an articulation with restricted mobility. The function of any articulation in the body that can be moved by voluntary muscle action, either directly or indirectly, can be influenced by muscle energy procedures. The amount of patient effort may vary from a minimal muscle twitch to a maximal muscle contraction. The duration of the effort may vary from a fraction of a second to a sustained effort lasting several seconds.

TYPES OF MUSCULAR CONTRACTION

There are four different types of muscle contraction in muscle energy technique. They are

1. Isometric
2. Concentric isotonic
3. Eccentric isotonic
4. "Isolytic"

During an isometric contraction, the distance between the origin and the insertion of the muscle is maintained at a constant length. A fixed tension develops in the muscle as the patient contracts the muscle against an equal counterforce applied by the operator, preventing shortening of the muscle from the origin to the insertion.

A concentric isotonic contraction occurs when the muscle tension causes the origin and insertion to approximate.

An eccentric isotonic contraction is one in which the muscle tension allows the origin and insertion to separate. In fact, the muscle lengthens.

An "isolytic" contraction is a nonphysiologic event in which the contraction of the patient attempts to be concentric with approximation of the origin and insertion, but an external force applied by the operator occurs in the opposite direction.

With the elbow as an example, let us see how each of these contractions operates. With the patient's elbow flexed, the operator holds the distal forearm and shoulder. The patient is instructed to bring the wrist to the shoulder while the operator holds the wrist and shoulder in the same relative position. The force inserted by the patient's contracting biceps has an equal counterforce applied by the operator. This results in isometric contraction of the biceps brachii muscle. Muscle tone increases but the origin and insertion do not approximate.

A concentric isotonic contraction occurs during the process of holding a weight in the hand and bringing it to the shoulder by increasing the flexion at the elbow. The concentric isotonic contraction of the biceps brachii increases muscle tone, and the origin and insertion are approximated.

An eccentric isotonic contraction occurs when the weight brought to the shoulder is now returned to the starting position by increasing the amount of elbow extension. There is tone within the biceps brachii allowing the origin and insertion to separate in a smooth and easy fashion as the elbow extends and the weight is taken away from the shoulder.

An isolytic contraction occurs when the elbow is flexed at 90 degrees and the patient attempts to increase the flexion of the elbow while the operator holding the shoulder and wrist forcefully extends the elbow against the effort of the patient to concentrically contract the biceps brachii. An isolytic procedure must be used cautiously to lengthen a severely contractured or hypertonic muscle because rupture of the musculotendinous junction, insertion of tendon into bone, or muscle fibers themselves can occur.

MUSCLE PHYSIOLOGY AND PRINCIPLES

It is beyond the scope of this volume to describe all of the elements of muscle physiology that underlie muscle energy technique. The reader is referred to a physiology text for those details. Knowledge of a few principles of muscle physiology is necessary for the manual medicine practitioner to use these techniques appropriately.

Muscles are made up of multiple fibers including intrafusal and extrafusal. The alpha neurons innervate the extrafusal fibers. During normal resting tone, some extrafusal fibers are contracting while others are relaxed so that not all fibers are contracting at the same time. The intrafusal fibers, or spindles, lie in parallel with the extrafusal fibers and their function is to monitor the length and tone of the muscle. The spindle is innervated by gamma fibers that set the length and tone of the spindle. The spindle is sensitive to change in length and in rate of change. With stimulation of the spindle by stretch or muscle contraction, afferent type II fibers project information to the spinal cord. Through complex central control systems, the spindle is preset for the anticipated action of the muscle. If the muscle action and the spindle are not congruent, abnormal muscle tone can result. Muscle imbalance of hypertonic muscle tone has become one of the hypothetic constructs of somatic dysfunction. The Golgi tendon apparatus lies in series with the extrafusal fibers of the muscle and is sensitive to muscle tension. As the muscle contracts or is passively stretched, the tension buildup in the Golgi apparatus provides afferent information to the cord through 1B fibers that inhibit alpha motor neuron output.

The control of muscle tone is a complex nervous system activity that takes information from the mechanoreceptors of the articulation and periarticular structures, the muscle spindle, and the Golgi tendon apparatus and processes this information in the spinal cord, brainstem, and higher centers. The cord processes many activities through local reflexes and propriospinal tracts that have been preprogrammed. The cord has the capacity to learn good and bad muscle behavior. Complex ascending and descending spinal pathways integrate conscious and subconscious motor behavior.

Muscle fibers are of two types: fast twitch that contract and relax rapidly and slow twitch that relax slowly. All muscles have combinations of fast- and slow-twitch fibers, and this composition is important in determining its tonic and phasic functions. Dysfunctional postural muscles become hypertonic, short and tight, whereas dysfunctional phasic muscles become weak and inhibited. Of major significance in vertebral somatic dysfunction is hypertonicity of the postural muscles of the fourth layer of the erector spinae group, the multifidi, rotators, and intertransversarii. These muscles are dense in spindles and function more as proprioceptors than prime movers. When dysfunctional, they alter joint mechanics locally and alter the behavior of the larger muscles of the erector spinae group.

Isometric muscle energy techniques primarily reduce the tone in a hypertonic muscle and reestablish its normal resting length. Shortened and hypertonic muscles are frequently identified as the major component of restricted motion of an articulation or group of articulations. The reflexes involved are somewhat complex (Fig. 8.1). Afferents from Golgi tendon receptors and gamma afferents from spindle receptors feed back to the cord; gamma efferents return to the intrafusal fibers resetting their resting length, and this changes the resting length of the extrafusal fibers of the muscle. There is a slight delay after the muscle isometric contraction before it can be taken to a new resting length. Simply put, after an isometric contraction, a hypertonic muscle can be passively lengthened to a new resting length.

When using isotonic procedures, two other muscle physiologic principles are considered. The first is the classic law of reciprocal innervation and inhibition (Fig. 8.2). When an agonist muscle contracts and

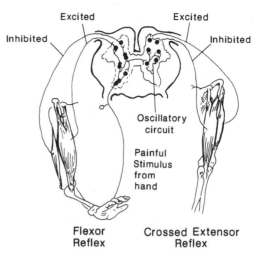

Figure 8.2.
Reciprocal inhabitation reflex arc.

shortens, its antagonist must relax and lengthen so that motion can occur under the influence of the agonist muscle. The contraction of the agonist reciprocally inhibits its antagonist allowing smooth motion. The harder the agonist contracts, the more inhibition occurs in the antagonist, in effect relaxing the antagonist. The second principle of isotonic muscle energy technique is that a series of muscle contractions against progressively increasing resistance increases the tone and improves the performance of a muscle that is too weak for its musculoskeletal function. Isotonic muscle energy procedures reduce hypertonicity in a shortened antagonist and increase the strength of the agonist.

All of these muscle contractions influence the surrounding fasciae, connective tissue ground substance, and interstitial fluids and alter muscle physiology by reflex mechanisms. Fascial length and tone are altered by muscle contraction. Alteration in fasciae influences not only their biomechanical function, but also the biochemical and immunologic functions. The patient's muscle effort requires energy and the metabolic process of muscle contraction results in carbon dioxide, lactic acid, and other metabolic waste products that must be transported and metabolized. It is for this reason that the patient will frequently experience some increase in muscle soreness within the first 12 to 36 hours after a muscle energy technique treatment. Muscle energy procedures provide safety for the patient because the activating force is intrinsic and the patient can easily control the dosage, but it must be remembered that this effort comes at a price. It is easy for the inexperienced practitioner to overdo these procedures, and, in essence, overdose the patient.

Stretch Reflex

Figure 8.1.
Muscle spindle reflexes.

ELEMENTS OF MUSCLE ENERGY PROCEDURES

The following five elements are essential for any successful muscle energy procedure:

1. Patient-active muscle contraction;
2. Controlled joint position;
3. Muscle contraction in a specific direction;
4. Operator-applied distinct counterforce; and
5. Controlled contraction intensity.

The patient is told to contract a muscle while the operator holds an articulation or portion of the musculoskeletal system in a specific position. The patient is instructed to contract in a certain direction with a specified amount of force, either in ounces or pounds. The operator applies a counterforce: one that prevents any approximation of the origin insertion (making the procedure isometric), one to allow yielding (for a concentric isotonic contraction), or one that overpowers the muscle effort (resulting in a isolytic procedure).

Patients commonly make the following errors during muscle energy procedures: They contract too hard, contract in the wrong direction, sustain the contraction for too short a time, or do not relax appropriately following the muscle contraction. The most common operator errors are the following: not accurately controlling the joint position in relation to the barrier to movement, not providing the counterforce in the correct direction, not giving the patient accurate instructions, and moving to a new joint position too soon after the patient stops contracting. The operator must wait for the refractory period following an isometric contraction before the muscle can be stretched to a new resting length.

Clinical experience has shown that three to five repetitions of muscle effort for 3 to 7 seconds each are effective in accomplishing the therapeutic goal. Experience will tell the operator when longer contraction or more repetitions are needed.

The isometric contraction need not be too hard (Table 8.1). It is important that it be sustained and that the muscle length be maintained as nearly isometric as possible. After the sustained but light con-

traction, a momentary pause should occur before the operator stretches the shortened and contracted muscle to a new resting length. Isotonic procedures require forceful contraction by the patient because the operator wants to recruit the firing of muscle fibers and make them work as hard as possible, resulting in relaxation of the antagonist. The muscle should contract over its total range. After any muscle energy procedure the patient should relax before repositioning against a new resistant barrier.

JOINT MOBILIZING MUSCLE EFFORT

There are three different ways a muscle contraction can be used to overcome joint restriction. Let us use as an example restriction of a segment to right rotation. The left rotator muscle is short and tight and the right rotator muscle weak. One approach (NMT 1) is to engage the restrictive barrier to right rotation and ask the left rotator muscle to contract isometrically. After the isometric contraction, the left rotator muscle can be stretched to a new resting length increasing right rotation. A second option would be to have the right rotator muscle contract concentrically against a yielding counterforce, pulling the articulation into right rotation (NMT 2). Although this might be effective, it is infrequently used because it is painful for the patient and difficult for the operator to control. A third option (NMT 3) would be to engage the restrictive barrier and have the right rotator muscle contract isometrically, causing inhibition of the tight left rotator and allowing more free right rotation.

MUSCLE ENERGY TECHNIQUES

In succeeding chapters, muscle energy techniques will be described for specific regions. Here we shall use the elbow as an example. Assume there is restriction of elbow movement into full extension, that is, the elbow is flexed. One cause of restricted elbow extension is hypertonicity and shortening of the biceps brachii muscle. The operator might choose an isometric muscle energy technique to treat this condition as follows:

1. Patient sits comfortably on the treatment table with the operator standing in front.
2. Operator grasps patient's elbow with one hand and distal forearm with the other hand (Fig. 8.3).
3. Operator extends the elbow until the first barrier to extension movement is felt.
4. Operator instructs the patient to attempt to bring the forearm to the shoulder using a few ounces of force in a sustained manner.
5. Operator provides equal counterforce to the patient's effort.
6. After 3 to 7 seconds of contraction, the patient is instructed to stop contracting and relax.

Table 8.1.
Comparison of Isometric and Isotonic Procedures

Isometric	Isotonic
1. Careful positioning	1. Careful positioning
2. Light to moderate contraction	2. Hard to maximal contraction
3. Unyielding counterforce	3. Counterforce permits controlled motion
4. Relaxation after contraction	4. Relaxation after contraction
5. Repositioning	5. Repositioning

7. Operator waits until the patient is completely relaxed after the contracting effort and extends the elbow to a new resistant barrier (Fig. 8.4).
8. Steps 2 through 7 are repeated three to five times until full elbow extension is restored.

The restriction of elbow extension might also be the result of length and strength imbalance between the biceps muscle as the elbow flexor and the triceps muscle as the elbow extender. A weak triceps could prevent full elbow extension. The operator might choose an isotonic muscle energy technique to treat this condition as follows:

1. Patient sitting on table with operator in front.
2. Operator grasps elbow and distal forearm and takes elbow into full flexion (Fig. 8.5).
3. Patient is instructed to extend the elbow with as much effort as possible, perhaps several pounds.
4. The operator provides a yielding counterforce that allows the elbow to slowly but steadily extend throughout its maximal range (Fig. 8.6).

Figure 8.3.
Isometric muscle contraction, biceps.

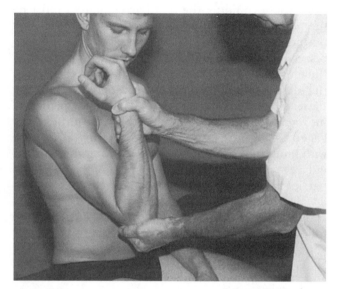

Figure 8.5.
Concentric isotonic contraction.

Figure 8.4.
Full elbow extension.

Figure 8.6.
Full range of elbow extension.

5. Operator returns elbow to full flexion and the patient repeats the contraction of the triceps to extend the elbow, but this time the operator provides increasing resistance to elbow extension.

6. Several repetitive efforts are accomplished with the operator providing increasing resistance each time and with the patient endeavoring to take the elbow through full extension with each effort.

7. Approximately three to five repetitions are usually necessary to achieve full elbow extension.

In any of these muscle energy procedures, it is important to accurately assess the resistant barrier. With an isometric technique, the first barrier sensed must be the point where the operator carefully holds the joint position. If the operator "crashes into" the muscle-resistant barrier in positioning the joint, an increase in the muscle hypertonicity will result, just the opposite of the desired therapeutic effort. Second, when using these procedures in a joint with multiple planes of movement available, each motion barrier must be engaged in the same fashion. In the vertebral column with motion restriction around and along three different axes, precision in the engagement of the restrictive barrier is essential for therapeutic effectiveness.

Successful muscle energy technique can be ensured if the operator will constantly keep in mind the following three words:

    Control
    Balance
    Localization

Both the operator and patient must be balanced and the operator must be in control of the localization against the resistant barrier. There must be continued control of the muscle effort by the patient and the yielding or unyielding counterforce by the operator. Each element is essential with each effort during the procedure.

CONCLUSION

In this author's opinion, muscle energy is one of the most valuable forms of manual medicine treatment because many therapeutic effects result from a single procedure and the procedures are physiologically and anatomically quite safe. It is possible to achieve increased joint movement, normalization of muscle strength and length, stretch of shortened fascia, and removal of passive congestion, all during a single procedure. Not only has muscle effort been used to move a joint, but also physiology that is more normal has been restored to the muscle.

SUGGESTED READINGS

Davidoff RA. Skeletal muscle tone and the misunderstood stretch reflex. *Neurology* 1992;42: 951–963.

Korr I. Muscle spindle and the lesioned segment. In: Proceedings of the International Federation of Orthopedic Manipulative Therapists; 1977; Vail, CO. 45:53.

Mitchell FL Jr, Moran PS, Pruzzo NA. *An evaluation and treatment manual of osteopathic muscle energy procedures.* Valley Park, MO: Mitchell, Moran & Pruzzo Associates, 1979.

Mitchell FL. Structural Pelvic Function. Yearbook of the American Academy of Osteopathy. Carmel, Ca. 1958, 71–90.

Pvorak J, Dvorak V. Manual Medicine, Therapeutic, New York. Thieme-Stratton, Inc, 1983.

9

MOBILIZATION WITH AND WITHOUT IMPULSE TECHNIQUE

The field of manual medicine continues to have difficulty with the use of the term "manipulation." For many years, and continuing in many circles today, the term is used for a manual procedure resulting in the popping sound accompanying the cavitation phenomenon. Dorland's Medical Dictionary defines manipulation as "the skillful or dexterous treatment by the hands." The Foundations of Osteopathic Medicine text defines it as "therapeutic application of manual force." The Chiropractic and much German language literature still refer to manipulation as "high-velocity, low-amplitude thrust technique." "Mobilization" is the term commonly used for a manual medicine procedure that does not include the thrusting that results in the "popping" sound. The scientific advisory committee of the International Federation of Manual Medicine, during its work in the 1980s, recommended the term "mobilization with impulse" to designate a procedure with an operator-applied extrinsic thrusting force and mobilization without impulse having a repetitive, graded operator-applied extrinsic force applied without a thrust.

Mobilization without impulse, or articulatory, procedure is an extension of range-of-motion testing. The techniques use a repetitively applied force at the motion barrier with the goal of increasing the range of motion in an articulation with hypomobility. The operator needs to be precise with localization with both mobilizations with and without impulse. The operator constantly monitors the end feel of the motion range and attempts to return a more normal end feel with enhanced range. A graded series of mobilizing efforts from 1 to 4 are made depending upon the amount of motion introduced (1 = limited, 4 = maximum). Some systems refer to grade 5 as mobilization with impulse. Mobilization without impulse procedures can be applied regionally to a group of segments or individually to a single vertebral motion segment. The primary effect is on the stretch of the connective tissue with mobilization of the passive congestion associated with immobility. One might also anticipate modulation of neural activity to relieve pain and discomfort and restore more normal neural activity in spinal cord

segments. Mobilizations with and without impulse are direct-action techniques and differ only in the external activating force used. They are frequently combined, beginning without impulse for several repetitions and finally applying an impulse.

These procedures have long been deemed the treatment of choice for the "manipulable lesion." Terms such as "joint lock," "joint blockage," and "chiropractic subluxation" all emphasize alteration in articular function.

The use of an extrinsic applied force has been found useful in overcoming restricted articular movement. Despite recent developments in manual medicine procedures (e.g., muscle energy technique, functional and indirect technique, myofascial release, craniosacral technique, etc.), high-velocity, low-amplitude thrust remains one of the most frequently used forms of manual medicine. Because it is commonly used, there is the danger of inappropriate usage yielding poor or no therapeutic result and the risk of complications. As with all therapeutic interventions, these procedures should be applied after an appropriate diagnosis and in a proper manner.

JOINT PLAY

John Mc. Mennell, M.D., is credited with contributing the concept of joint play to manual medicine. Joint play is defined as movement within a synovial joint that is independent of, and cannot be introduced by, voluntary muscle contraction. The movements are small (less than $\frac{1}{8}$ in. in any plane), with a precise range that depends on the contour of the opposing joint surfaces. These joint-play movements are deemed essential for the normal, pain-free, nonrestricted, movement of the particular articulation. If these movements are absent, normal voluntary movements are restricted and frequently painful. Mennell defines joint dysfunction as loss of joint-play movement that cannot be recovered by the action of voluntary muscle, that is, joint dysfunction is loss of joint play. These principles apply to all synovial joints and are applicable in the spine and the extremities. Mennell's diagnostic system tests for normal joint-play movements in each articulation and introduces therapeutic joint manipulation to restore movement and function. Mennell's 10 rules of therapeutic manipulation are as follows:

1. Patient must be relaxed.
2. Operator must be relaxed. Therapeutic grasp must be painless, firm, and protective.
3. One joint is mobilized at a time.
4. One movement in a joint is restored at a time.
5. In performance of movement, one aspect of joint is moved upon the other, which is stabilized.
6. Extent of movement is not greater than that assessed in the same joint on opposite unaffected limb.
7. No forceful or abnormal movement must ever be used.
8. The manipulative movement is a sharp thrust, with velocity, to result in approximately $\frac{1}{8}$-in. gapping at the joint.
9. Therapeutic movement occurs when all of the "slack" in the joint has been taken up.
10. No therapeutic maneuver is done in the presence of joint or bone inflammation or disease (heat, redness, swelling, etc.).

These 10 rules are applicable to all procedures described as high-velocity; low-amplitude thrust techniques or mobilization with impulse.

THEORIES OF JOINT DYSFUNCTION

Many theories have been proposed for the cause of joint dysfunction and the therapeutic effect of mobilization with impulse. They include alteration in the relationship of the opposing joint surfaces, the articular capsules, and associated meniscus and on neural mechanisms from the mechanoreceptors and nociceptors and the resultant effect on segmentally related muscle function. At this time, all of these are considered working hypotheses. Theories involving joint surfaces include "lack of tracking" of opposing joint surfaces and "hitching within the joint." It has been suggested that a change in the thixotropic property of the synovial fluid might make it more "sticky." It has been postulated that a fringe of synovium from the articular capsule might be caught between the two opposing joint surfaces. It has been demonstrated that menisci are present in the zygapophysial joints of the spine and contain innervation by C-fibers. It seems reasonable that they might become entrapped between the opposing joint surfaces, and gapping of the joint might release the entrapped meniscus resulting in enhanced function. This theory remains controversial and to date has not been demonstrated in a research study. More recently, it has been postulated

that stress on the capsule of the involved joint alters the afferent nerve traffic from the type I mechanoreceptors so that central control of motion cannot determine the joint's spatial relationship. This alteration in neural control is postulated to affect the length and tone of the segmentally related muscles, further restricting normal joint movement.

CAVITATION PHENOMENON

Research into the mechanisms of mobilization with impulse (high-velocity, low-amplitude thrust) has demonstrated the cavitation phenomenon. Cavitation occurs at the time of the audible joint pop. A radiographic negative shadow appears within the joint with the density of nitrogen. This gaseous density remains present for a variable period of time, usually less than 20 minutes. The cavitation phenomenon suggests that the synovial fluid changes from a liquid to a gaseous state. The exact effect on the synovial fluid is unknown at this time. An additional observation in a spinal zygapophysial joint undergoing a mobilization procedure involves the segmentally related musculature. After the thrust, there is temporary electrical silence of the segmental muscles, with a refractory period before electrical activity returns. It is hypothesized that the segmentally related muscles return to function that is more normal after the thrusting procedure and contribute to the positive therapeutic response. Another observation of a neural relationship to a segmental vertebral dysfunction has been inhibition of segmentally related muscles. Mobilization with impulse of these vertebral dysfunctions results in increased strength and control of the inhibited muscles. This observation is particularly related to stacked, nonneutral (type II) dysfunctions of the extended, rotated, and side bent (ERS) type in the midscapular thoracic spine and the serratus anterior and rhomboid muscles. Much more research is needed, but clinical experience shows that joint dysfunction (somatic dysfunction) responds positively to the application of mobilization with impulse technique.

INDICATIONS FOR THE USE OF MOBILIZATION WITH IMPULSE

These procedures appear to be most effective in somatic dysfunction when the restriction is in and closely around the joint itself, the so-called "short restrictors." They are usually applied as precisely as possible to a single joint level and for specific joint motion loss. Although Mennell states that a therapeutic procedure should occur in only one plane, it is possible to influence all three planes of vertebral movement simultaneously by specific localization and leverage application. These procedures appear to be much more effective in subacute and chronic conditions than in acute somatic dysfunction. Although most are designed for a single joint and its motion loss, some of the procedures can be applied in a regional fashion. Zink advocated their use with his respiratory–circulatory model, which was designed to mobilize regions of the body to enhance fluid circulation, rather than overcoming specific joint restriction. The difference between specific and nonspecific mobilizations with impulse lies with the principle of localization and locking described below.

Mobilization with impulse (high-velocity, low-amplitude thrust) and mobilization without impulse procedures are used in direct and exaggeration methods. The most common usage is direct, with engagement of the restrictive barrier, and applying an external activating force to the barrier to achieve joint motion that is more normal. Some authors advocate the exaggeration method (also called "rebound thrust") in which the thrust is against the normal physiologic barrier in the direction opposite the motion loss. This author uses only the direct method and would use something other than an exaggeration thrust if a direct action thrust was not possible. Other assisting forces are gravity (patient seated or standing versus recumbent) and patient respiratory efforts, both for relaxation and for influence on joint position desired.

PRINCIPLES OF TECHNIQUE APPLICATION

Joint Gapping

All thrusting procedures result in gapping of the joint, requiring that the operator know the anatomic joint contour and the movement possible at that articulation. The gapping can be in the plane of the joint, at right angles to the plane, or with joint distraction. Any successful mobilization with impulse procedure contains an element of joint distraction and gapping. The audible joint pop or click appears to coincide with joint gapping. It must be remembered that the production of joint noise is not the therapeutic goal. In fact, Kimberly states that the goal of a successful thrusting procedure is "painless and noiseless restoration of maximum joint function."

Localization

Localization limits the thrusting procedure to the joint needing treatment but other joints receive the mobilizing impulse. This relates to Mennell's principle of holding one bone of the articulation and moving the other bone in relation to it.

It is essential that the operator have a good understanding of vertebral mechanics, both normal and dysfunctional, before using mobilization with impulse techniques. Using impulse without appropriate localization and understanding of vertebral mechanics can result in damage to the tissues including fracture of zygapophysial joints and herniation of the intervertebral disc. One localization principle that is most useful is the introduction of convexities in two different planes localized to the segment under treatment. The first convexity introduced is into the forward-bending or backward-bending arc of movement. The objective is to engage the forward-bending (flexion) or backward-bending (extension) component of the nonneutral vertebral somatic dysfunction. The goal is to place the segment under treatment at the apex of the convexity introduced either through a forward-bending and backward-bending overturning movement or an anteroposterior or posteroanterior translatory movement. For example, if L1 has forward-bending restriction in relation to L2, forward bending of the trunk is introduced from above downward through the thoracic spine to L1. Flexion of the lower extremities, pelvis, and lumbar spine from below upward is introduced up to L2. The L1 through L2 interspace becomes the apex of the forward-bending curve introduced and is localized against the forward-bending (flexion) barrier. This localization can also be performed by translation from anterior to posterior at the L1 through L2 level. The second convexity introduced is that of side bending, creating a convexity right or left. Introduction of side bending while forward bent (flexed) or backward bent (extended) couples the rotation to the same side (nonneutral vertebral mechanics). If in our example of L1 through L2 the side bending and rotation restrictions are to the right, side bending to the right establishes a convexity of the thoracolumbar spine to the left with the apex of the L1 through L2 interspace. This left convexity can be established by a right-to-left translatory movement as well as right side bending from above or below. The introduction of two convexities, one from front to back and the other through side bending with the apex of each convexity at the segment to be treated, is the principle used for a nonneutral (type II) vertebral dysfunctions in which there is either forward-bending or backward-bending restriction, together with side-bending and rotation restriction to the same side.

In the neutral group (type I), vertebral dysfunctions localization is accomplished by the introduction of side bending and rotation to opposite sides from above downward and from below upward to the segment requiring treatment. Forward bending and backward bending are introduced only to place the joint(s) under treatment at the point of maximum ease in the forward-bending or backward-bending arc of movement that is "neutral" at that level. This is best demonstrated when using the lateral recumbent (lumbar roll) technique. With the patient in the left lateral recumbent position, the apex of the group curve is placed in the neutral position of the forward-bending and backward-bending arc. With L1 through L2 as our example, forward bending and backward bending are introduced until L1 through L2 is in its neutral position in the anteroposterior curve. The operator pulls the patient's left upper extremity anteriorly and caudally, introducing left side bending and right rotation of the vertebral column down to the L1 level. With the other hand, the operator rolls the patient's pelvis anteriorly, introducing rotation to the left from below upward until L2 is reached. This results in neutral group localization at L1 through L2 and any articulatory or thrusting force summates at that level. The goal is to localize so that the transverse processes of the segment under treatment are maintained in the coronal (xy) plane. The lower in the lumbar spine that localization is desired, the more movement is introduced from above downward and less from below upward. Higher in the lumbar spine and into the lower thoracic spine, less movement is introduced from above downward and more from below upward.

Levers

Levers are classified as short or long. A short lever is one in which a portion of one vertebra (spinous process) is firmly held while force is applied to a bony process of the adjacent vertebra (spinous process, transverse process, mamillary process) and the resultant applied force is sufficient to move one segment on the other. Long levers are established by using one of the extremities, or multiple segments within the vertebral column, in a "locking" maneuver. Long levers have the advantage of reducing the force required and increasing the distance the force travels. Long-lever technique requires precise localization and limitation of force. A vertebral column long lever involves the principles of ligamentous or bony lock. A ligamentous lock occurs when the spine is sufficiently forward bent to place maximum tension on the posterior ligamentous structures surrounding the zygapophysial joints. A joint lock occurs when the spine is backward bent with engagement of the zygapophysial joints. Both of these maneuvers reduce joint mobility. Levers can also be established using concept III of vertebral motion in which introduction of motion in one direction reduces vertebral motion in all others. The introduction of a neutral (type I) vertebral movement (side bending and rotation to opposite sides) limits the movement of the vertebra involved and can include as many segments of the vertebral column as desired. Long levers are used to establish localization at any specific vertebral segmental level. Segments above and below the dysfunctional vertebral segment are "locked" in a long lever while the segment to be treated is "free" to receive the activating force applied. It is not uncommon for the neophyte practitioner to use excessive force to a joint that is inappropriately locked through poor localization.

Fulcrum

A fulcrum is used in many mobilizations with impulse techniques, particularly in the cervical and thoracic spines. The role of the fulcrum is to assist in localization of the activating force to the appropriate segment. There are firm rubber blocks or wedges of varying sizes and shapes that some practitioners use. This author prefers the use of hand position to establish a fulcrum. The advantage of using fingers or hand combinations for a fulcrum is the ability to sense localization at the segment under treatment. In the cervical area, a finger-pad pressure against a zygapophysial joint line serves as fulcrum around which the vertebrae can be moved to overcome restriction of the opposite zygapophysial joint. In the thoracic spine, various hand positions can be used to block the lower segment of the vertebral motion segment under treatment, allowing the operator to move the superior segment in any direction necessary to engage the restrictive barrier. In rib dysfunctions, the thenar eminence above or below a dysfunctional rib can serve as an appropriate fulcrum against which an activating force can be localized.

Velocity

Velocity means speed of application not force. In mobilization with impulse technique, the velocity is high. The maneuver should have quickness. The common mistake made is that the maneuver is a "push" rather than a "quick thrust." The thrusting maneuver should be applied only when all of the "slack" within the joint is removed. One must engage the restriction at its elastic barrier so that the thrusting procedure reestablishes the residual joint play available until one reaches the firm anatomic barrier. Remember that additional force does not make up for poor localization and poor velocity. The neophyte practitioner frequently "backs off" from the barrier in an attempt to get a "running start" against the barrier. This must be avoided by careful localization against the elastic barrier of the restriction and moving with velocity from that point in the direction of motion loss.

Amplitude

Mobilization with impulse technique attempts to create movement of $\frac{1}{8}$ in. at the joint under treatment. The thrusting force should be applied quickly and for a short distance. With short lever technique, the amplitude of the thrust to achieve $\frac{1}{8}$-in. at the joint is considerable less than that with long-lever technique. When two long levers are used, a great deal of movement is introduced by the operator to the patient. What must be remembered is that the summation of all of that movement results in a thrust amplitude at the joint under treatment of $\frac{1}{8}$ in.

Balance and Control

As in any successful manual medicine procedure, both the operator and the patient must be in body positions that are comfortable, easily controlled, and balanced. The patient can be completely relaxed so that the operator can apply the thrust with maximum efficiency. The table must be at the appropriate height for the patient's and the operator's sizes. If the table is too high, the operator's ability to control the patient is compromised. The patient should be appropriately placed on the table, not too far away, not too close to the operator, so that localization can be accurate and the patient does not fear falling. The thrust is most appropriately provided by weight transfer of the operator's body rather than by a specific muscle action. In lateral recumbent lumbar roll technique, some operators attempt to introduce the thrust by an adduction movement of the arm placed on the pelvis, rather than with a total body movement. It is most difficult to provide appropriate velocity, amplitude, and direction with an adductor muscular movement of the operator's upper extremity. It is much easier to apply the proper thrust by the weight transfer of the operator's body (with the arm contacting the patient being incorporated as part of the operator's body) or with the arm fully extended, and the thrust applied by a balanced movement of the operator's body in the right direction.

Therapeutic Goals of Mobilization with Impulse Technique

These procedures are useful in increasing range of movement of an articulation that has dysfunction (loss of joint play). Although the motion loss seemed to be only in one direction, a successful thrust procedure will increase range of movement in all possible directions. While moving the joint, one might attempt to realign the skeletal parts in their normal anatomic relationship, intending to restore normal joint receptor activity at that level. An additional outcome is reduction of muscle hypertonicity and/or spasm in an attempt to restore balance to the segmentally related musculature. Another therapeutic outcome might be the stretching of shortened connective tissues surrounding the articulation. The fascial connective tissues may be shortened and tightened as the result of the altered position of the articulation, the healing of the inflammatory process following injury. As suggested earlier, the therapeutic goal might be the movement of fluid, both intra- and extravascular, by "wringing out" the tissues. One or more of these therapeutic goals might be the objective of a procedure, but many of the others would be operative simultaneously. These procedures seem most effective for subacute and chronic dysfunctions that appear to be due to short restrictors.

Contraindications

As in all forms of manual medicine, accurate diagnosis is essential, and precision and accuracy of thera-

peutic intervention are required. When these criteria are met for mobilization with impulse, the contraindications become fewer. However, these procedures have more contraindications, both absolute and relative, than others. Absolute contraindications for mobilization with impulse are hypermobility and instability of an articulation and the presence of inflammatory joint disease.

There are many relative contraindications and authors classify them differently. For example, in the cervical spine there is a major concern about these procedures and the vertebral artery. The vertebral artery is anatomically at risk at the craniocervical junction, and movements of extension and rotation will narrow normal arteries. In the presence of disease of the vertebral arteries, these movements become even potentially more dangerous. The need for precision of diagnosis and application of technique becomes crucial in the presence of disease of the vertebral arteries. The cervical spine is also a site of developmental and congenital conditions that might contraindicate a thrusting procedure. These include agenesis of the odontoid process and Down syndrome. Throughout the vertebral column there is concern for metabolic and systemic bone disease, particularly osteoporosis and metastatic carcinoma. With careful and precise localization and the appropriate amount of force, mobilization with impulse technique can restore the lost joint play despite the alteration in osseous architecture. Degenerative joint diseases of the zygapophysial and uncovertebral joints of Luschka are also relative contraindications. Degenerative joint disease alters the capacity of the zygapophysial joints to function and an inappropriate mobilization with impulse technique could damage these joints. However, somatic dysfunction of these joints can complicate the degenerative joint process. The joint dysfunction can be successfully treated with a mobilization with impulse procedures if the aforementioned principles are applied properly. The thrusting impulse can be appropriately applied to the elastic barrier of the joint dysfunction even in the presence of altered anatomic barrier because of degenerative joint disease.

Of major concern is the use of mobilization with impulse procedures in the presence of intervertebral disc disease, particularly in the acute phase. Some authors believe that it is the treatment of choice, whereas others believe it is contraindicated. The concern is the possibility of exacerbating the disc pathology into increased herniation and sequestration with entrapment of neural elements. This author has used mobilization with impulse procedures with successful therapeutic results in the presence of known disc herniation demonstrated by appropriate imaging. It is interesting to note that little change has occurred in the imaging of the disc by the procedure. It has been reported that an acute cauda equina syndrome has followed the use of mobilization with impulse technique in the presence of lumbar disc disease. This potential danger should always be considered.

CONCLUSION

Mobilizations with and without impulse techniques are valuable in the armamentarium of the manual medicine practitioner. They require accuracy of diagnosis and precision of therapeutic intervention. They differ only in the form of mobilizing force. In mobilization with impulse technique, the application of velocity rather than force is a necessary skill to be mastered.

SUGGESTED READINGS

Bogduk N, Jull G. The theoretical pathology of acute locked back: aA basis for manipulative therapy. *Man Med* 1(3):78–82, 1985.

Brunarski DJ. Clinical trials of spinal manipulation: a critical appraisal and review of the literature. *J Manip Physiol Ther* 1984;4:243–249.

Cassidy JD, Mierav Dr, Noftal et al. A quantitiative study of joint mobilization and manipulation. Presented to Back Pain Research Society. Boscombe, Bournemouth. Nov 1, 1985.

Dorland's Medical Dictionary, 23rd Edition, W.B. Saunders Co. Philadelphia, 1959.

England R, Deibert P. Electromyographic studies, I: consideration in the evaluation of osteopathic therapy. *J Am Osteopath Assoc* 1972;72:221–223.

Foundations for Osteopathic Medicine, Ward RC Exec Ed, Baltimore, Williams & Wilkins, 1997.

Grice AA. Muscle tonus changes following manipulation. *J Can Chiropractic Assoc* 1974;19:29–31.

Kimberly PE. Personal Communication. MSU/COM Tutorial on Mobilization with Impulse Technique. East Lansing, Mi, 1984.

Mennell, J MCM. Joint Pain. Boston, Little Brown & Co., 1964.

Shekelle PG. Spinal update: spinal manipulation. *Spine* 1994;19:858–861.

Walton WJ. *Osteopathic diagnosis and technique procedures*, 2nd ed. Colorado Springs, CO: American Academy of Osteopathy, 1970.

Unsworth A, Dowson D, Wright V. Cracking in the metacarpophalangeal joint, *Ann Rheum Dis*, 1971 30:348–351.

10
PRINCIPLES OF INDIRECT TECHNIQUE

Indirect techniques are not as well known as the direct action techniques, particularly mobilization with impulse (high-velocity thrust). There are a number of variations of indirect technique with different names and terminology, but they all seem to have a common mode of action. They all move away from, rather than into, the barrier (indirect technique). The mechanism of action seems to be through a neural reflex with reduction of aberrant afferent impulses to the spinal cord resulting in more normal motor behavior. They might well be called afferent reduction techniques. Many people view them as being highly complex, although the principles are relatively simple and straightforward. These procedures focus more on the functional than the structural aspect in the structure-function interface.

HISTORY

Indirect techniques have a rich history developing primarily within the osteopathic profession beginning in the 1940s and 1950s. William Garner Sutherland, D.O., the developer of the craniosacral concept and techniques (see Chapter 12), treated the vertebral column and extremity articulations with balanced membranous tension. He did not address the restriction in a direct fashion but held the articulation in a position of balance. He believed the balance was within the ligaments, but subsequent study has found that the underlying principle is more likely through complex neural control of motor function. Several groups of osteopathic physicians in different areas of the country built on this work and developed the functional approach to technique. Hoover led one group in the Pacific Northwest and focused on the principle of the dynamic neutral point of joint motion. Bowles, Johnston, and other members of the New England Academy of Osteopathy on the east coast developed a study group and refined these concepts, emphasizing "ease" and "bind" as terms for the variations of palpatory sensation. Laughlin, of Kirksville, Missouri, developed his variation of this technique building on the balanced membranous tension concepts of Sutherland.

Jones developed the system he called "strain–counterstrain" in 1955 after observing relief of pain and improved function after the patient assumed a pain-free position. He further observed the relation of tender points on the anterior and posterior aspects of the body with various somatic dysfunction patterns. His technique evolved by associating the behavior of the tender points and their response to a pain-free position and the subsequent slow return to normal posture.

Schiowitz and his colleague DiGiovanni developed a variation called "facilitated positional release" in 1977. This system focuses on localized tissue texture abnormalities instead of tender points and identifies body positions that facilitate reduction of the tissue tension and improved function. This system also adds compression or torsion of the part under treatment at the balanced point. The position is held for 3 to 4 seconds instead of the 90 seconds recommended for the strain–counterstrain technique of Jones.

As can be seen, there are multiple varieties of these techniques that have gained in popularity and now are included in the manual medicine practitioner's armamentarium.

STRUCTURE-FUNCTION INTERFACE

The interrelationship of structure and function in the body, and the body's tendency to self-regulation, are well-recognized basic principles. Indirect (functional) techniques build on these principles, particularly from the perspective of function. In viewing a dysfunctional vertebral segment, the thought is not that the bone is out of place but that it has abnormal behavior in relation to the rest of the organism. The classic structural approach would attempt to "put the bone back in place," whereas the functional approach would attempt to restore coordinated activity with other segments of the vertebral column and the related soft tissues. A helpful analogy is to imagine a rank of soldiers marching in a parade. One soldier in the rank is out of step. Because he is out of step, he is easily visible. The soldier is in line in the rank, he is not out of place, but he is highly visible because he is "out of step." He does not function in a coordinated manner with his fellow soldiers. The soldier's commanding officer would not take the soldier out of the rank and put him elsewhere, but would change his stride so that it matched the remaining soldiers in the rank. The practitioner using functional technique focuses on restoring coordinated activity in an involved vertebral dysfunction in a similar fashion to the change in behavior in the soldier who is out of step in the rank.

BARRIER CONCEPTS

Chapter 3 described normal and restrictive barriers. In the absence of dysfunction, there is a midrange neutral point of maximum ease or freedom within the total range of motion. In the presence of somatic dysfunction, the neutral point is no longer in midline but is found as the point of maximum ease or freedom between the restrictive barrier in one direction and the normal physiologic and anatomic barriers in the opposite direction. Direct action techniques, such as muscle energy and mobilization with and without impulse, are interested in engaging the restrictive barrier and applying an activating force in the direction of motion loss. Functional technique is more interested in the behavior of the motion present than in its specific relationship to the barrier. The practitioner is more interested in the quality of motion, rather than the quantity, and how the dysfunctional segment behaves when motion is introduced. Functional diagnosis looks for the normal and reasonably expected coordination of movement and the quality and ease of movement in any given area or segment.

NEUROLOGIC HYPOTHESIS

The working hypothesis for indirect functional technique is the premise that dysfunction results in altered neural activity. The abnormal dysfunction stimulates aberrant afferent impulses from mechanoreceptors and nociceptors. These impulses are transmitted to the spinal cord for processing, locally at the cord level and centrally through ascending and descending neural pathways. This abnormal neural traffic results in abnormal efferent signals to the final common pathway of the alpha motor neuron to muscle. Hypothetically, restoration of more normal afferent signals to the central nervous system returns the neural traffic at the spinal cord to more normal levels, resulting in restoration of more normal neural activity to the muscle. Functional techniques can be described as afferent reduction procedures. The functional diagnostic process is extensive in that it searches for alteration in behavior of all segments within the musculoskeletal system, attempts to restore them to more normal behavior, and requires that each dysfunctional segment is given appropriate attention.

FUNCTIONAL DIAGNOSIS

Functional diagnosis begins by identifying areas of tenderness, tissue tension, and/or the areas of most restriction. One diagnostic process has the operator percussing with fingertips over vertebral motion segments and their adnexal tissues. Loss of tissue resilience is identified in areas of significant dysfunction. A second diagnostic method has the operator looking for areas of tender points and localized tension points. A third method finds the operator passively introducing ranges of motion throughout the vertebral axis in a symmetric fashion seeking for areas of resistance to the induced motion. A fourth process is to identify vertebral somatic dysfunction by the biomechanical method described in Chapter 6 and then assess the functional characteristics of the dysfunction.

EASE-BIND CONCEPT

In functional technique, the practitioner searches for the quality of movement rather than range. Is the movement easy and free (ease), or is the movement restricted and difficult (bind)? The spectrum runs from maximum ease to maximum bind with many gradations between. Functional diagnosis searches for the ease–bind interface.

The procedure to identify ease and bind is as follows. A palpating hand is placed over the suspected segmental dysfunction and is called the "listening hand." Contact is maintained in a quiet and noninvasive fashion, focusing on changes that occur at the dysfunctional segment and its adnexal tissues. The listening hand seldom introduces movement or energy. It is a "receiver" of information. The operator's other hand contacts some area of the musculoskeletal system distant from the dysfunctional segment and either introduces motion or monitors the motion the patient performs under verbal cues. This hand is called the "motor hand." It introduces the movement that the listening hand monitors, responding as ease or bind. The process requires a motion demand and a response. The motion hand initiates the demand, and the listening hand monitors the response.

Functional technique has a constant diagnostic and treatment interaction. The motor hand introduces diagnostic and therapeutic motions and the listening hand monitors the response, giving constant feedback as the outcome. The diagnosis–treatment can be viewed as a cybernetic loop of continuous input and output with feedback assessment throughout the process. Because of the dynamic process involved in functional technique, the practitioners may look as though they are performing many different things with little standardization. In fact, the processes are quite standard in that there is motion introduced by one hand and constantly monitored by the other.

THERAPEUTIC USE

Acute Conditions

Functional technique is particularly useful in acute conditions because it is nontraumatic and can be performed repeatedly and frequently. Functional technique does not seek a major structural change but a tissue response. Reprogramming of aberrant afferent stimulation is important in acute and chronic conditions. Acute conditions appear to respond quite favorably and rapidly to functional technique. Special equipment is not necessary and it can be performed in any location, even in an intensive care unit.

Chronic Conditions

Functional technique is also effective in chronic conditions because it overcomes the abnormally programmed neural response and not just altered position. Restoring the position of a dysfunctional vertebral segment is of little value without restoring the neuromuscular mechanisms that control its function. The diagnostic component of functional technique is useful in chronic conditions as it monitors tissue response and behavior regardless of the therapeutic intervention.

Prognostic Value

Functional diagnostic technique is of prognostic value. It assesses the therapeutic response of a dysfunctional level regardless of the therapeutic intervention. For example, lift therapy for an anatomically short lower extremity and pelvic tilt mechanism (a structural intervention) will change the functional capacity of the entire musculoskeletal system. Functional diagnosis helps to determine if the structural intervention of the lift has accomplished improvement in musculoskeletal function both locally and distantly.

TYPES OF INDIRECT (FUNCTIONAL) TECHNIQUE

All functional techniques can be classified as afferent reduction procedures. Most functional techniques can be placed in one of the following categories: balance and hold, dynamic functional procedures, strain–counterstrain, and release by positioning.

Balance and Hold

These procedures are performed in any body position: standing, sitting, supine, prone, or lateral recumbent. Each hand has a particularly important role in performing balance-and-hold functional technique. The listening hand monitors at the dysfunctional segment as the motor hand introduces motion passively or the patient assumes body positions under the practitioner's verbal commands.

Motion is sequentially introduced in six different directions seeking the balance point of maximum ease within each range. Each is then held in that position while stacking one on top of the other. The stacking sequence makes little difference. The ranges introduced are forward bending–backward bending; side bending right–side bending left; rotation right–rotation left; anteroposterior (AP) translation; translation laterally, both right and left; and. translation cephalic–caudad.

The last movement introduced is respiration. Once each of the ranges within the dysfunctional segment has been "stacked" at the point of maximum ease, inhalation and exhalation effort is introduced. The phase of respiration found to be the freest is then held as long as comfortably possible. This is usually for 5 to 30 seconds. At the end of the comfortable holding of the breath, the patient is instructed to breath normally and naturally. A new balance point is sought for each of the motion directions. The respiratory effort is repeated. The entire process is repeated until release of restriction is felt and increased mobility is obtained. The usual operator sense is that the neutral point is returning more and more toward normal and that range is increasing.

Dynamic Functional Procedures

The second category of functional technique is described as "dynamic functional." The focus is on the restoration of normality to the apparently abnormal tracking of the dysfunction. The process follows the inherent tissue motion. Inherent tissue motion is a function of many physiologic phenomena, particularly the cranial rhythmic impulse, contraction–relaxation of muscle tone, and the dynamic effects of respiration and circulation. In dynamic functional technique the listening hand monitors the response to motion introduced by the motor hand and directs the motion demand along the path of increasing ease. The goal is to restore more normal movement patterns and the operator attempts to "ride out" the dysfunction. The operator continually seeks ease and avoids bind. These techniques look quite varied because of the dynamic motion patterns introduced. They can be standardized by the formula C-C-T-E-T.

C (1)—Contact over the adnexal tissue of the dysfunctional segment
C (2)—Control of the induced motion by the motor hand
T (1)—Test the adnexal tissue response
E–Evaluate the compliance of the segment as normal or abnormal
T (2)—Treatment by constantly monitoring the bind–ease point of the dysfunctional segment.

Strain-counterstrain Technique

The third category of functional technique is "strain–counterstrain." This system was originated and developed by Jones. There are three cardinal features of this system. The first is the identification and monitoring of palpable tender points on the anterior and posterior aspects of the body. They are similar in location to diagnostic points identified by other authors: Travell trigger points, Chapman reflexes, and acupuncture (see Chapter 7). The second element has the patient assuming a body position that is the most comfortable and has the least pain. The position is held for 90 seconds while the operator monitors the tender point for reduction of tenderness and tension. Clinical experience has found that 90 seconds is the ideal: Less is usually not effective and more does not increase the response. The third element is the slow operator-assisted movement of the patient to a normal posture. This is crucial for success.

There are more than 200 Jones tender points (Figs. 10.1 and 10.2) and each correlates with a somatic dysfunction in the musculoskeletal system. Anterior tender points seem related to flexed dysfunctions and respond best to a flexion body position. Posterior tender points relate to extended dysfunctions and respond best to extension body position. The more lateral the tender point, the more side bending and rotation are necessary in the held body position.

The diagnostic process is to systematically assess the patient for tender points in the usual locations, particularly looking for "hot'" (most tender and reactive) and clusters of tender points.

The treatment by counterstrain usually involves five or six tender points. It is recommended that the most "hot" be treated first and clinical experience will show that many of the minor points will resolve spontaneously. There is a common posttreatment reaction despite the apparent nontraumatic nature of the procedure. It usually occurs from 12 to 36 hours after treatment and the patient should be advised of the possibility. Caution is advisable to prevent overtreatment. Counterstrain can be used in combination with other techniques. It is recommended that a text specific to this system be studied before attempting to use this technique (Jones LH, Kusunose RS, Goering EK. *Jones strain-counterstrain.* Boise, ID: Jones Strain-counterstrain, Inc., 1995).

Release by Positioning

This system has many similarities to the strain–counterstrain approach. The diagnosis of a somatic dysfunction is made by any of a variety of ways. Of particular value is the role of palpation of tissue texture change associated with the dysfunction. Once identified, the vertebral segment is started at the neutral point of flexion–extension and the part is taken to a point of ease in rotation and side bending by operator guiding while monitoring the response of the tissue texture. Instead of using pain and tenderness as in strain–counterstrain, resolving of the tissue texture change is the goal. When the point of ease is found, a small amount of compression or torsion is added and held for 3 to 5 seconds and reassessment is made. Theoretically, the positional release changes the behavior of the spindle system resulting in change of cord-level control of muscle hypertonicity. It is nontraumatic, quickly applied and can be combined with other procedures.

FUNCTIONAL PALPATION EXERCISE

The following exercise is useful in learning the principles of functional diagnosis and treatment.

1. Patient sits on examining table in an erect position with arms folded across the chest, each hand holding the opposite shoulder.
2. Operator stands behind and to the side of the patient placing fingertips of the listening hand over the upper thoracic region. The listening hand should be as quiet as possible.
3. Operator's other hand becomes the motor hand and is placed on top of the head. This hand leads the patient through certain movements in the fashion of the use of the reins on the bridle of a horse. The motor hand introduces passive movement and monitors the response of a patient movement from operator verbal commands.
4. Operator introduces forward bending in a slow and smooth fashion attempting to identify (with the listening hand) changes in ease and bind from maximum ease to maximum bind. Operator reverses the procedure into backward bending. Several repetitions are made, constantly evaluating the range of ease to bind motion in both directions.
5. With the patient in the neutral starting position, the motor hand introduces side bending to the right and rotation to the left of the head and neck on the trunk. This introduces neutral (type I) vertebral motion. Operator monitors the range of this coupled movement through the ease and bind phenomena. Reverse the movement to side bending left and rotation right. Is there symmetry to the ease and bind? As you modulate side bending and rotation, is there difference in the ease and bind of each component of the motion?
6. Beginning at the neutral position, the operator introduces a small amount of forward bending, right-side bending, and right rotation of the head and neck on the trunk. This introduces nonneutral (type II) coupled movement. The

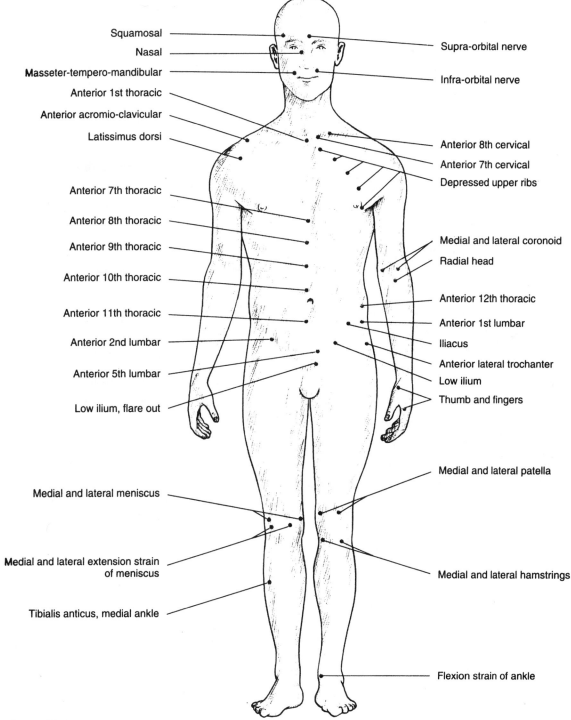

Squamosal
Nasal
Masseter-tempero-mandibular
Anterior 1st thoracic
Anterior acromio-clavicular
Latissimus dorsi

Anterior 7th thoracic
Anterior 8th thoracic
Anterior 9th thoracic
Anterior 10th thoracic
Anterior 11th thoracic
Anterior 2nd lumbar
Anterior 5th lumbar
Low ilium, flare out

Medial and lateral meniscus

Medial and lateral extension strain
of meniscus

Tibialis anticus, medial ankle

Supra-orbital nerve
Infra-orbital nerve

Anterior 8th cervical
Anterior 7th cervical
Depressed upper ribs

Medial and lateral coronoid
Radial head

Anterior 12th thoracic
Anterior 1st lumbar
Iliacus
Anterior lateral trochanter
Low ilium
Thumb and fingers

Medial and lateral patella

Medial and lateral hamstrings

Flexion strain of ankle

Figure 10.1.

listening hand monitors for ease and bind of this motion. Repeat to the left side. Are they symmetric in the quality of ease and bind and in each component of the motion?

This exercise can be repeated throughout the vertebral axis in a number of positions. Diagnostically, the operator is attempting to classify each segment as normal, marginally dysfunctional, or significantly dysfunctional. The normal segment has a wide range of minimal signaling throughout the procedure. A significantly dysfunctional segment has a narrow range of rapid signaling in the ease–bind range. It is not uncommon to find a segment that is marginally dysfunctional and it is important to decide how significant it is within the total musculoskeletal complex. This deci-

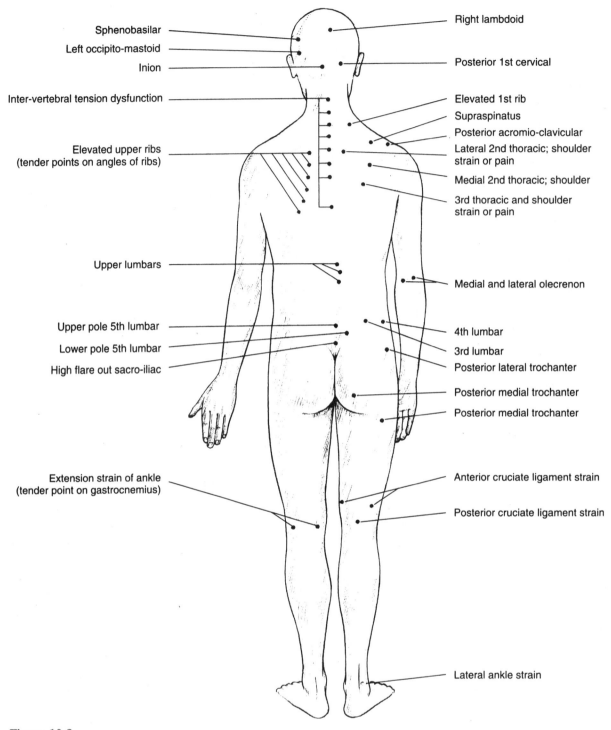

Sphenobasilar
Left occipito-mastoid
Inion
Inter-vertebral tension dysfunction
Elevated upper ribs
(tender points on angles of ribs)
Upper lumbars
Upper pole 5th lumbar
Lower pole 5th lumbar
High flare out sacro-iliac
Extension strain of ankle
(tender point on gastrocnemius)

Right lambdoid
Posterior 1st cervical
Elevated 1st rib
Supraspinatus
Posterior acromio-clavicular
Lateral 2nd thoracic; shoulder strain or pain
Medial 2nd thoracic; shoulder
3rd thoracic and shoulder strain or pain
Medial and lateral olecrenon
4th lumbar
3rd lumbar
Posterior lateral trochanter
Posterior medial trochanter
Posterior medial trochanter
Anterior cruciate ligament strain
Posterior cruciate ligament strain
Lateral ankle strain

Figure 10.2.

sion can only be achieved through experience that is the only and best teacher.

FUNCTIONAL TECHNIQUES

The following techniques demonstrate the system of functional technique attributed to Laughlin, of Kirksville, Missouri. These techniques have been refined and standardized by Stiles, who had the oppor- tunity to study extensively with Laughlin. There are many systems of functional (indirect) technique. These techniques are examples of the balance-and-hold and the dynamic functional principles. The diagnosis attributed to these techniques follows the postural structural model for terminology purposes, but to successfully use these techniques, the principles identified previously need to be implemented.

Functional Technique

Lumbar Spine
Sitting
Diagnosis: Nonneutral dysfunctions: extended, rotated, and side bent (ERS) and Flexed, rotated, sidebent (FRS)

1. Patient sitting on table.
2. Operator sits behind patient.
3. Operator's listening hand is placed over dysfunctional segment with index finger on superior vertebra and thumb on inferior vertebra (Fig. 10.3).
4. Operator's motion hand placed on patient's shoulder to control side bending and rotation from above (Fig.10.4).
5. Operator places head at the patient's thoracolumbar region to control flexion and extension through AP translation (Fig.10.5).
6. Operator introduces side bending and rotation through the motion hand, and flexion-extension through AP translation to the balance point of ease in all six degrees of freedom (Fig.10.6).
7. Inhalation/exhalation efforts are used to find point of maximum ease and held until release occurs (balance and hold).
8. A dynamic indirect approach can be implemented by applying a load from the motion hand to the listening hand at step 6 and following the unwinding inherent motion in the tissues as they seek balance.

Figure 10.3.

Figure 10.5.

Figure 10.4.

Figure 10.6.

Functional Technique

Pubes
Supine
Diagnosis: Superior or inferior pube

1. Patient supine, knees flexed, and dropped into abduction with the soles of feet together.
2. Operator stands at side of table and palpates right and left side of the pubic symphysis with index fingers above and thumbs below (Fig. 10.7).

3. Operator introduces cephalic to caudad motion to point of maximum ease (Fig.10.8).
4. Balance-and-hold approach uses respiratory force assist until balance of symmetric position and motion occurs.
5. A dynamic approach introduces motion in the direction of ease and follows inherent motion until balance of function is achieved.

Figure 10.7.

Figure 10.8.

Functional Technique

Sitting
Sacroiliac
Diagnosis: Left-on-left torsion.

1. Patient sitting on table.

2. Operator sits behind patient with the right hand over the right sacral base as the listening hand (Fig.10.9), and the left hand on the left shoulder as the motion hand (Fig.10.10).

3. Operator's head is placed in the thoracolumbar region to control flexion–extension by AP translation (Fig.10.11).

4. Operator's right thumb is over the sacral base while the right index finger exerts lateral distraction on the medial side of the posterior superior iliac spine (PSIS) sensing for ease at the upper pole of the right sacroiliac joint.

5. Operator's head introduces AP translation and flexion–extension to ease at the listening hand.

6. Operator's (left) motion hand introduces left side bending and right rotation of the patient's trunk to ease at the listening hand (Fig.10.12).

7. The balance-and-hold approach fine-tunes ease at the listening hand then introduces respiratory effort to achieve release of tension and return of function. Several repetitions may be necessary with fine-tuning after each respiratory assist.

8. The dynamic indirect approach initiates motion in the direction of ease and follows the inherent tissue response as the tissues "unwind." The thumb of the right hand may be moved to the left inferior lateral angle to initiate and assist the process.

Figure 10.9.

Figure 10.11.

Figure 10.10.

Figure 10.12.

Functional Technique

Sacroiliac
Sitting
Diagnosis: Left sacrum (flexed) anterior nutated

1. Patient sitting on table.

2. Operator sits behind patient with the left hand over the left sacral base as the listening hand with the thumb over the sacrum and the index finger medial to the left PSIS (Fig.10.13).

3. Operator's right hand is placed on the patient's right shoulder as the motion hand (Fig.10.14).

4. Operator's head is placed at the thoracolumbar junction.

5. Operator introduces flexion–extension, AP translatory motion through the head until ease is felt at the listening hand (Fig.10.15).

6. Operator motion hand introduces right-side bending and left rotation until ease is felt at the listening hand (Fig.10.16).

7. The balance-and-hold approach maintains the point of ease and uses respiratory action to achieve release of restriction in the tissues.

8. The dynamic indirect approach initiates motion in the direction of ease through the motion hand and follows the inherent tissue motion as it seeks ease and balance of tension. The operator's left thumb can be moved to the left inferior lateral angle to assist in release. The motion hand controls the trunk as ease is sought in all dimensions.

Figure 10.13.

Figure 10.15.

Figure 10.14.

Figure 10.16.

Functional Technique

Sacroiliac
Sitting
Diagnosis: Right sacrum (extended) posterior nutated

1. Patient sitting on table.
2. Operator sitting behind patient with the right hand over the upper pole of the right sacroiliac joint as the listening hand. The thumb is over the right sacral base and the right index finger provides lateral distraction on the right PSIS.
3. Operator's left hand is on patient's left shoulder as the motion hand (Fig. 10.17).
4. Operator's head is at the thoracolumbar junction.

5. Operator introduces a little flexion, posterior translation, and right-side bending/rotation until ease is felt at the listening hand. The patient's weight is shifted to the right ischial tuberosity (Fig.10.18).
6. The balance-and-hold approach maintains the point of maximum ease at the right sacral base by fine-tuning and then using respiratory effort to achieve balance of tissue tension.
7. The dynamic indirect approach initiates motion at the right sacral base through the motion hand and follows the balance point until tissue release occurs and function restored.

Figure 10.17.

Figure 10.18.

Functional Technique

Sacroiliac
Sitting
Diagnosis: Left-on-right torsion

1. Patient is sitting on the table.
2. Operator sitting behind patient with the left hand over the upper pole of the left sacroiliac joint as the listening hand. The thumb is on the sacral base and the index finger gives lateral distraction on the left PSIS.
3. Operator's right hand is placed on the patient's right shoulder as the motion hand (Fig.10.19).
4. Operator's head is placed at the thoracolumbar junction.

5. Operator introduces flexion and posterior translation to localize to the listening hand.
6. Operator's motion hand introduces side bending and rotation to the left to balance at the left sacral base. The patient's weight is usually on the left ischial tuberosity (Fig. 10.20).
7. The balance-and-hold approach localizes ease in all dimensions at the left sacral base and initiates respiratory action to achieve tissue balance.
8. The dynamic indirect approach initiates motion through the motion hand in the direction of ease at the listening hand and follows the inherent tissue motion in the direction of ease to tissue balance.

Figure 10.19.

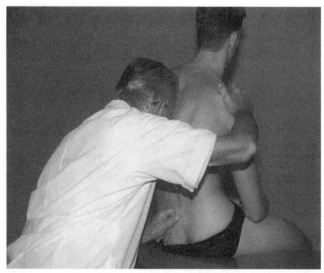

Figure 10.20.

Functional Technique

Iliosacral
Sitting
Diagnosis: Right anterior ilium

1. Patient is sitting on the table.
2. Operator sitting behind the patient.
3. Operator's right hand lies over the right iliac crest with the thumb over the sacrum at the lower pole of the sacroiliac joint as the listening hand.
4. Operator's left hand contacts the patient's left shoulder as the motion hand (Fig 10.21).
5. Operator's head is placed at the thoracolumbar junction.

6. Operator introduces AP translation until the right ilium starts to move forward, then left-side bending and rotation until ease is felt over the upper pole of the right sacroiliac joint. The patient's weight is usually on the left ischial tuberosity (Fig.10.22).
7. The balance-and-hold approach seeks ease in all dimensions, adds respiratory effort, and fine-tunes until balance of tissue tension occurs.
8. The dynamic indirect approach is initiated by loading through the motion hand in the direction of the listening hand and following the inherent tissue motion until tissue balance is achieved.

Figure 10.21.

Figure 10.22.

Functional Technique

Iliosacral
Sitting
Diagnosis: Left posterior ilium

1. Patient sitting on the table.
2. Operator sitting behind patient.
3. Operator's left hand contacts the left iliac crest with the thumb over the sacrum at the lower pole of the left sacroiliac joint as the listening hand.
4. Operator's right hand contacts the patient's right shoulder as the motion hand (Fig. 10.23).
5. Operator head is at the thoracolumbar junction.

6. Operator introduces AP translation to localize to the lower pole left sacroiliac joint (Fig. 10.24), then introduces left-side bending until the left ilium moves to ease in posterior rotation (Fig. 10.25).
7. The balance-and-hold approach seeks ease in all dimensions and adds respiratory effort to achieve balanced tissue tension.
8. The dynamic indirect approach introduces motion through the motion hand toward the left sacroiliac joint and follows inherent tissue motion until balanced tissue tension is achieved.

Figure 10.24.

Figure 10.23.

Figure 10.25.

Functional Technique

Pelvis
Sitting
Diagnosis: Pelvic compression

1. Patient sitting on table.
2. Operator sitting behind patient.
3. Operator's two hands grasp the ilia with the thumbs over the sacral base and the fingers along the iliac crests (Fig. 10.26).
4. Operator's head contacts the thoracolumbar junction.

5. Operator introduces AP translatory motion until ease is felt at the two sacroiliac joints (Fig. 10.27).
6. Operator's two hands compress the pelvis and rotate anteriorly and posteriorly on each side to the point of ease (Fig. 10.28).
7. The balance-and-hold approach holds the two ilia at the point of maximum ease and using respiratory effort seeks release and balance of tissue tension.
8. The dynamic indirect approach introduces motion through both hands and follows inherent tissue motion until balance in three dimensions is achieved.

Figure 10.27.

Figure 10.26.

Figure 10.28.

Functional Technique

Thoracolumbar Spine
Sitting
Diagnosis: Vertebral dysfunction either ERS or FRS

1. Patient sitting on the table, arms folded across chest.

2. Operator sitting behind patient.

3. Operator's right hand contacts the thoracolumbar spine as the listening hand.

4. Operator's left hand grasps patient's left elbow as the motion hand (Fig. 10.29).

5. Operator's listening hand introduces flexion and extension through AP translation and adds cephalic distraction to the point of ease.

6. Operator's motion hand introduces side bending and rotation of the trunk, plus cephalic distraction, to the point of maximum ease (Fig. 10.30).

7. The balance-and-hold approach introduces motion to maximum ease in all dimensions and adds respiratory effort until balance in tissue tension is achieved.

8. The dynamic indirect approach introduces motion through the motion hand in the direction of ease and follows inherent tissue motion until balance of tissue tension is achieved.

Figure 10.29.

Figure 10.30.

Functional Technique

Upper Thoracic Spine
Sitting
Diagnosis: Vertebral dysfunction either ERS or FRS

1. Patient sitting on the table.
2. Operator standing behind patient with the patient's trunk against the operator for control.
3. Operator's left hand contacts the dysfunctional segment as the listening hand with fingers on each vertebra.
4. Operator's right hand contacts the top of the patient's head as the motion hand (Fig. 10.31).

5. Operator introduces flexion (Fig. 10.32) and extension (Fig. 10.33) through AP translation to maximum ease at the listening hand.
6. Operator's motion hand introduces side bending and rotation to the dysfunctional segment, seeking maximum ease at the listening hand (Fig. 10.34).
7. The balance-and-hold approach seeks balance in all dimensions, then adds respiratory effort until tissue tension balance is achieved.
8. The dynamic indirect approach introduces motion through the motion hand in the direction of the listening hand and follows inherent tissue motion until tissue tension balance is achieved.

Figure 10.31.

Figure 10.33.

Figure 10.32.

Figure 10.34.

Functional Technique

Middle and Lower Thoracic Spine
Sitting
Diagnosis: Vertebral dysfunction, either ERS or FRS

1. Patient sitting on the table.
2. Operator stands behind patient with the patient's trunk against the operator's torso for control.
3. Operator's left hand contacts the dysfunctional segment with a finger contact on each of the two vertebrae as the listening hand.
4. Operator's right hand lies over the patient's right shoulder with the hand behind the patient's neck as the motion hand (Fig 10.35).
5. Operator introduces flexion (Fig. 10.36) or extension (Fig. 10.37) through AP translation to ease at the listening hand.
6. Operator's motion hand introduces side bending and rotation to ease at the listening hand (Fig. 10.38).
7. The balance-and-hold approach seeks ease in all dimensions and adds respiratory effort until balance of tissue tension is achieved.
8. The dynamic indirect approach initiates motion through the motion hand in the direction of ease at the listening hand and follows inherent tissue motion until balance of tissue tension is achieved.

Figure 10.35.

Figure 10.37.

Figure 10.36.

Figure 10.38.

Functional Technique

Thoracic Spine and Ribs
Sitting
Diagnosis: Combined vertebral and rib dysfunction

1. Patient sitting on the table with the left hand on the back of the neck.
2. Operator stands behind patient with the left hand grasping patient's left elbow as the motor hand (Fig. 10.39).

3. Operator's right hand is placed in the medial groove adjacent to the spinous processes over the restricted segments and serves as the listening hand. The thumb lies over the zygapophysial joints and the palm over the costotransverse articulation of the rib (Fig. 10.40).
4. Operator introduces flexion (Fig. 10.41) and extension (Fig. 10.42) through AP translation to ease at the listening hand.

Figure 10.39.

Figure 10.41.

Figure 10.40.

Figure 10.42.

5. Operator introduces side bending and rotation to ease at the listening hand (Fig. 10.43).

6. The balance-and-hold approach seeks ease in all dimensions and adds respiratory effort until balance in tissue tension is achieved.

7. The dynamic indirect approach initiates motion through the motion hand to ease at the listening hand and follows inherent tissue motion until three-dimensional tissue tension balance is achieved.

8. A variant of this technique has the patient's left hand grasping the right shoulder, the operator's left hand becoming the listening hand over the thoracic vertebra and ribs, and the operator's right hand grasping the patient's left elbow as the motion hand (Fig. 10.43). The rest of the procedure follows as above. This variant allows for different combinations of flexion–extension and side bending/rotation to the listening hand (Fig. 10.44).

Figure 10.43.

Figure 10.44.

Functional Technique

Mid and Lower Ribs
Sitting
Diagnosis: Structural or respiratory rib dysfunction

1. Patient sitting on the table.
2. Operator stands behind patient with the trunk supporting the patient's torso.
3. Operator's right hand is placed over the medial side of the rib angle with the fingers along the rib shafts of the dysfunctional rib(s) as the listening hand (Fig. 10.45).
4. Operator's left arm reaches across the patient's upper trunk and grasps the right shoulder as the motion hand.

5. Flexion–extension is introduced through AP translation to ease at the listening hand.
6. Operator's motion hand introduces side bending and rotation to ease at the listening hand (Fig. 10.46).
7. The balance-and-hold approach localizes ease in all dimensions at the listening hand and uses respiratory effort until balance of tissue tension is achieved.
8. The dynamic indirect approach introduces movement through the motion hand in the direction of ease at the listening hand and follows inherent tissue motion until balance in tissue tension is achieved. Occasionally, compression is useful in initiating the inherent tissue motion.

Figure 10.45.

Figure 10.46.

Functional Technique

First Rib
Sitting
Diagnosis: Respiratory dysfunction, first rib

1. Patient sitting on the table with right hand grasping back of neck.

2. Operator stands behind patient with the listening left hand palpating the patient's right first rib with the thumb on the posterior aspect and the fingers on the anterior aspect (Fig. 10.47).

3. Operator's motion right hand grasps the patient's right elbow.

4. Operator introduces AP trunk translation and internal–external rotation of the patient's right arm localizing ease at the listening hand (Fig. 10.48).

5. The balance-and-hold approach localizes ease in all directions and adds respiratory effort until balance of tissue tension occurs.

6. The dynamic indirect approach initiates a compressive action in the direction of ease through the motion hand and follows inherent tissue motion until tissue tension is relieved and motion reestablished.

Figure 10.47.

Figure 10.48.

Functional Technique

Upper Ribs
Sitting
Diagnosis: Respiratory rib dysfunction

1. Patient sitting with left hand grasping the right shoulder.
2. Operator stands behind patient with thorax supporting the patient's torso.
3. Operator's left listening hand contacts the upper left ribs (Fig. 10.49) with the thumb behind and the fingers over the anterior aspect.
4. Operator's right motion hand controls the patient's left upper extremity through the elbow.

5. Operator's body introduces AP translation; the motion hand introduces flexion, adduction, and abduction of the patient's upper arm to maximum ease at the listening hand (Fig. 10.50).
6. Additional ease may be obtained by the patient side bending and rotating the head to the right.
7. The balance-and-hold approach maintains ease in all dimensions and adds respiratory effort until tissue balance and motion is restored.
8. The dynamic indirect approach initiates motion through the motion hand in the direction of ease at the listening hand and following the inherent tissue motion until tissue tension is relieved and motion is restored.

Figure 10.49.

Figure 10.50.

Functional Technique

Single Rib (Variation 1)
Sitting
Diagnosis: Respiratory or structural rib dysfunction

1. Patient sitting on table.
2. Operator stands or sits at side of patient and identifies dysfunctional rib (Fig. 10.51).
3. Operator places both thumbs at the mid-axillary line of the dysfunctional rib with the middle fingers spanning and holding the rib shaft anteriorly and posteriorly (Fig. 10.52).

4. Patient is instructed to lean toward the operator's hands and gently side bend and rotate the trunk away (Fig. 10.53).
5. Operator translates the patient until the rib appears to "float" then initiates respiratory effort until release of tissue tension and restoration of motion occurs.

Figure 10.52.

Figure 10.51.

Figure 10.53.

Functional Technique

Single Rib (Variation 2)
Sitting
Diagnosis: Respiratory or structural rib dysfunction

1. Patient sitting on table.
2. Operator stands behind patient with thorax supporting the patient's torso.
3. Operator's listening hand is placed over the posterior aspect of the dysfunctional rib with the thumb near the costotransverse articulation and the fingers along the rib shaft.
4. Operator's motion hand reaches across anterior upper thorax of the patient and grasps the shoulder on the side of dysfunction (Fig. 10.54).

5. Operator introduces translation of the patient's body and moves the shoulder through elevation, depression, and anterior and posterior rotations until ease is felt at the listening hand (Fig. 10.55).
6. The balance-and-hold approach seeks ease in all dimensions and adds respiratory effort until release of tissue tension and restoration of motion are achieved.
7. The dynamic indirect approach initiates motion in the direction of ease and follows the inherent tissue motion until tissue tension is released and motion is restored.

Figure 10.54.

Figure 10.55.

Functional Technique

Single Typical Rib Dysfunction
Supine
Diagnosis: Respiratory or structural rib dysfunction

1. Patient supine on the table.
2. Operator sits at side of dysfunction [hand position shown with patient sitting (Fig. 10.56)].
3. Operator's posterior hand slides under patient and contacts the posterior shaft while the anterior hand contacts the anterior shaft of the dysfunctional rib (Fig. 10.57).
4. Operator introduces AP compression and seeks point of maximum ease.
5. Balance-and-hold approach adds respiratory effort to achieve tissue tension balance and restored function.
6. The dynamic indirect approach initiates motion through both hands in the direction of ease and follows inherent tissue motion until tissue tension is relieved and motion is restored.

Figure 10.56.

Figure 10.57.

Functional Technique

Sternum
Supine
Diagnosis: Manubrioglodiolar sternal dysfunction

1. Patient supine on the table.
2. Operator stands at side of the patient.
3. Operator places one hand over the sternum (Fig. 10.58) with the other hand overlying the first and pointed in the opposite direction (Fig. 10.59). A variant of the hand position has one hand over the body of the sternum pointed vertically and the other horizontally across the manubrium with the two hands adjacent to the angle of Louis (Fig. 10.60).
4. Operator introduces slight compression followed by cephalic–caudad, clockwise, (Fig.10.61) and counterclockwise compressions (Fig. 10.62), shifting side to side, with AP rocking movements seeking point of maximum ease.

5. The balance-and-hold approach seeks the point of maximum ease and introduces respiratory effort until balanced motion is achieved.
6. The dynamic indirect approach initiates motion by added compression and follows the inherent tissue motion until tissue tension is relieved and motion is restored.

Figure 10.60.

Figure 10.58.

Figure 10.61.

Figure 10.59.

Figure 10.62.

Functional Technique

Occipitoatlantal Junction (C0–C1)
Sitting
Diagnosis: Flexion–extension C0–C1 dysfunction

1. Patient sitting on table.

2. Operator stands behind patient with chest wall and abdomen supporting the patient's posterior torso.

3. Operator's two hands grasp the skull with the thumbs along the occipital protuberance (Fig. 10.63).

4. Operator's arms contact the patient's shoulders and a cephalic lift to the head is applied until ease is felt.

5. Operator fine-tunes ease with head flexion–extension, rotation, and side bending to maximum (Fig. 10.64).

6. The balance-and-hold approach holds ease in all dimensions and adds respiratory effort until tissue tension is relieved and motion is restored.

7. The dynamic indirect approach initiates motion in the direction of ease and follows inherent tissue motion until release is felt and motion established.

Figure 10.63.

Figure 10.64.

Functional Technique

Upper Cervical Spine (C1–C2)
Sitting
Diagnosis: Dysfunction at C1–C2

1. Patient sitting on table.

2. Operator stands behind patient with chest wall and abdomen supporting the patient's posterior torso.

3. Operator's left hand is placed over the front of the skull and the right hand under the occiput with the thumb and index fingers in contact with the atlas/axis region (Fig. 10.65).

4. Operator introduces cephalic distraction followed by flexion–extension and side bending/rotation seeking the point of maximum ease.

5. The balance-and-hold approach would hold the point of maximum ease and apply respiratory effort until tissue tension is released and motion is restored.

6. The dynamic indirect approach initiates motion in the direction of ease through combined motion of both hands and follows the inherent tissue motion until tissue tension is released and motion is restored.

Figure 10.65.

Functional Technique

Occipitoatloid Junction (C0–C1)
Supine
Diagnosis: Flexion–extension dysfunction

1. Patient supine on the table arms at sides.
2. Operator sitting at head of table.
3. Operator's left hand cradles the occiput with the thumb and index finger in contact with the posterior arch of the atlas (Fig. 10.66).
4. Operator's right hand contacts the frontal area (Fig. 10.67).
5. Operator introduces small AP nodding movements of the skull until the atlas is at maximum ease.

6. Operator applies compression\distraction through the occiput and right–left translation through the atlas to the point of maximum ease (Fig. 10.68).
7. The balance-and-hold approach holds the point of maximum ease and applies respiratory effort until tissue tension releases and motion is restored.
8. The dynamic indirect approach initiates motion in the direction of ease through both hands and follows inherent tissue motion until tissue tension releases and motion is restored.

Figure 10.67.

Figure 10.66.

Figure 10.68.

Functional Technique

Typical Cervical Spine
Sitting
Diagnosis: ERS or FRS

1. Patient sitting on table.
2. Operator standing behind patient with chest and abdomen supporting patient's posterior torso.
3. Operator's listening left hand is placed over the dysfunctional segment of the lower cervical spine. The thumb and index finger span the posterior pillars or the transverse processes (Fig. 10.69).
4. The motion right hand is placed on the patient's forehead.
5. Operator introduces flexion–extension, side bending, and rotation through the motion hand to maximum ease at the listening hand (Fig. 10.70). AP translatory movement can be introduced through the operator's trunk. Cephalic-to-caudad translation can be introduced through combined movement of both hands.
6. The balance-and-hold approach maintains the point of maximum ease and applies respiratory effort until tissue tension releases and motion is restored (Fig. 10.71).
7. The dynamic indirect approach introduces motion through the right hand in the direction of ease and follows inherent tissue motion until tissue tension releases and motion is restored.

Figure 10.70.

Figure 10.69.

Figure 10.71.

Functional Technique

Typical Cervical Spine
Supine
Diagnosis: ERS or FRS

1. Patient supine on the table.
2. Operator sitting at head of table.
3. Operator hands support patient's head and upper cervical spine with the index and middle fingers over the articular pillar of the dysfunctional segment (Fig. 10.72).
4. Operator introduces flexion–extension, AP translation, side bending, and rotation through combined movement of both hands seeking point of maximum ease under finger tips (Fig. 10.73).
5. The balance-and-hold approach maintains the point of maximum ease and applies respiratory effort until tissue tension is released and motion is restored (Fig. 10.74).
6. The dynamic indirect approach initiates motion in the direction of ease and follows the inherent tissue motion until tissue tension releases and motion is restored.

Figure 10.73.

Figure 10.72.

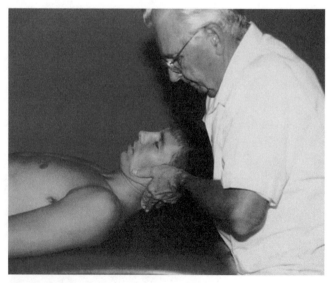

Figure 10.74.

Functional Technique

Shoulder Girdle
Step 1

1. Patient supine on the table.
2. Operator sits at the side of the shoulder to be treated.
3. Operator's listening hand is placed over the patient's clavicle with the little finger along the shaft and the fourth and fifth finger pads over the sternoclavicular joint. The heel of the hand is over the acromioclavicular joint (Fig. 10.75).

4. Operator's motion hand grasps the patient's arm either above or below the elbow and abducts to about 90 degrees (Fig. 10.76).
5. Operator's motion hand introduces adduction–abduction, internal–external rotation, and compression–distraction along the humerus to ease at the listening hand.
6. The balance-and-hold approach maintains the point of ease and adds respiratory effort until release of tissue tension occurs.
7. The dynamic indirect approach introduces motion in the direction of ease and follows the inherent tissue motion until tissue tension is relieved.

Figure 10.75.

Figure 10.76.

Functional Technique

Shoulder Girdle
Step 2

1. Operator and patient position as in step 1.

2. Operator's listening hand is placed over the gleno-humeral joint with the thumb behind and the fingers in front (Fig.10.77).

3. Operator's motion hand grasps the patient's arm in the same fashion as step 1 and introduces abduction to 80 to 90 degrees then fine-tunes through the listening hand by internal–external rotation, compression–decompression until maximum ease is obtained (Fig. 10.78).

4. The balance-and-hold approach maintains ease and adds respiratory effort until release of tissue tension is achieved.

5. The dynamic indirect approach initiates motion in the direction of ease through the motion hand and follows inherent tissue motion until tissue tension is released and motion is restored.

Figure 10.77.

Figure 10.78.

Functional Technique

Shoulder Girdle
Step 3

1. Operator and patient position as in steps 1 and 2.

2. Operator switches hands with the listening hand over the pectoral region in the direction of the fibers of the pectoralis minor. The motion hand controls the arm and introduces abduction so that the arm is in the direction of the pectoral muscle fibers (Fig. 10.79).

3. Operator's motion hand introduces compression–decompression, internal–external rotation, and adduction–abduction until the point of maximum ease is felt at the listening hand.

4. The tissues are balanced between the two hands.

5. The balance-and-hold approach maintains the point of maximum ease and adds respiratory effort until tissue tension is relieved and motion is returned.

6. The dynamic indirect approach initiates motion in the direction of ease and follows inherent tissue motion until tissue tension is relieved and motion is restored.

Figure 10.79.

Functional Technique

Acromioclavicular and Glenohumeral Joints
Sitting

1. Patient sitting on table.

2. Operator stands behind patient and supports patient's trunk against operator's body.

3. Operator's foot is placed on table on side being treated and drapes patient's relaxed arm over knee with medial hand placed over the patient's acromioclavicular and glenohumeral areas (Fig. 10.80).

4. Operator's lateral hand grasps the patient's elbow.

5. Operator introduces AP and medial–lateral translation and rotation of the patient to ease at both the shoulder and the elbow (Fig. 10.81).

6. The balance-and-hold approach identifies the point of maximum ease and adds respiratory effort until tissue tension is relieved and motion is restored.

7. The dynamic indirect approach introduces motion in the direction of ease, frequently with a compression–decompression maneuver in the long axis of the arm, and follows the inherent tissue motion until tissue tension is relieved and motion is restored.

Figure 10.80.

Figure 10.81.

Functional Technique

Radial Head
Sitting

1. Patient sitting.

2. Operator stands in front of patient with listening hand over the dysfunctional elbow with the thumb over the anterior aspect and the index finger over the posterior aspect of the radial head (Fig. 10.82).

3. Operator's motion hand grasps the patient's distal forearm and introduces flexion–extension, internal–external rotation, adduction–abduction, compression–decompression to the point of maximum ease (Fig. 10.83).

4. The balance-and-hold approach maintains the point of maximum ease and introduces respiratory effort until tissue tension is relieved and motion is restored.

5. The dynamic indirect approach introduces motion in the direction of ease and follows inherent tissue motion until tissue tension is relieved and motion is restored.

Figure 10.82.

Figure 10.83.

Functional Technique

Wrist and Hand
Sitting

1. Patient sitting on table.

2. Operator stands in front of patient grasping the dysfunctional wrist and hand with the proximal hand over the distal forearm (Fig. 10.84).

3. Operator's distal hand grasps the patient's hand either with a handshake hold (Fig. 10.85) or with the fingers interdigitating (Fig. 10.86).

4. Operator's distal hand introduces flexion–extension, internal–external rotation, adduction–abduction and compression–decompression to the point of maximum ease (Fig. 10.87).

5. Balance-and-hold technique maintains the point of ease and adds respiratory effort until tissue tension is relieved and motion is restored.

6. The dynamic indirect approach introduces motion in the direction of ease and follows inherent tissue motion until tissue tension is relieved and motion is restored.

Figure 10.84.

Figure 10.86.

Figure 10.85.

Figure 10.87.

Functional Technique

Hip and Leg
Supine

1. Patient supine on table.

2. Operator stands at side of table on side of dysfunctional leg and one foot on the table.

3. Operator flexes patient's leg to about 90 degrees of hip and knee flexion with the leg draped over the operator's thigh.

4. Operator's proximal hand is on the patient's knee with the distal hand holding the patient's foot (Fig. 10.88).

5. Operator introduces compression–decompression through the thigh and/or leg until ease is obtained. Fine-tuning is done by medial–lateral rotation, adduction–abduction, and flexion–extension of the hip and knee (Fig. 10.89).

6. The balance-and-hold approach maintains the point of maximum ease and adds respiratory effort until tissue tension is relieved and motion is restored.

7. The dynamic indirect approach initiates motion in the direction of ease and follows the inherent tissue motion until tissue tension is relieved and motion is restored.

Figure 10.88.

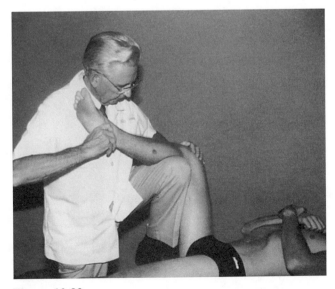

Figure 10.89.

Functional Technique

Knee and Fibular Head
Sitting

1. Patient is sitting on the table with legs dangling.
2. The operator sits in front of the patient.
3. Operator's listening hand palpates the knee with the thumb over the medial meniscus and the fingers on the fibular head (Fig. 10.90).
4. Operator's motion hand holds the foot and ankle and introduces compression–decompression to loose pack the tibia on the femur.

5. Operator fine-tunes ease at the listening hand by introducing abduction–adduction, internal–external rotation, and flexion–extension (Fig. 10.91).
6. The balance-and-hold approach maintains maximum ease and adds respiratory effort until tissue tension is relieved and motion is restored.
7. The dynamic indirect approach initiates motion in the direction of ease and follows inherent tissue motion until tissue tension is relieved and motion is restored.

Figure 10.90.

Figure 10.91.

Functional Technique

Foot and Ankle

1. Patient sitting or supine on table.
2. Operator's listening hand grasps the heel of the patient (Fig. 10.92).
3. Operator's motion hand grasps the forefoot and initiates motion through compression (Fig. 10.93).
4. Operator fines-tunes maximum ease through the introduction of dorsi and plantar flexion, inversion–eversion, and adduction–abduction (Fig. 10.94).
5. The balance-and-hold approach maintains maximum ease and uses respiratory effort until tissue tension is relieved and motion is restored.
6. The dynamic indirect approach initiates motion primarily through compression–distraction and follows inherent tissue motion until tissue tension is relieved and motion is restored.

Figure 10.93.

Figure 10.92.

Figure 10.94.

CONCLUSION

Indirect (functional) techniques are based on a common neurologic model in which reducing the flow of abnormal afferent impulses into the central nervous system reprograms the "central computer" to more normal function. These procedures focus on the quality of movement, particularly the quality on the initiation of motion, rather than the amount of range or the feel of its end point. They are primarily nontraumatic and easily used in a variety of patient conditions and health care settings. They require considerable practice to educate the senses to the ease-and-bind phenomena and to the point of maximum pain-free position for the tissues of the musculoskeletal system. The value of these procedures in patient care warrants the expenditure of time and effort needed for the student to acquire proficiency.

SUGGESTED READINGS

Hoover HW. *Functional technique.* Carmel, CA: Yearbook of the Academy of Applied Osteopathy, 1958; 47–51.

Johnston WL, Friedman HD. *Functional methods.* Indianapolis, IN: American Academy of Osteopathy, 1994.

Johnston WL, Robertson JA, Stiles EG. *Finding a common denominator for the variety of manipulative techniques.* Carmel, CA: Yearbook of the American Academy of Osteopathy, 1969; 5–15.

Jones LH. *Strain and counterstrain.* Colorado Springs, CO: American Academy of Osteopathy, 1981.

Stiles EG. Manipulative techniques: four approaches. *Osteopathic Med* 1975;1:27–30.

Stile EG, Shaw HH. Functional techniques based upon the approach of George Andrew Laughlin DO. Course syllabus. Michigan State University, College of Osteopathic Medicine, Continuing Education, 1991.

11
PRINCIPLES OF MYOFASCIAL RELEASE AND INTEGRATED NEUROMUSCULOSKELETAL TECHNIQUE

Robert C. Ward, D.O., F.A.A.O., is credited with developing these release techniques as one of the newer additions to the field of manual medicine. He describes these myofascial release techniques as a "bridging" technique spanning the spectrum of manual medicine procedures. It combines many of the principles of soft-tissue technique, muscle energy technique, indirect technique, and inherent-force craniosacral technique. They are classified as combined procedures as they influence the biomechanics of the musculoskeletal system and the peripheral and central neural control mechanisms. There are multiple authors and teachers of myofascial release technique with many similarities and differences.

Fascia has received the attention of many individuals including the osteopathic physician Neidner who used twisting forces on the extremities to restore fascial balance and symmetry. Rolf was famous for deep pressure and stretching of the fascia from the top of the head to the tips of the toes. Rolfing requires extensive investment in time and energy, both by the patient and operator, and the process is not always comfortable.

The myofascial release technique described here can be classified as direct or indirect, and frequently is used in a combined fashion. It applies the principles of biomechanical loading of soft tissue and the neural reflex modifications by stimulation of mechanoreceptors in the fascia. The resistant barrier may be engaged directly with tissue stretching, or loading can occur in the direction away from the resistant barrier in an indirect fashion. These are frequently called direct and indirect barriers. Frequently the barriers are addressed in a combined fashion in each direction.

Myofascial release technique builds on inherent tissue motion. Living tissues have an inherent motion that continues at various rates and amplitudes. The inherent tissue motion of the musculoskeletal system is thought to be the result of rhythmic changes in tone of muscle, pulsating forces of arterial circulation, the effects of respiration, and the inherent force of the cranial rhythmic impulse.

Activating forces in myofascial release technique are both intrinsic and extrinsic. The intrinsic forces include inherent tissue motion, inherent body rhythms, respiration, muscle contraction, and eye movement. Extrinsic activating forces applied by the operator include the application of loads primarily of compression, traction, and twisting to apply the appropriate tension in the soft tissues to effect biomechanical and reflex change. This technique is used for regional and local dysfunctions. It shares the common goal of all manual medicine procedures to achieve symmetric, pain-free motion of the musculoskeletal system in postural balance.

FASCIA

The clinician using myofascial release technique must have a thorough working knowledge of the continuity and integration of fascia. The fascia of the body is continuous from region to region and totally invests all other elements of the body. Various portions of fascia carry individual names but all fasciae are continuous.

Fasciae can be described as consisting of three layers. The superficial fascia is attached to the undersurface of the skin and is loosely knit, fibroelastic, areolar tissue. Within the superficial fascia are fat, vascular structures (including capillary networks and lymphatic channels), and nervous tissues, particularly the pacinian corpuscles referred to as skin receptors. The skin can be moved in many directions over the deeper structures because of the loosely knit nature of superficial fascia. Within the superficial fascia is potential space for the accumulation of fluid and metabolites. Many of the palpatory changes of tissue texture abnormalities are the result of changes within the superficial fascia.

Deep fascia is tough, tight, and compact. It compartmentalizes the body. It envelops and separates muscles, surrounds and separates internal visceral organs, and contributes greatly to the contour and function of the body. The peritoneum, the pericardium, and the pleura are specialized elements of the deep fascia. The tough, resistant, and confining characteristics of deep fascia can create problems such as the compartment syndromes. Trauma with hemorrhage in the anterior compartment of the lower leg can cause

155

swelling that is detrimental to the sensitive nerve structures within the compartment. Frequently, surgical fasciectomy is necessary to relieve the compression on neural elements.

The subserous fascia is the loose areolar tissue that covers the internal visceral organs. The many small circulatory channels and fluids within this fascia lubricate the surfaces of the internal viscera.

Function of Fascia

Fascia provides support for vessels and nerves throughout the body. It enables adjacent tissues to move on each other while providing stability and contour. It provides lubricating fluid between structures for movement and nutrition. The pacinian corpuscles in the superficial fascia provide afferent information for many complex reflexes involving the neuromuscular system. The fascia described is continuous with specialized elements such as ligaments and tendons. These tissues have unique characteristics, but share with the general fascia collagen fibers, elastic fibers, cellular elements, and ground substance. Specialized mechanoreceptors and proprioceptors are found within these specialized elements of fascia that report information to the spinal cord and brain on body position and movement, both normal and abnormal. Within the ground substance of the fascia are many of the substances that contribute to immune mechanisms within the body.

Biomechanics of Fascia

Fascia's intimate connection with muscle provides the opportunity for contraction and relaxation. Fascia has elasticity that allows it to both retain its shape and respond to deformation. Elastic deformation is the capacity of fascia to recover its original shape when the load is removed. If the load is great and applied for a longer period, fascia may not be able to recover its original size and shape, resulting in plastic deformation. When subjected to an extension load and held constant, fascia has the capacity to "creep." The relaxation of the tissue that accompanies creep allows for less resistance to a second application of load. This phenomenon has clinical significance when the clinician observes the effects of acute and repetitive injury and long-term stress on connective tissues. Fascia has the capacity to change when subjected to stress and lose energy. This phenomenon, called "hysteresis," is used therapeutically in myofascial release technique.

Fascial Injury

Fascia responds to acute injury or chronic recurrent microtrauma (such as postural imbalance due to anatomic short leg) in a variety of ways. The first is the inflammatory process of injury that spans the spectrum from acute to chronic changes. Inflammatory fluid can be easily contained and absorbed in the superficial fascia, but when within the tight compartments of deep fascia it becomes quite detrimental. These fascial changes are palpable by the trained hand and are contributors to the tissue texture abnormalities characteristic and diagnostic of somatic dysfunction.

Fascia under stress responds biomechanically. Depending on the amount and type of load, deformation may be temporary or permanent. The number and type of collagen and elastic fibers within the connective tissue and the type of load applied determine the fascial change that occurs under biomechanical stress. The biomechanical stress of fascial injury causes the receptors to send afferent information to the central nervous system for processing. The ability or inability of these receptors to adapt and the facility of the central nervous system to adjust determine the short- and/or long-term effect on neural integration resulting from the connective tissue injury.

Biochemical and immunologic changes occur within the ground substance of the fascia and have general systemic effects that seem quite far removed from the injury to the soft tissues. Scarring during the healing process frequently interferes with the functions of support, movement, and lubrication. Many detrimental symptoms result that are difficult to objectify. Soft-tissue changes lead to persistent symptoms long after there has been healing of the acute tissue injury. Victims of flexion–extension type cervical injuries (whiplash injury) from motor vehicle and other accidents frequently have persistent symptoms that are difficult to explain. Recent research indicates that some of these people have fatty replacement of deep cervical muscles that may reflect the effects of "soft-tissue injury" accompanying the trauma (see Chapter 21).

MUSCLE

Muscle is the second focus of myofascial release technique. Muscles can be classified as those that maintain posture, the so-called "static muscles," and those that provide movement, the so-called "phasic muscles." Muscles can perform both functions, but usually one will predominate. Clinically, the muscles that have postural function respond by facilitation, hypertonicity, and shortening. In the lower half of the body these include the iliopsoas, rectus femoris, tensor fascia lata, quadratus lumborum, adductors, piriformis, hamstrings, and erector spinae. In the upper half of the body, the postural muscles that respond by facilitation, hypertonicity, and shortening are the levator scapulae, upper trapezius, sternocleidomastoid, pectorals, scalenes, latissimus dorsi, subscapularis, and flexors of the upper extremity. Dynamic phasic muscles respond by inhibition, hypotonicity, and weakness. In the lower half of the body, these include the gluteus maximus, medius, and minimis; rectus abdominous; internal and external abdominal obliques; peroneals; vasti of the thigh; and tibialis anterior. In the upper half of the body, they include the middle and lower trapezius, serratus anterior, rhomboids, supra- and infraspinatus, deltoids, deep neck flexors, and extensors of the upper extremity.

Each muscle action has an equal and opposite muscle reaction, the agonist–antagonist principle. Sherrington's law of reciprocal innervation and inhibition balances the tone and function of agonist and antagonist muscles on the ipsilateral and contralateral sides. Sophisticated neuromuscular reflexes constantly maintain body posture, prepare for, initiate, and continue movement patterns.

Function of muscle in the musculoskeletal system is an integrated and highly complex process. Motor control through the central nervous system from the premotor cortex through the brainstem, cerebellum, spinal cord, and finally to the final common pathway, the alpha motor neuron to skeletal muscle. This control system for muscle function is highly complex and has voluntary and involuntary components. This complex motor programming is altered by afferent impulses coming from the mechanoreceptors within the articular and fascial systems. When this central control system is working efficiently, movement patterns are symmetric, coordinated, and free. When altered, inefficient and uncoordinated movement results. One need only contrast the performance of an Olympic-level runner and a patient with advanced Parkinson disease. Between these two extremes are gradations of hypertonicity, hypotonicity, and altered integrative coordination, particularly noted in patients with minimal brain dysfunction.

Muscle injury interferes with its anatomy and function. Acute trauma results in muscle tears, disturbances at the myotendinous junction, and alterations of insertion of tendon into bone. These injuries undergo fibrosis as part of the healing process similar to other injuries of soft tissues. Functional loss can result. Injury not only alters the anatomy of the muscle, but also interferes with its neuroreflexive response to motor control and contributes to persistent long-term symptoms.

CONCEPTS IN MYOFASCIAL RELEASE TECHNIQUE

The first concept is "tight–loose." Within the myofascial system, tightness creates and weakness permits asymmetry. There are biomechanical and neural reflexive elements to the tight–loose concept. Increased stimulation causes an agonist muscle to become tight, and the tighter it becomes, the looser its antagonist becomes because of reciprocal inhibition. The fascia surrounding a hypertonic, contracted muscle short-ens and requires loosening of the fascia in the opposite direction for accommodation. One cannot step a mast on a boat by pulling on the forestay if the backstay is not sufficiently loose to permit movement. In acute conditions, the cycle can be described as continuing spasm–pain–spasm. The result is tightness that progresses from the acute condition of muscle contraction to muscle contracture, leading to chronicity. In chronic conditions, the cycle is described as pain–looseness–pain. Manual medicine practitioners are familiar with the painful symptoms of hypermobility. The practitioners using myofascial release procedures apply the fundamental tight–loose concept on a continuing basis.

The second concept is the use of "palpation" in myofascial pain syndromes. Many diagnostic and therapeutic systems build on peripheral stimulation and include acupuncture, acupressure, Chapman reflexes, Travell trigger points, and Jones tender points. Skilled palpation of myofascial elements frequently identifies locations of myofascial pain that can be therapeutically addressed by the hands. Frequently noted is the occurrence of myofascial pain in areas of soft-tissue looseness. Sensitivity of the myofascial elements, particularly in the chronic state, frequently has a burning quality. Recall that the sympathetic division of the autonomic nervous system is the only division that innervates the musculoskeletal system. Sympathetic nervous system reflexes probably mediate many symptoms found in myofascial pain syndromes.

The third concept is "neuroreflexive change" occurring with the application of manual force on the musculoskeletal system. Hands-on application of force to the musculoskeletal system results in afferent stimulation through mechanoreceptors that require central processing at the spinal cord, brainstem, and cortical levels. Afferent stimulation frequently results in efferent inhibition. When afferent stimulation of a stretch is applied during a myofascial release procedure, the operator waits for relaxation in the tight tissues by efferent inhibition. The neuroreflexive response is highly variable and modified by the amount of pain, the patient's pain behavior, the level of wellness, the nutritional status, the stress response, and the basic lifestyle of the individual including the use/abuse of alcohol, tobacco, and drugs, including prescription medications.

The fourth concept is the "release" phenomenon. The sensation of release occurs in other forms of manual medicine, particularly in craniosacral technique and the ease–bind of indirect (functional) technique. When using myofascial release technique, appropriate application of stress on tissue results in tissue relaxation in fascia and in muscle. Tightness "gives way" or "melts" under the application of load. Release of tightness is sought to achieve improvement in symmetry of form and function. The release phenomenon is both an enabling and a terminal objective when applying a myofascial release procedure. Release can occur in several directions and through different levels of tissue during a myofascial release procedure. The release phenomenon is one that guides the practitioner through the treatment process.

PRINCIPLES OF MYOFASCIAL RELEASE EVALUATION

Ward has expanded his mnemonic M A I (N) 4 to B E M A I (N) 4.

B stands for behavior, particularly the patient's response to stress. Behavioral response to stress is modified by many factors including race, education, family, financial status, religion, and many others. Patients respond differently to the stress of their injuries as well as to the hands-on process of the patient–provider interaction. Behavioral issues, particularly in patients with chronic pain, are significant in any therapeutic outcome.

E stands for endocrine status. The endocrine system influences all of the other systems of the human organism. It has major influence on the musculoskeletal system and responds to stress within the musculoskeletal system. Alterations in thyroid function and carbohydrate metabolism in diabetes alter the response of the musculoskeletal system to stress and injury and its response to treatment interventions. Assessment of the musculoskeletal system by palpation identifies tissue texture abnormalities that may be associated with disturbances of the endocrine system. Therapeutic interventions used within the myofascial release technique system will alter the stimulation to the endocrine system and its close linkage with the nervous system.

M stands for mechanical analysis of the musculoskeletal system for its symmetry–asymmetry, looseness–tightness, and its response to postural balance or imbalance. Mechanical loading is important in the injury process and in the therapeutic process.

A stands for anatomy and the overall functional capacity of the body. Assessment is made in a three-dimensional sense of all of the anatomy of the body with particular reference to muscle function, joint mechanics, and nervous system control. The practitioner should have a working knowledge of the integration of all elements of the musculoskeletal system, particularly the integrating aspects of fascia and the motor control of the musculoskeletal system. The examiner assesses both symmetry or asymmetry of form and function, recognizing that asymmetry is the rule whereas symmetric function is the goal of any treatment outcome.

I stands for the immune system and the patient's response to stress. The immune system is highly complex and responds to many factors beginning with the general health status of the patient and the response to stressors in the internal and external environments. Altered immune function, particularly that associated with rheumatologic conditions, strongly influences the musculoskeletal system and its response to stress and to treatment interventions.

N stands for altered neurologic function. The central nervous system is highly complex and is subject to functional and pathologic changes. Assessment of the patient's nervous system function by traditional neurologic examination assists in differentiating functional from organic pathologies of the central nervous system. There are many other neurologic considerations, including the assessment of autonomic nervous system function. Are there palpable changes in the musculoskeletal system that may reflect alteration in autonomic nervous system balance and tone? The patient's lifestyle and psychologic status influence nervous system responses. As part of the neurologic response, the examiner is interested in the nociceptive behavior of the patient. A patient's response to pain, pain behavior, and lifestyle will influence the patient's response to a nociceptive episode. The patient's nutritional status strongly affects the nervous system. Poor nutrition, particularly of the inadequacy of B-complex vitamins, results in abnormal nervous system function. Nutritional status, alcohol and tobacco use or abuse, and prescribed medications as well as street-drug use strongly influence response of the patient's nervous system.

The assessment of the patient using the myofascial release system must be viewed from a total integrative perspective. Consider all of these behavioral, anatomic, and physiologic factors when assessing the patient and when providing the therapeutic intervention.

MYOFASCIAL RELEASE TREATMENT CONCEPTS

Ward has coined another mnemonic to describe the principles of myofascial release treatment. It is **P O E (T)²**. **P O E** stands for *point of entry* into the musculoskeletal system. Entry may be made from anywhere in the musculoskeletal system including the lower extremity, the upper extremity, the thoracic cage, the abdomen, and the vertebral complex from the cranial cervical junction to the pelvis. The two **T**'s stand for *traction and twist*. Traction and twist are but two of the applications of load that are of assistance in the diagnostic and treatment process. Traction produces stretch along the long axis of myofascial elements that are short and tight. Stretch should always be applied in the long axis rather than transversely across myofascial elements. Twisting force provides the opportunity to localize the traction, not only at the point of contact with the patient, but also at points some distance away. Compressive and shear forces are also used to localize to different levels of the myofascial system and to provide different loads. The practitioner should develop the ability to sense change locally at the point of contact as well as at some distance away. For example, when grasping the lower extremity near the ankle, the operator should attempt to feel through the extremity to the knee, thigh, hip, sacroiliac joint, and into the vertebral column sensing changes that occur at each level. This is all perceived through the contact point at the ankle. This skill requires concentration, practice, and an appreciation for the three-dimensional aspects of the musculoskeletal system.

The treatment process includes assessment of tightness and looseness throughout the system and the application of loads, both into the direct and indirect barriers, seeking the release phenomena. Tightness and looseness can be different between the superficial and deep layers of the musculoskeletal system. Frequently, tightness in the superficial layers is found overlying the looseness in the deeper structures surrounding the articular elements. This may be compensatory in nature, but the superficial tightness and the deep-level looseness should both be approached appropriately so that the result is more symmetric function throughout the system.

Patient activity during the treatment process can assist in the achievement of the therapeutic goal. These *enhancers* include muscle contraction, joint motion of the upper and lower extremities, respiration, and eye movement. Any activity that increases the central nervous system processing, particularly of the cranial nerves, seems to enhance the effectiveness of the practitioner-applied loading forces. One or more enhancers may be used throughout the treatment process. The process of adding enhancers has led Ward to call this "integrated neuromuscular release." The enhancers add the neural-challenging component to the biomechanical challenge of the soft tissues.

Following treatment by these techniques, patients are given specific exercises that are individualized for their problem. Stretching exercise maintains the added length of the tight tissues and strengthening exercise restores the functional capacity of the weaker inhibited muscles. In treatment of muscle imbalance, first stretch the short, tight muscle groups and follow with strengthening exercise for the weaker, loose muscle groups. Exercise programs should also enhance the integrative function of muscle balance. Such exercises as cross-pattern pep walking, swimming, square dancing, rebounding, and so forth can be used. The goal is to increase mobility and strength and enhance muscular coordination.

These procedures are more than biomechanical and neuroreflexive. They address the total patient.

General health issues such as lifestyle, coping mechanisms, appropriate use of alcohol and other medications, discontinuance of tobacco, adequate and appropriate nutrition, and weight control are all issues that need to be addressed concurrently with the myofascial release treatment program.

EXERCISES IN PALPATION

Myofascial release procedures require skill at palpating the musculoskeletal system for something other than one bone moving on the other. One must learn to "read the tissues" for their tightness–looseness, their inherent mobility, and the usual soft tissue texture abnormalities of hard–soft, cool–warm, smooth–rough, and so forth (see Chapter 2). One needs to develop increased sensitivity to the patient's tissues both at point of contact and at some distance. There are many exercises in palpation that can be useful and the following are but a few.

Place the fingertips of all five fingers together without contact with the rest of the hand. Introduce force from one hand to the other and then reverse. Sense what goes on with the hand generating the force and the one receiving the force. Are they different from side to side? Now take one hand and stroke with the finger pads down the volar surface of the fingers and palms, first with light stroking and then with increased pressure. Repeat using the other hand as the motor hand. Sense the difference in the sensitivity of the hand being stroked, as well as the sensation of touch by the finger pads of the motor hand. To properly sense what goes on in the patient, you must have an awareness of your own palpatory skills and sensations and your own self-body awareness.

Fold your hands together, interlacing all your fingers. You will find that either the right or the left second metacarpophalangeal joint is on top. Now reverse the position so that the other metacarpophalangeal joint is on top. Sense the difference, with one appearing to be more comfortable than the other does, and with the less comfortable one feeling tighter.

Stretch your arms out ahead of you, crossing them at the wrist and pronating both hands until the palmer surfaces meet. Interlace your fingers and raise the extended arms over your head. As you reach toward the ceiling, feel the difference in tension between the right and left sides of your body. Return to the starting position, reverse the way in which your wrists are crossed, and repeat the procedure. Again, note the difference in tension from side to side and the difference introduced by altered crossing of the wrists.

Working with a patient partner, return to the forearm described in Chapter 2. This time, start with your palpating hand some distance from the forearm and slowly move toward the forearm until you begin to feel radiant energy from the patient. This is usually sensed as heat. Repeat the procedure several times with your eyes closed to see if you can repeatedly stop at the point where you first feel the sensation and if the distance from your palpating hand to the forearm is consistent. Continue to approach the forearm until you are palpating just the superficial hair, and course up and down over the forearm, attempting to sense what is going on under your hand. See if you can identify differences in the proximal forearm, distal forearm, wrist, and hand. Place your hand in contact with the skin and concentrate, applying no motion of your own, but attempt to sense the inherent movement of the patient's tissues under your hand. It takes several seconds to several minutes to begin to sense an inherent oscillatory movement within the forearm.

When you have mastered the ability to apply pressure but not movement and the ability to sense inherent movement within your patient, place the palm of your hand in contact with the bony sacrum. This should be done both in the supine and prone positions. The contour of the sacrum fits nicely in the palm of your hand. In the prone position it is sometimes necessary to use a slight compressive force to begin to feel the inherent motion of the sacrum. In a supine position the patient's body weight on your hand is sufficient to initiate inherent sacral movement. Try to follow the sacrum in the directions in which it wishes to move. Do not attempt to direct it. What are the rhythm, amplitude, and direction of the sacrum moving in space? When you have been able to identify inherent soft-tissue and bony movement, you are well on your way to being able to use myofascial release technique.

A simple exercise to begin with is to perform the old "Indian burn" to your partner's forearm. Grasp your partner's forearm with both hands close together, apply enough pressure to control the skin and superficial fascia down to the deep fascia, then twist each hand in opposite directions sensing for a barrier, then reverse the direction of your hand-twisting to sense the difference. Is one direction tight and the other loose? Now twist into the tight direction and hold it there. Do you feel it begin to loosen? That is the sensation of hysteresis and creep.

EXAMPLES OF MYOFASCIAL RELEASE TECHNIQUE

Wide varieties of myofascial release techniques are in use by many practitioners. They are highly individualized to the skill of the practitioner and to the needs of the patient at the treatment visit. The following examples are those taught by Ward but have been found most effective in this author's hands. They provide the reader with only a small sample of the total system.

Myofascial Release Technique

Lumbosacral Spine: One

Prone with longitudinal traction

1. Patient prone with arms off side of table, feet over the end, with head turned to the most comfortable side.

2. Operator stands at side of patient, facing foot of table. If right-handed, on patient's left, if left-handed, on patient's right.

3. Operator places distal hand over sacrum with heel of hand at lumbosacral junction. Operator's proximal hand is placed in the midline over the thoracolumbar junction with fingers pointing caudally (Fig. 11.1).

4. Operator introduces compression and separates both hands in a longitudinal fashion sensing for symmetry or asymmetry (Fig. 11.2).

5. Operator follows inherent tissue motion, sensing direct and indirect barriers, constantly searching for balance of tightness and looseness.

6. Operator applies twisting and torsional loads as necessary to achieve balance while the patient uses enhancing maneuvers.

7. After release(s) are achieved, reassess for enhanced motion and balance.

Figure 11.1.

Figure 11.2.

Myofascial Release Technique

Lumbosacral Spine: 2

Prone with transverse traction

1. Patient prone on table with arms at side, feet off end, and head turned to most comfortable position.

2. Operator stands at side of table with cephalic hand transversely across the thoracolumbar junction and the caudal hand transversely across the lumbosacral junction and sacral base (Fig. 11.3).

3. Operator applies compression and introduces transverse shear in opposite directions sensing for tightness and looseness (Fig. 11.4).

4. Operator may apply a twisting force as barriers are engaged (Fig. 11.5).

5. Operator follows inherent tissue motion, sensing for balance of tightness and looseness while patient performs enhancing maneuvers.

6. After release(s) are achieved, reassess for enhanced motion and balance.

Figure 11.4.

Figure 11.3.

Figure 11.5.

Myofascial Release Technique

Thoracolumbar Junction and Posterior Diaphragm

Prone

1. Patient prone with arms off side of table, feet off the end, and head turned to the most comfortable side.

2. Operator stands at side of patient, facing toward the head.

3. Operator's hands are placed on each side of the thoracolumbar junction with the thumbs vertical along the spinous processes and the remainder of the hand along the lower ribs overlying the posterior diaphragm (Fig. 11.6).

4. Operator's whole hand introduces compressive load and the left moves clockwise while the right moves counterclockwise in a lateral and superior direction (Fig. 11.7).

5. Operator assesses direct and indirect barriers from superficial to deep, sensing for tissue balance while patient performs enhancing maneuvers.

6. Redness of the skin is frequently seen after this technique and is described as the "blush" phenomenon.

7. After release(s) are achieved, reassess for enhanced motion and balance.

Figure 11.6.

Figure 11.7.

Myofascial Release Technique

Prone

Sacral release

1. Patient prone with arms off side of table, feet off end of table, and head turned to the most comfortable side.
2. Operator places hand over sacrum with heel over base and fingers over the apex including the inferior lateral angles (Fig. 11.8).
3. Operator's other hand is placed on top (Fig. 11.9).

4. Operator's hand pressure is anterior and inferior with a rocking motion from side to side, forward and backward, and across the oblique axes.
5. Operator follows the inherent sacral motion, sensing for indirect barriers (looseness) and direct barriers (tightness) until release(s) occur.
6. Patient performs enhancing maneuvers to assist in treatment procedure.
7. Treatment goal is balance of the sacrum between the innominates

Figure 11.8.

Figure 11.9.

Myofascial Release Technique

Prone

Sacrotuberous ligament and urogenital diaphragm release

1. Patient prone with arms off side of table, feet off end of table, and head turned to the most comfortable side.
2. Operator at side of table facing cephalad places hands over buttocks area with the thigh in contact with the sacrotuberous attachments at the inferior lateral angles of the sacrum (Fig. 11.10).

3. Tension in the sacrotuberous ligaments is tested for symmetric balance.
4. Operator's hands twist in clockwise and counterclockwise directions, sensing for tightness and looseness (Fig. 11.11).
5. Operator applies load to balance tension in the sacrotuberous ligament while the patient performs enhancing maneuvers.
6. Treatment goal is balance of the sacrotuberous ligaments and urogenital diaphragm.

Figure 11.10.

Figure 11.11.

Myofascial Release Technique

Supine or Sitting

Thoracic inlet (necklace) technique

1. Patient sitting on table with operator standing behind with both hands encircling the thoracic inlet (Fig. 11.12) with the thumbs on each side of the spinous process of T1 (Fig. 11.13).

2. Patient supine on table with operator sitting at head of table and hands placed on thoracic inlet as above (Fig. 11.14).

3. Operator's hands in contact with thoracic inlet with palms over trapezius and fingers contacting the medial end of the clavicle and upper sternum introducing compression followed by twisting and traction load seeking direct and indirect barriers (Figs. 11.15 and 11.16).

4. Operator, using a steering-wheel action, rotates the thoracic inlet to symmetry of anteroposterior and rotary balance.

5. Various patient arm positions are used to enhance load application. Patient performs enhancing maneuvers to increase release(s).

Figure 11.14.

Figure 11.12.

Figure 11.15.

Figure 11.13.

Figure 11.16.

Myofascial Release Technique

Sitting

Thoracic spine

1. Patient sitting on table with operator sitting facing away from the patient with the trunk against the patient for stability.

2. Operator's anterior hand is vertically placed over the sternum with the fingertips covering the manubriosternal junction (Fig. 11.17).

3. Operator's posterior hand is placed vertically over the spinous processes of the lower to mid-thoracic spine (Fig. 11.18).

4. For the upper thoracic spine, the operator's left hand is transversely placed across the sternum, upper ribs, and medial end of the clavicles (Fig. 11.19).

5. Operator's posterior hand is transversely placed across the upper thoracic spine (Fig. 11.20).

6. Operator's hands apply compression, cephalic to caudad shear, transverse shear, and clockwise and counterclockwise twisting loads, seeking direct and indirect barriers.

7. Patient performs enhancing maneuvers to assist in the enhancement of release(s).

These are but a few examples of myofascial release technique. They can be used as the primary manual medicine intervention or as a terminal technique to assess the success of other manual medicine interventions to ensure that myofascial balance has been achieved. Some practitioners find these techniques fatiguing and time-consuming, whereas others find them easy and efficient.

Figure 11.17.

Figure 11.19.

Figure 11.18.

Figure 11.20.

CONCLUSION

Myofascial release and integrated neuromuscular release techniques use direct and indirect actions with activating forces that are extrinsic and intrinsic. They influence the biomechanics of the musculoskeletal system and the reflexes that direct, integrate, and modify movement. The goal is restoring functional balance to all of the integrative tissues in the musculoskeletal system, and the techniques are useful in acute, subacute, and chronic conditions, with simple and complex problems. The techniques can be used in multiple patient positions. They usually consist of symmetric placement of the operator's hands, introducing some twisting force to engage the tissues, and following directly or indirectly along fascial planes to sense areas of tightness and looseness. Traction is placed on the tight area awaiting the sensation of release. Release is hypothesized as following reflex neural efferent inhibition and biomechanical hysteresis within the tissues. The techniques are highly individualized to the patient's needs and the operator's training and experience.

SUGGESTED READINGS

Ward RC. Integrated neuromusculoskeletal release and myofascial release: an introduction to diagnosis and treatment. In: Ward RC, et al., eds. *Foundations for osteopathic medicine.* Baltimore, MD: Williams & Wilkins, 1997.

Ward RC. Tutorial on level I myofascial release technique. Course syllabus. Michigan State University College of Osteopathic Medicine, 1986.

Section **//**

TECHNIQUE PROCEDURES

12

CRANIOSACRAL TECHNIQUE

William G. Sutherland, D.O., is credited with extending the osteopathic concept, and osteopathic manipulative treatment, above the craniocervical junction. His curiosity was raised when viewing the temporoparietal suture in the anatomy laboratory and thought it resembled the gills of a fish. He further reasoned that it might relate to respiration in some fashion. Thus began many years of study, research, and self-manipulation. Sutherland began to teach the principles of craniosacral technique in the mid 1940s. Craniosacral technique procedures were initially not readily received in the professional community but have become increasingly popular through the work of Sutherland and his many students.

Sutherland extended the principles of Andrew Taylor Still to the articulations of the skull. He reasoned that the sutures functioned as joints between the bones of the skull and were intricately fashioned for the maintenance of motion. The sutures are present throughout life and consistently have similar areas of bevel change. Skulls can be disarticulated by "explosion" (filling with beans through the foramen magnum, then immersing in water) and the bones consistently separate at the sutures. The bone does not fracture, the sutures separate. Sutherland reasoned that the skull would have normal mobility during health and show restrictions in response to trauma or systemic disease. Clinical observations were consistent with his hypothesis. Since Sutherland's time, there has been an increasing body of clinical evidence and research supporting some of the basic premises of his concept. Craniosacral technique requires the practitioner to make an intense study of the osseous cranium, sutures, and meninges and to finely tune the palpatory sense necessary to perceive inherent mobility within the craniosacral mechanism. Application of manual medicine procedures to the cranium and sacrum requires precision and dexterity.

ANATOMY

The skull can be divided into three elements: (a) the vault, consisting of portions of the frontal bone, the two parietal bones, the occipital squama, and the temporal squama that develop from membrane; (b) the base, consisting of the body of the sphenoid, the petrous and mastoid portions of the temporals, the basilar and condylar portions of the occiput that form in cartilage; and (c) the facial bones. The bones of the skull can be further divided into those that are paired and unpaired. The unpaired midline bones are the occiput, sphenoid, ethmoid, and vomer. The paired bones include the parietals, temporals, maxillae, zygoma, palatines, nasals, and frontal. The frontal is viewed as a paired bone because of the functional characteristics it provides, and the fact that the metopic suture frequently remains open during life. The mandible has both paired and unpaired characteristics. It is bilaterally related to the temporal bones, but when the teeth are present and approximated, they serve as a long suture between the mandible and the two maxillae.

MOTION

The sphenobasilar junction appears to fuse after the late teens but the motions perceived from contact on the skull exterior can be best described as having taken place at the sphenobasilar junction. There appears to be residual pliability of bone at the sphenobasilar junction throughout life similar to the pliability of bone in the remaining bones of the skeleton. The motion of the midline bones is primarily flexion and extension with an overturning moment around a transverse (x) axis. Flexion–extension movement is described as occurring when the sphenoid and occiput rotate in opposite directions. During sphenobasilar flexion, the sphenoid rotates anteriorly with the basisphenoid being elevated and the pterygoid processes moving inferiorly. Concurrently, the occiput rotates posteriorly with the basiocciput being elevated, and the squamous portion and condylar parts being depressed caudally. During sphenobasilar flexion, the ethmoid rotates in the opposite direction to the sphenoid and in the same direction as the occiput. During sphenobasilar flexion, the vomer is carried caudad as the anterior portion of the sphenoid moves in that direction. During sphenobasilar extension, all of the motions are reversed. The paired bones move into internal and external rotations as they accompany sphenobasilar flexion and extension. During sphenobasilar flexion, there is external rotation of the paired bones. During sphenobasilar extension, the paired bones move into internal rotation.

The combination of flexion–extension of the midline unpaired bones and the internal–external rotation of the paired bones causes observable change in cranial contour. With flexion, the transverse diameter of the skull increases, the anteroposterior (AP) diameter decreases, and the vertex flattens. With sphenobasilar extension, the transverse diameter decreases, the AP diameter increases, and the vertex becomes more prominent. The facial bones can be viewed as being suspended from the frontal bone. The paired bones consist of the parietal, temporal, frontal, zygoma, maxilla, palatine, and nasal bones. Their motion is described as internal and external rotation and is normally synchronous with sphenobasilar flexion and extension. During sphenobasilar flexion, there is external rotation of the paired bones. The sphenoid determines the motion characteristics of the paired facial bones. Dysfunction of the front half of the cranium, particularly of the facial bones, is related to altered function of the sphenoid. Dysfunction of the posterior half of the cranium relates to dysfunction of the occipital bone.

MENINGES

The dura is attached at the foramen magnum, continues down the spinal canal with attachment to the upper two or three cervical vertebrae, and continues freely within the spinal canal until attachment at the second segment of the sacrum. This membrane attachment appears to link the sacral component with the occiput in the craniosacral mechanism. As one of many movements, the sacrum has an involuntary nutation–counternutation movement that is synchronous with flexion–extension at the sphenobasilar junction. During sphenobasilar flexion the foramen magnum is elevated and the tension on the dura causes the base of the sacrum to move posteriorly and the apex anteriorly. This counternutational movement is described as craniosacral flexion. During sphenobasilar extension, the foramen magnum moves inferiorly, reducing tension on the dura, resulting in the sacral base moving anteriorly and the apex posteriorly. This nutational movement is called "craniosacral extension." The terms "flexion" and "extension" are the reverse of that used in a postural–structural model for sacral mechanics. Despite the terminology confusion, the concept to be understood is the relationship of the movement of the occiput and the sacrum that normally occurs in synchronous directions.

The dura also is continuous with the spinal nerve roots as they emerge from the spinal canal and forms the perineurium. Traction on peripheral nerves can influence the central dura as well.

SUTURES

The sutures are joints that join the bones of the skull. At birth there are no sutures and the vault bones are separate plates on the dura. The skull is like a bag filled with fluid and under tension. As the skull bones grow and mature, they develop the sutures as articulations. The sutures develop their shape and contour depending on the motion occurring at the area during growth. It is fascinating to see the marked similarity of sutures and their beveling across a number of different specimens. There are many different types of sutures that are designed to permit and direct specific types of movement between opposing cranial bones. The sutures contain extensions of the dura and other connective tissue, primarily Sharpey fibers. Anatomic and histologic study of the sutures demonstrate that fiber direction is not haphazard and random, but specific at each sutural level. The sutures contain blood vessels with accompanying nerves for vasomotor control. Free nerve endings with unmyelinated C-fibers are found within the sutures suggesting the possibility of pain perception and transmission. A detailed description of the cranial sutures is beyond the scope of this text. The reader is strongly urged to study the classical anatomic work as well as the sutures found on each bone of a disarticulated skull.

SUTURE PALPATION EXERCISE

The following palpation exercise identifies palpable sutures in a living subject and the location of anatomic parts used in diagnosis and treatment of cranial dysfunctions (Fig. 12.1).

1. Palpate the depression at the base of the nose and between each orbit. This is the junction of the two nasal bones and the frontal bone and is called "nasion."
2. Proceed laterally over the upper margin of the orbit and follow it laterally and inferiorly to the upper outer portion and feel the frontozygomatic suture.
3. Continuing inferiorly along the lateral aspect of the orbit and beginning to move medially one feels the zygomaticomaxillary suture.
4. Continuing medially along the inferior aspect of the orbit and up its medial way, palpate the suture of the maxillonasal junction and the maxillofrontal suture.
5. Returning to the nasion, move upward between the two supraorbital ridges of the frontal bone, the midline of which is a point called "glabella." Moving superiorly from glabella along the midline the palpator may feel the remnant of the metopic suture as a depression or a ridge.

Temporal lines

Temporal fossa

Zygomatic arch

Posterior border of
ramus of mandible

Angle of mandible

Inferior border of mandible

Mental tubercle

Remains of
metopic suture

Glabella

Nasion

Internasal suture

Perpendicular plate
of ethmoid

Vomer

Anterior nasal spine

Intermaxillary suture

Symphysis menti (line of
union of mandibular
halves)

Mental protuberance

Figure 12.1.
Skull, frontal view.

6. Continuing toward the vertex of the skull in the midline, one strikes a depression approximately one third of the way posteriorly on the vertex. This depression is the junction of the sagittal and coronal sutures and is the remnant of the anterior fontanel and is called "bregma."

7. Moving posteriorly from bregma along the midline, the sagittal suture is palpable and by moving the finger pads from side to side one can feel the serrated sutural contour (Fig. 12.2).

8. Starting from bregma, palpate bilaterally along the coronal suture feeling the junction

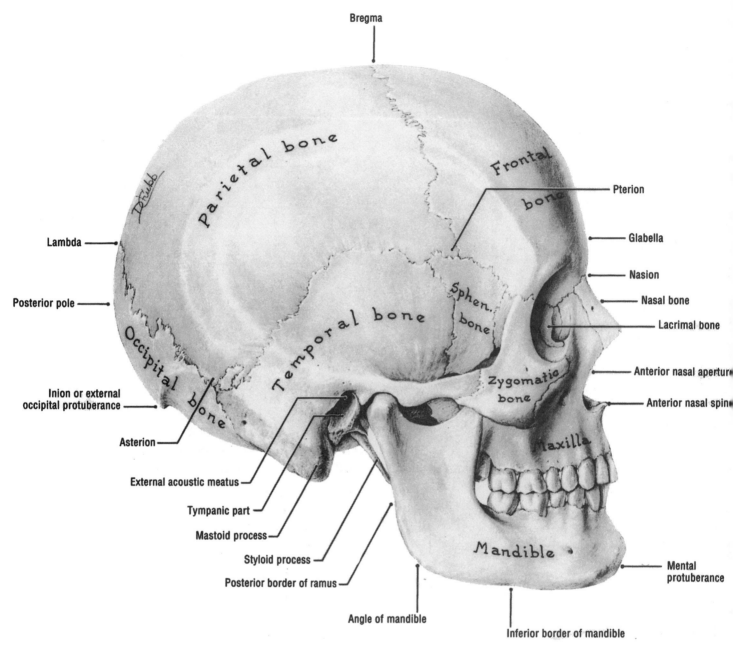

Figure 12.2.
Skull, lateral view.

of the frontal and the parietal bone on each side. At the lower extremity of the coronal suture, the palpating finger moves somewhat deeper and palpates the junction of the sphenoid, frontal, parietal, and temporal bones. This junctional area is called "pterion." The inferior aspect of this junction is the palpable tip of the great wing of the sphenoid, which is used extensively for craniosacral diagnosis and treatment.

9. From the pterion, follow the suture line posteriorly along the junction of the parietal and temporal squama. This suture courses over the top of the ear in a circular fashion and ends just posterior to the ear.

10. Moving straight posteriorly from the posterior inferior aspect of the suture between the parietal and the temporal squama is a short suture between the parietal bone and the mastoid portion of the temporal. At the posterior aspect of this suture is a slight depression at the junction of the parietal bone, mastoid portion of the temporal, and the occiput called the "asterion."

11. From the asterion, move inferiorly along the posterior aspect of the mastoid process following the occipital mastoid suture. The lower portion of this suture is lost in the soft tissues of the muscular attachment of the head to the neck (Fig. 12.3).
12. From the asterion on each side, course medially and superiorly along the lambdoidal suture separating the parietal bone from the occipital squama. The point at which the two sutures join with the sagittal suture is called "lambda." The lambdoidal sutures are frequently asymmetric and occasionally contain extra bony structures called "wormian bones."

This exercise should be repeated on multiple patients until the examiner is confident of his or her ability to palpate the sutures of the skull and identify landmarks used to control the bones of the skull during the examination and the treatment process. The pterion and asterion are the two most frequently used in the craniosacral technique system.

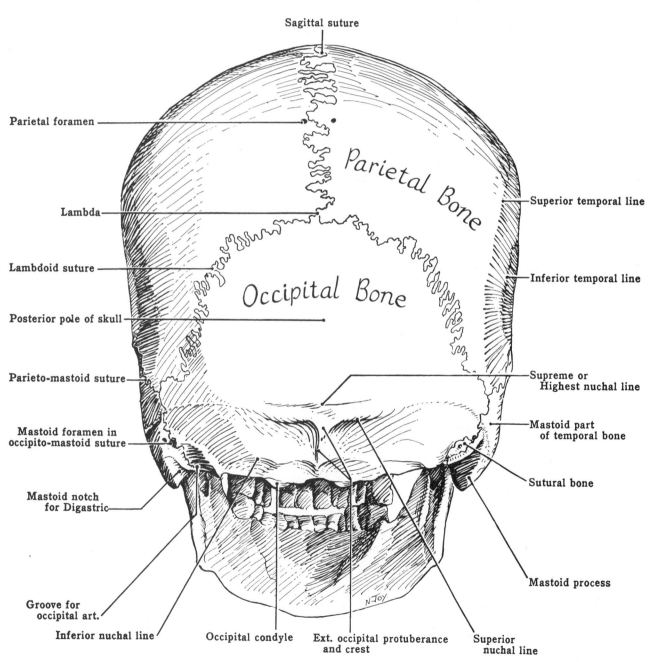

Figure 12.3.
Skull, posterior view.

CRANIAL MENINGES

The meninges are divided into three layers: the pia, arachnoid, and dura. The external layer of the dura is continuous with the periosteum and the cranium. The internal layer has several duplications that separate segments of the brain and encircle the venous sinuses (Fig. 12.4).

There are three duplications of the dura with intricate fiber directions in each and are named the falx cerebri, tentorium cerebelli, and falx cerebelli. The falx cerebri is attached anteriorly to the crista galli of the ethmoid, the frontal bone, both parietal bones, and the occipital squama. It encloses the superior sagittal sinus at its osseous attachment. At its free border is found the inferior sagittal sinus. The falx cerebri separates the two cerebral hemispheres. The tentorium cerebelli separates the cerebrum and cerebellum and attaches to the sphenoid, occiput, both parietals, and temporal bones. It attaches to the petrous ridges of the temporal bones and along the occipital squama where it encloses the transverse sinus. It is attached to the posterior inferior corner of each parietal bone where the transverse sinus starts into sigmoid sinus. At the junction of the falx cerebri and the tentorium cerebelli is found the straight sinus. This junction is of significance as the location of

the reciprocal tension membrane called the "Sutherland fulcrum." The falx cerebelli separates the two hemispheres of the cerebellum. The diaphragm sellae covers the sella turcica of the sphenoid and is penetrated by the stalk of the pituitary. These dural membranes are under constant dynamic tension so that increased tension in one requires relaxation in another and vice versa. During sphenobasilar flexion there is shortening of the falx cerebri from before backward because of the overturning of the sphenoid and occiput in opposite directions. This is accompanied by flattening of the tentorium cerebelli resulting from external rotation of the two temporal bones. During sphenobasilar extension, the reverse occurs with the lengthening of the AP diameter of the skull by rotation of the sphenoid and the occiput and elevation of the tentorium cerebelli because of internal rotation of the temporal bones. Craniosacral motion combines articular mobility and change in tension within the membranes. The membranous attachment at the foramen magnum of the occiput and at S2 of the sacrum determines the synchronous movement of the cranium and the sacrum. This dural attachment allows the examiner to influence the cranium through the sacrum and the sacrum through the cranium.

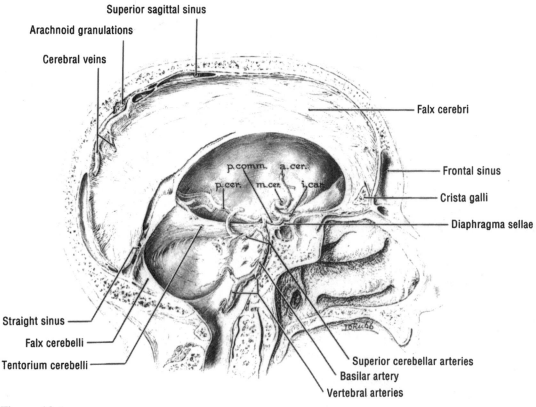

Figure 12.4.
Cranial meninges.

RESPIRATION AND THE THREE DIAPHRAGMS

Sphenobasilar flexion and extension are related to and influenced by voluntary respiratory activity. Inhalation enhances sphenobasilar flexion, and exhalation enhances sphenobasilar extension. The tentorium cerebelli can be viewed as the diaphragm of the craniosacral mechanism. It descends and flattens during inhalation similar to the thoracoabdominal diaphragm. The pelvic diaphragm is intimately related to the sacrum within the osseous pelvis. The pelvic diaphragm also descends during inhalation. One can then view the body from the perspective of the three diaphragms: the tentorium cerebelli, the thoracoabdominal diaphragm, and the pelvic diaphragm. In health these diaphragms should function in a synchronous fashion. If dysfunction interferes with the capacity of any of the three, it is reasonable to assume that the other two will be altered as well. This observation has been made in clinical practice. The thoracic inlet can also be viewed as a diaphragm as it participates in respiration and could be described as a fourth diaphragm.

PRIMARY RESPIRATORY MECHANISM

By placing both hands over the superior and lateral aspects of the skull like a wet towel and waiting for a sufficient period of time, the examiner experiences the palpatory sensation of widening and narrowing of the skull. This motion sensation occurs at a normal rate of 8 to 14 times per minute and is of relatively low amplitude. This sensation, called the "cranial rhythmic impulse" (CRI), is interpreted as the result of the five components of the primary respiratory mechanism. Sutherland postulated the existence of the primary respiratory mechanism as consisting of the following:

1. Inherent mobility of the brain and spinal cord. The living tissue of the brain appears to have an inherent mobility observable during a craniotomy procedure. The motion has been described as that of coiling and uncoiling of the cerebral hemispheres. During the uncoiling process, the cerebral hemispheres appear to swing upward and the unpaired bones move into flexion while the paired bones move into external rotation. During the coiling process, the cerebral hemispheres descend and the unpaired midline bones move into extension motion while the paired bones move into internal rotation. The cause of this inherent bone motility is unknown but is one of the biologic rhythms that cannot be artificially restored if lost.

2. Fluctuation of the cerebrospinal fluid (CSF). The CSF is formed in the vesicles in the lateral ventricles and flows through the third and fourth ventricles, into the cisterns of the skull, and throughout the spinal canal. Obstruction to the flow of CSF leads to pathologic conditions such as hydrocephalus. The site of exit of the CSF from the system is not well known, but CSF follows dural attachments to the spinal nerves and to the spinal nerves themselves. The coiling of the brain seems to increase the volume of the cerebral ventricles whereas uncoiling seems to compress them. This may explain some of the mechanism for the circulation of CSF. This fluctuation is easily observed when measuring intraspinal pressure through a manometer attached to an intraspinal needle. The level does not remain constant but fluctuates.

3. Motility of intracranial and intraspinal meninges. The falx cerebri, falx cerebelli, and tentorium cerebelli are all duplications of the intracranial dura. The membranes within the cranium have an intimate and intricate pattern suggestive of stress bands that seem to vary from specimen to specimen suggesting individual response to tension variations. The intracranial membranes are continuously under dynamic tension so that a change in one requires adaptive change in another. During sphenobasilar flexion, the tent descends and flattens and the falx cerebri shortens from before backward. In sphenobasilar extension the reverse occurs. The intracranial membranes connect with the intraspinal membranes through continuity from the firm attachment at the foramen magnum down the spinal canal to the upper two or three cervical vertebrae, and then to the attachment to the second sacral segment. Movement of the foramen magnum alters tension on the anterior and posterior aspects of the spinal dura resulting in motion of the sacrum between the two hip bones.

4. Articular mobility of cranial bones. There are no sutures present at birth. The sutures appear to develop to permit and guide certain types of movement between cranial bones. The cranial bones and sutures are intimately attached to the dura and contain vascular and nervous system elements. Sharpey fibers within the sutures have a consistent direction between anatomic specimens. These fibers appear to permit and yield to motion in certain directions. Sutural obliteration does not appear to occur normally during the aging process. Patent sutures in humans have been identified into

the ninth decade. The amount of motion across any individual suture is quite small, but when aggregated throughout the multiple bones of the skull with multiple sutures, there appears to be sufficient motion to be palpable clinically.

5. The involuntary mobility of the sacrum between the ilia. The sacrum is suspended between the two ilia by the ligaments of the sacroiliac joints. The posterior sacroiliac ligaments are thick and strong with multiple fiber directions. They can be viewed as analogous to the ropes of a child's swing. The anterior sacroiliac ligaments are inferior as well as anterior and appear to support the sacrum from below like the seat of a child's swing. The sacrum can be cupped in an examiner's hand in either the prone or supine position. With light palpatory compression, the examiner normally feels a to-and-fro oscillating movement of the base and apex of the sacrum synchronous with the flexion and extension motion palpated in the cranium.

The primary respiratory mechanism and its related CRI responds to trauma, disease processes, psychologic stress, exercise, respiration, and can be influenced by the skilled application of craniosacral manual medicine procedures. The normal rate of the CRI is 8 to 14 per minute, quite close to the patient's respiratory rate. A patient can voluntarily control diaphragmatic respiration but cannot directly influence the primary respiratory mechanism. Voluntary inhalation and exhalation can influence the CRI and the inherent mobility of the osseous and membranous cranium.

CRANIOSACRAL DIAGNOSIS

The diagnostic process begins with observation and palpation in a screening examination. The examiner looks for skull symmetry from the anterior, posterior, superior, and both lateral views. Observation is made for symmetry of the frontal bosses, orbits, nose, zygoma, maxillae, mandible, level of the ears, and overall cranial contour. The screening examination proceeds by palpation of skull contour in all dimensions and, in particular, palpation of the sutures as previously described. Palpation of the sutures looks for widening, narrowing, tension and other tissue texture changes, and tenderness. The skull is assessed by palpation for resiliency to see if it is harder and less resilient than normal. Normal bone has a pliability that is lost in the presence of motion restriction. Palpation over the parietotemporal region by the "wet towel" application of the two hands, ascertains the rate, rhythm, and amplitude of the CRI.

Another screening examination helpful for determining if there is asymmetric loss of cranial motion is the temporal lift (Fig. 12.5).

A five-finger hold for the temporal lift has the examiner grasp each temporal bone with the middle finger in the external auditory meatus, the thumb and index fingers on the superior and inferior aspects of the zygomatic process, and the ring and little finger in front and behind the mastoid process. With the patient supine on the table, the examiner pulls both temporal bones in a direction toward the vertex. Each temporal bone is then allowed to settle back to its neutral position. The examiner assesses the symmetry or asymmetry of the small amount of joint play motion available in each temporal bone. The horizontal portions of the sphenosquamous suture, the horizontal portion of the occipital mastoid suture, and the zygomaticotemporal sutures are beveled such that the temporal bone sits on top of the sphenoid, zygoma and occiput. The temporal lift procedure assesses the presence or absence of mobility of the temporal bones on each side.

The sacrum is screened for its anterior and posterior nutational movements between the two ilia in either prone or supine position. The examiner cradles the sacrum in the palm of the hand and assesses the sacral movement and its relation to the CRI palpated at the skull. A finding of exaggerated, depressed, or irregular movements instead of the normal anterior and posterior nodding movements requires additional diagnostic assessment. If the screening examination provides evidence of craniosacral dysfunction, additional scanning and segmental definition examinations are necessary.

Figure 12.5.
Temporal bone, lateral view.

ASSESSMENT OF SPHENOBASILAR MOTION

Evaluation of sphenobasilar mechanics (Fig. 12.6) is accomplished by placing the hands and fingers over the skull in a position that is called the "vault hold."

There are several variations of the vault hold, but each includes control of the great wings of the sphenoid at the pterion and the occiput at the asterion. The classic vault hold has the index finger on the sphenoid at the pterion and the little finger at the asterion, with the ear between the middle and ring fingers (Fig. 12.7). This four-point contact provides the examiner the opportunity to evaluate sphenobasilar mechanics. A second vault hold uses the thumbs on the sphenoid at the pterion with the little finger on the occiput at the asterion, with the ear between the index and middle fingers (Fig. 12.8). A third vault hold finds the examiner cradling the occiput in the palm of one hand holding posterior to the occipitomastoid suture and the other hand spanning the front of the skull with the thumb on one great wing of the sphenoid and the long finger on the opposite great wing (Fig. 12.9). Each of these vault holds has their uses. The beginning student should use the first vault hold described.

Sphenobasilar flexion and extension are described as occurring around two parallel transverse axes with each moving in the opposite direction. With sphenobasilar flexion, the index and little fingers separate as they move in a caudad direction. With sphenobasilar extension, the fingers on each side move closer together as the hands move cephalically.

Sphenobasilar side bending–rotation is described as motion of the sphenoid and occiput along two different axis systems. They both rotate in the same direction around an AP axis and in opposite directions around two parallel vertical axes. With sphenobasilar side bending–rotation to the right, the fingers of the right hand separate and move in a caudad direction while the fingertips on the left side narrow and move cephalically, resulting in the right side of the skull appearing to become more convex. Sphenobasilar left-side bending–rotation results in similar findings on the opposite side.

Sphenobasilar torsion movement is described as movement of the sphenoid and occiput in opposite directions along an AP axis. The motion is introduced through the four-point vault hold contact, by alternately

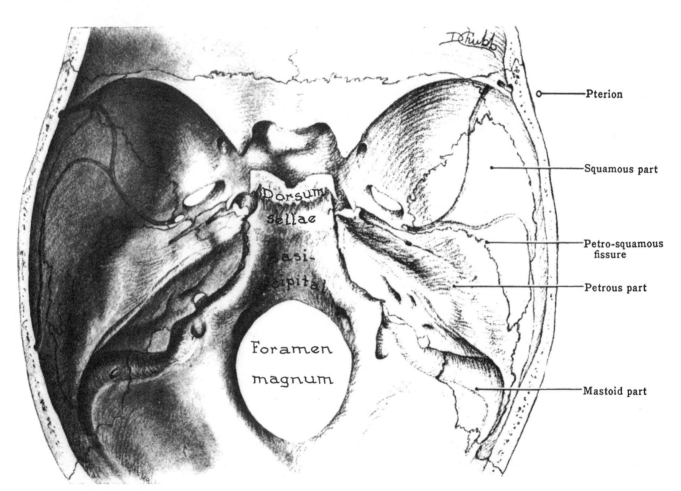

Figure 12.6.
Sphenobasilar junction from above.

Figure 12.7.
Vault hold, index and little finger.

Figure 12.8.
Vault hold, thumb and little finger.

Figure 12.9.
Two-handed vault hold.

turning one hand forward while the other turns backward. The hand moving anteriorly carries the sphenoid caudad and elevates the occiput on that side. The hand that rotates posteriorly carries the sphenoid high and the occiput low on the same side. This torsional movement should be bilaterally symmetric, but if restricted, the dysfunction is named for the side in which the sphenoid is held in a cephalic (high) position.

Sphenobasilar flexion–extension, side bending–rotation, and torsion are all present physiologically. Other altered movements of the sphenobasilar junction usually result from trauma include lateral strain, vertical strain, and sphenobasilar compression. Traumatic episodes can include birth trauma, childhood falls, sports injuries, motor vehicle collisions, industrial accidents, altered muscle balance from chronic postural deficit, abnormal chewing from poor dental hygiene, and many others.

Sphenobasilar compression can be anterior–posterior resulting from injury to the skull from before backward and behind forward. If present, the compression restricts the midline sphenobasilar movement patterns. The skull usually compensates for this restriction by increased internal and external rotation of the paired lateral bones. Lateral compression can occur with trauma from right to left or left to right resulting on impaction of the temporal bone on that side.

Sphenobasilar lateral strain results from trauma from left to right or right to left in front of, or behind, the sphenobasilar junction altering the relation of the sphenoid and occiput in the horizontal plane. Lateral strain is described as movement of the sphenoid and occiput in the same direction around two parallel vertical axes. To test for a lateral strain with the patient supine using the vault hold, one hand lifts one side of the head toward the ceiling, allows it to return, and reverses it on the opposite side. This introduces side-to-side translatory movement. If this motion test is asymmetric, it is described as a lateral strain to the side in which the basisphenoid moves freely. A skull with a lateral strain pattern has a quadrilateral appearance.

Vertical strain results with trauma from above or below, in front or behind, the sphenobasilar junction altering the relation of the sphenoid and occiput in the sagittal plane. Vertical strain is described as rotation of the sphenoid and occiput in the same direction around two parallel transverse axes. If asymmetric, a vertical strain is named for the position of the basisphenoid and are superior or inferior. To test for vertical strain, both hands of the vault hold rotate forward and backward symmetrically. As both hands rotate forward, they carry the sphenoid into flexion with elevation of the basisphenoid and the occiput into extension. As both hands rotate backward, they carry the sphenoid into extension with depression of the basisphenoid and flexion of the occiput. Both of these strain mechanisms alter the central axis through the sphenobasilar junction. Traumatic lateral and vertical strains and compressions significantly alter the craniosacral mechanism. Sphenobasilar compression is identified by reduction in the rate and amplitude of the CRI and the overall reduction of cranial mobility.

Interference with symmetric sphenobasilar function leads the operator to assess articular causes of the restriction. After assessment of abnormal sphenobasilar mechanics, the operator needs to decide whether the restriction is in the anterior or posterior aspects of the skull and whether it is more on the right or left. This leads to "four-quadrant" diagnosis. The decision is based on the operator's judgment of the location of the major restrictor while assessing the sphenobasilar strain patterns. The operator also makes an assessment of the nature of the restriction. Is it articular? Is it membranous from the meninges? Is it reduced fluid fluctuation? The answers to these questions determine the therapeutic strategy. Comprehensive specific sutural motion testing is beyond the scope of this volume and the reader is referred to standard texts in the field. However, the major, more common articular restrictor of the anterior and posterior quadrants will be subsequently described.

PRINCIPLES OF CRANIOSACRAL TECHNIQUE

The goals of craniosacral technique are to improve motion in sphenobasilar mechanics, remove articular restrictions, reduce membranous tension restrictions, improve circulation (particularly of the venous system), reduce potential neural entrapment from exit foramen at the base of the skull, and increase the vitality of the CRI. These techniques have local effects within the head and neck region, distal effects throughout the body, and all are directed toward enhancing the level of wellness of the patient. All of these goals can be accomplished by the restoration of balanced membranous tension. Normal dynamic reciprocal tension of the falx cerebri and tentorium cerebelli is absent in the presence of restriction or alteration in relationship of cranial bones and their sutures. Alteration in membranous tension affects the venous sinuses within the skull resulting in the reduction of venous drainage and overall intracranial congestion. The dura is intimately attached to the periosteum on the internal surface of the skull and at each exit foramen. Abnormal dural tension might contribute to neural entrapment and result in altered neural function. Restoring maximum mobility to the osseous cranium restores balanced membranous tension, enhances venous flow, reduces neural entrapment and permits normal CRI rate, rhythm, and amplitude.

Treatment of the craniosacral system can begin at either the sacrum or the cranium or can be done concurrently. A sequence for treatment that has proven to be clinically effective begins by screening the cranium and identifying if the skull is rigid or nonrigid. If rigid, the approach is to decongest the head by venous sinus release and enhance the cranial rhymthic impulse (CRI) by compression of the 4th ventricle (CV4) procedures. Following the reduction of rigidity within the skull, the sphenobasilar mechanics are assessed and appropriately treated. If sphenobasilar compression is identified, it should be addressed so that the remaining sphenobasilar motions can be more efficient. Treatment of sphenobasilar strain patterns may include approaches both from the cranial and sacral ends of the system. Temporal bone rotational capability is then assessed, and, if asymmetric, appropriate sutural evaluation and treatment are performed to restore symmetry of internal and external temporal rotations. The facial component is then assessed and treated as appropriate. Successful craniosacral treatment restores functional balance to the cranial and sacral limbs of the mechanism, enhances mobility of the cranial bones, balances membranous tension, and enhances the vitality of the CRI.

METHODS OF CRANIOSACRAL TECHNIQUE

Craniosacral technique shares with other forms of manual medicine the approach to barriers. In addition to the usual methods of direct action, indirect, and exaggeration technique, there are two others, namely disengagement and molding. In the direct action method, the barrier is engaged and an activating force is applied in the direction of motion loss. The exaggeration method moves in the opposite direction to motion loss against the physiologic barrier and applies an activating force. The indirect method finds the neutral point between the area of

normal motion in one direction and restricted motion in the opposite and holds that position while activating forces are applied. This is described as "balanced membranous tension." The disengagement method applies an activating force to separate sutures particularly at pivot areas. Molding technique modifies resiliency and contour of bone by the application of external force while waiting for intrinsic activating forces to alter the contour and resiliency of bone. The most commonly applied procedures in craniosacral technique are indirect balanced procedures and exaggeration. Direct action technique is used more commonly in infants and children prior to the full development of the sutural components to the cranial bones. Direct action technique in adults can be helpful but requires very precise indication and localization.

ACTIVATING FORCES

The primary activating force in craniosacral technique is the inherent primary respiratory mechanism. Fluctuation of CSF is a potent intrinsic activating force that is easily directed from the exterior of the skull. The normal fluid fluctuation is in an anterior-to-posterior midline direction, but can be altered for intrinsic activating force purposes by being directed with finger contact exactly opposite the area of skull restriction. This principle is frequently used in V-spread technique. As an example, in the presence of restriction of the left occipitomastoid suture, the operator's left index and middle fingers are placed on each side of the occipitomastoid suture. The index finger of the right hand is placed over the right frontal bone directly opposite the left occipitomastoid suture (Fig. 12.10). Following sep-

Figure 12.10.
V spread.

aration of the two fingers of the left hand, an attempt is made to direct the fluid from the right frontal to the left occipitomastoid regions. Minimal compression on the right frontal area results in a sensation of surflike pounding against the restricted joint until release occurs. The same fluid-fluctuation activating force is used in some of the molding method techniques.

Respiratory assistance is a second activating force. Voluntary inhalation enhances flexion and external rotation movements of the craniosacral mechanism and voluntary exhalation enhances extension and internal rotation movements. The use of forced inhalation or exhalation, and holding respiration at the extreme of movement, can be used as an activating force to enhance motion in any direction.

A third activating force is enhancement of dural tension by application of effort at the sacrum and from the feet. Enhancement of flexion and extension movement can be made directly from the sacrum by the operator's hand in either direction as desired. Dorsiflexion and plantar flexion of the foot, either voluntarily by the patient or passively by an operator, enhances the intrinsic activating force. Dorsiflexion appears to enhance flexion at the sphenobasilar junction, whereas plantar flexion enhances extension. Dorsiflexing or plantar flexing the right foot when working on the left side of the skull and using the left foot when working on the right side, use the principle of the longest diagonal.

The fourth activating force is the procedure called "CV4." This procedure is performed by the operator cradling the skull in the hands with the thenar eminence of against the occiput just medial to the occipitomastoid suture (Fig. 12.11). During normal craniosacral flexion, this portion of the occipital bone appears to become fuller and wider, and during exhalation less full and more narrow. After tuning into the CRI, the operator resists the occiput during the flexion phase until a "still point" is reached. The sensation experienced is that no motion is felt. The operator holds the occiput in this position for several cycles, awaiting the return of fluid fluctuation that is perceived by the inherent force pushing the hands away. The operator then allows restoration of the normal flexion and extension movement through the occipital bone. The outcome seems to be the enhancement of fluid movement, change in the rhythm of the diaphragms, and increased temperature in the suboccipital region. A still point can be achieved by a similar process of compression in places other than the occiput that results in a temporary period of reduced motion in the CRI.

CRANIOSACRAL TECHNIQUES

The preceding are all methods of enhancing activating forces in craniosacral technique. The main activating force continues to be the inherent mobility of

Figure 12.11.
CV4

the brain, meninges, and CSF. This can be termed "inherent force technique" and is intrinsic in nature. Enhanced fluctuation of the CSF by respiratory assistance, sacral or extremity force applications, or by the CV4 maneuver all ultimately depends on the intrinsic inherent force reestablishing normal mobility. The other main activating force is operator guiding where the operator applies external force to the skull by directing action to a suture, membranous tension, or the sphenobasilar junction. Another ancillary activating force can be through dural mobilization of the upper or lower extremities.

The operator needs to make a decision about the major restrictor in order to choose the appropriate technique. Is the restrictor articular? If so, a direct action articular technique is indicated. Is the restrictor membranous? If so, a membranous technique, such as, a frontal or parietal lift, temporal rocking, sacral technique, or the use of extremity dural mobilization technique is in order. Is the restrictor lack of fluid fluctuation? If so, V spread, CV4, or venous release technique is indicated. In most instances, a combination of techniques is required to reach the therapeutic goal.

Venous Sinus Technique

The goal of venous sinus technique is to enhance the flow of venous blood through the venous sinuses to exit from the skull through the jugular foramen. It is particularly useful when the initial palpatory screening examination reveals a hard, rigid skull with loss of resiliency. Venous congestion is believed to contribute to this hard, rigid sensation, and the operator attempts to enhance venous return to the central venous circulation.

The operator performs this procedure by sitting at the head of a supine patient and placing fingertip contact with the middle fingers over the external occipital protuberance of the occipital bone. The weight of the head is carried on these finger pads and the operator awaits a softening sensation of bone and beginning of a sensation of freer mobility. The fingers are moved sequentially along the midline of the occiput in the direction of the foramen magnum, awaiting the same softening sensation. The examiner returns to the external occipital protuberance and applies firm pressure with the pads of all four fingers along the superior nuchal line with increasing pressure from medial to lateral until softening is felt. This reduces congestion within the transverse sinus. Returning to the external occipital protuberance, the examiner places a thumb on each side of the occiput addressing the superior sagittal sinus while applying a pressure with the palmar surface of the thumb in a separation manner. The operator continues from posterior to anterior along the superior sagittal sinus working one thumb breadth at each application until reaching the bregma. From the bregma forward, the operator places the pads of four fingers on each side of the midline of the frontal bone and applies compression and lateral distraction waiting for the sensation of softening and release. Venous sinus technique is frequently used before approaching specific articular restrictions.

Condylar Decompression

The patient lies supine with the operator sitting at the head of the table cradling the skull in the palms of the hands. The middle finger pads are placed along the inferior aspect of the occiput beginning at the inion and sliding forward as far as possible. By flexing the distal interphalangeal joints of the middle fingers, the operator applies cephalic and posterior traction on the occiput. The operator's elbows are brought together, resulting in supination of both hands and separation of the middle fingers. The resultant force vector is cephalic and posterolateral on each side of the

occiput posterior to the foramen magnum. This pressure is continued until release of tension is felt, particularly the sensation of equal softening on each side of the occipital bone (see description in Chapter 13).

CV4: Bulb Compression

This technique has been previously described under activating forces. It is used independently or in combination with other approaches to restore function to the craniosacral mechanism. CV4 technique is particularly valuable in the enhancement of the amplitude of the CRI.

Sphenobasilar Symphysis

Dysfunctions at the sphenobasilar symphysis, both physiologic and traumatic, are addressed by one of the vault holds. The operator controls the greater wings of the sphenoid at the pterion and the occiput at the asterion and determines the sphenobasilar strain patterns present. Addressing the sphenobasilar strain pattern that appears to be the most restricted is frequently a valuable first approach. The operator addresses the dysfunction in either a direct, exaggeration, or indirect method. The most commonly used is the indirect method of balanced membranous tension. The operator finds the point of maximum ease within the range of the strain pattern and holds the mechanism at a balanced point until some release is achieved. Respiratory assistance and membranous enhancement from the sacrum and lower extremities are frequently concurrently used. Finding the balanced point of each of the strain patterns in a stacked fashion and applying a distraction force by separating the finger contact on the sphenoid and occiput in an AP direction accomplish decompression of the sphenobasilar symphysis.

Temporal Rocking

With the patient supine on the table and the operator sitting at the head, the skull is supported in the palms of the hand with each thumb behind the ear in front of the mastoid process with the interphalangeal joint at the apex and the metacarpophalangeal at the mastoid portion. This thumb placement allows control of the temporal bones on each side. Pressure by the distal phalanx of the thumb in a posteromedial direction on the inferior aspect of the mastoid process introduces external rotation. Compression in a posteromedial direction with the base of the thumb on the mastoid portion of the temporal bone enhances internal rotation. Movement of the thumbs can rock the temporal bones into internal and external rotations, either synchronously (both temporals into internal rotation or external rotation), or asynchronously (one temporal moving into internal rotation and the other external rotation). Asynchronous rocking of the temporals through several cycles appears to change the fluid fluctuation from an AP to-and-fro movement to a side-to-side, to-and-fro movement. Once asynchronous rocking is symmetric on each side, synchronous rocking is reintroduced to restore the normal AP to-and-fro fluid fluctuation. The operator should never leave a patient with asynchronous motion of the temporals because an adverse reaction of dizziness and nausea can result. Enhancement of synchronous rocking of the two temporals appears to have a beneficial effect on membranous balance. It is also of value in the temporomandibular joint function because asymmetric relationship of temporal movement interferes with symmetric temporomandibular joint function.

V Spread

This procedure is useful to separate restricted and impacted sutures wherever present. The principle is to place two fingers on each side of the restricted suture

with distraction and separation using fluid fluctuation as the activating force by applying pressure with the opposite hand at a point of greatest distance and opposite to the suture under treatment. The occipito-mastoid suture is one frequently treated by means of V spread ("Activating Forces") but the principles can be applied to any suture within the skull or face.

Lift Technique

Frontal and parietal lift technique is commonly used to aid in the balance of membranous tension. To perform a frontal lift, the patient is supine on the table with the operator sitting at the head. The operator grasps the inferior and lateral corners of the frontal bone on each side with one hand spanning the frontal bone or with two hands interlaced with the pisiforms on the frontal bone (Fig. 12.12). The hands apply a medial compression force to disengage the frontal, which is then lifted toward the ceiling sensing for a release. A frontal lift

Figure 12.12.
Frontal lift.

puts longitudinal traction on the falx cerebri as it lifts the frontal from the sphenoid. When the frontal bone appears to be in the midline and has been released anteriorly, it is slowly allowed to settle back to its normal relationship. It is not uncommon during this procedure to have the sensation that the frontal bone is wobbling from side to side when being distracted.

A parietal lift is performed by a four-finger contact on the two anteroinferior and posterior inferior corners of the parietal bones (Fig. 12.13). Compressive force is applied through the tips of the four fingers and each parietal bone is lifted toward the vertex. The four-corner compression disengages the parietal bone allowing for the lift that results in external rotation of the two parietal bones. The parietal lift places a transverse stress on the tentorium cerebelli balancing its tension from right to left. As with the frontal lift, when balance is achieved, the operator reduces the lifting force and allows the parietals to settle back into the skull. Lift techniques distract one bone from the other and apply loads to the meninges to achieve membranous balance.

SEQUENCE OF TREATMENT

Sequence of treatment varies from practitioner to practitioner, from patient to patient, and from one treatment to the next. There are several general principles that can be useful, applied, and adapted individually for the patient need. First and foremost, the craniosacral mechanism must be viewed within the context of the total musculoskeletal system. Craniosacral dysfunction may be primary, secondary, or of little significance in the patient's overall status. Secondary cranial dysfunction resulting from altered functional capacity elsewhere in the system will not respond well until the primary dysfunction is identified and appropriately treated. Conversely, continued treatment to dysfunction of the musculoskeletal system elsewhere in the system, without addressing the craniosacral dysfunction, will lead to less than satisfactory results.

Treatments that the craniosacral mechanism can follow are noted on page 181 (principles of craniosacral treatment). The goal should be to reduce venous congestion, mobilize articular restrictions, balance the sphenobasilar symphysis, and enhance the rate and amplitude of the CRI.

Craniosacral treatment, like all manual medicine, needs to be prescribed in the dosage appropriate for the individual patient's need. These procedures do not appear to be aggressive and forceful, but are powerful and if inappropriately applied can result in a poor outcome for the patient.

COMPLICATIONS AND CONTRAINDICATIONS

Complications to craniosacral treatment are fortunately quite rare, but do occur. The brainstem with its many control functions for the total body is intimately related to the sphenobasilar junction. Craniosacral treatment, particularly that which addresses sphenobasilar strain patterns, might lead to alteration in nervous system control of systemic function resulting in symptom exacerbation. This may include alterations in heart rate, blood pressure, or respiration and gastrointestinal irritability with nausea, vomiting, and diarrhea. These exacerbated symptoms appear to result from an alteration in autonomic nervous system control. A second area of potential symptom exacerbation and complications comprises the cervicocranial syndromes with headache, dizziness, and tinnitus. The vestibular system is highly sensitive to balance or imbalance of the temporal bones. Overly aggressive or improperly applied temporal rocking of the synchronous and asynchronous nature, may exacerbate symptoms of dizziness, vertigo, nausea, and vomiting. Care must be exercised in using craniosacral technique in

Figure 12.13.
Parietal lift.

individuals with psychologic and psychiatric problems. These procedures can cause significant emotional change in response to the patient's environment. Neurologic complications and symptom exacerbation can occur in patients with seizure states and dystonia of the central nervous system. Traumatic brain injury is a common, but frequently unrecognized, patient problem. Great care must be used in applying craniosacral technique to patients with traumatic brain injury, because it is difficult to predict the outcome of craniosacral treatment in these patients. The practitioner must be aware of and be prepared to deal with symptom exacerbation or onset of new symptoms in the patient under craniosacral treatment.

Contraindications are few but include suspicion for acute intracranial bleed or increase in intracranial pressure. These should be evaluated by appropriate diagnostic testing before implementing craniosacral treatment. Skull trauma requires adequate investigation to rule out fractures of the cranial base, depressed fractures of the vault, or subarachnoid hemorrhage. Seizure states are not an absolute contraindication but are relative depending upon the control of the seizure status.

Although the complications and contraindications are few, the admonition of *primum non nocere* (first do not harm) applies when using craniosacral technique.

CRANIAL TECHNIQUES

Condylar Compression (CV4)

1. Patient supine on table with operator sitting at head.
2. Operator's two hands cradle patient's occiput with the thenar eminences in contact with occipital squama palpating cranial rhythm (Fig. 12.11).
3. Operator resists occipital flexion movement until motion temporarily ceases (still point).
4. Operator gradually releases compression on occiput when cranial rhythm begins again until returned to normal.
5. Operator observes for change in respiration and increased perspiration of cervical area and forehead.

Frontal Lift

1. Patient supine on table with operator sitting at head.
2. Operator interlaces fingers of hands and grasps frontal bone with each pisiform in contact with inferior lateral angle (Fig. 12.12).
3. Operator lifts frontal bone anteriorly following any side-to-side fluctuation until lift appears to be midline.
4. Operator allows frontal to return to neutral.

Parietal Lift

1. Patient supine on table with operator sitting at head.
2. Operator applies each index finger on the anteroinferior corner and each little finger on the posterior-inferior corner of the parietal bone (Fig. 12.13).
3. Operator interlaces thumbs over vertex of the skull without touching and compresses medially with all four fingers.
4. Traction is applied toward the vertex until tension is felt to be symmetric in all four corners.
5. Operator gently releases traction allowing the parietals to return to neutral.

The following are the four most commonly found restrictors of the four quadrants of the skull: two posteriorly, the occipitomastoid and parietal notch, and two anteriorly, the sphenosquamous and palatines. There are numerous other sutural restrictions in the vault, base, and face that may need attention. The reader should pursue further study of these in a comprehensive text of the craniosacral system.

Occipitomastoid Suture

1. Operator sits at head of supine patient and controls the occiput in the right hand and the left hand controls the left temporal bone with the five-finger hold (Fig. 12.14).

2. Operator introduces external and internal rotations of the temporal and monitors the response in the occiput. If the occiput moves into extension rather than flexion when the temporal is externally rotated, there is restriction of the left occipitomastoid suture.

3. Treatment begins with establishing the longest diameter of dural tension by dorsiflexing the right foot.

4. The operator's right hand holds the occiput in flexion while the left hand externally rotates the temporal to the external rotation barrier while the patient fully exhales.

5. The operator instructs the patient to fully inhale rapidly or use a series of step breathing while the operator enhances temporal external rotation against the stabilized occiput.

6. The procedure may be repeated until normal motion between the temporal and occiput is restored.

7. Reassess.

Note: This dysfunction is the most common articular restriction of the posterior quadrant and is frequently related to dysfunction of the upper cervical vertebral complex.

Figure 12.14.
Occipitomastoid suture.

Parietal Notch

1. Operator sits at the head of the supine patient. Diagnosis is by medial springing of the posterior inferior corner of the parietal sensing for loss of mobility unilaterally.

2. Operator's left thumb is in contact with the mastoid process of the left temporal and the operator's right hand lies over the parietal bone with the thumb over the posterior inferior corner of the parietal (Fig. 12.15).

3. After establishing the longest diagonal by dorsiflexing the right foot, the operator presses medially with the right thumb and rotates the right hand counterclockwise on the parietal while the left thumb externally rotates the temporal to the barrier and the patient fully exhales.

4. The patient is instructed to take a rapid deep breath, or step breathe, while the operator's left thumb increases temporal external rotation and the right hand lifts the parietal superiorly and anteriorly, disengaging the parietal notch suture.

5. Reassess.

Figure 12.15.
Parietal notch suture.

Sphenosquamous Suture

1. Operator stands at right side of supine patient with one knee stabilizing right side of head.

2. Operator's left hand controls the left temporal with the thumb in front of the mastoid process.

3. Operator's gloved right hand places the little finger against the left lateral pterygoid plate of the sphenoid while the middle finger is placed on the left great wing and the right thumb on the right great wing if possible (Fig. 12.16).

4. After establishing the longest diameter by dorsiflexing the right foot, the operator engages the barrier by externally rotating the left temporal and pulling the left great wing anteriorly and having the patient fully exhale.

5. The patient takes a rapid deep breath and the operator simultaneously externally rotates the temporal while increasing the rotation of the sphenoid to the right and slightly into flexion.

6. Reassess.

Note: Dysfunction of this suture is one of the most common restrictors of the anterior quadrant.

Figure 12.16.
Sphenosquamous pivot suture.

Palatine

1. Operator stands at side of supine patient with the left hand grasping the sphenoid at the pterion bilaterally.

2. Operator's gloved right hand places little finger pad against the palatine just posterior to the left second molar (Fig. 12.17).

3. Operator flexes and extends sphenoid and monitors response at the palatine. During flexion, palatine should move laterally and during extension, it should move toward the vertex.

4. If restricted, the longest diameter is established and the sphenoid taken into marked flexion to disengage the pterygoid processes from the palatines.

5. If external rotation is restricted, the little finger presses laterally on the palatine as the patient takes a deep breath in.

6. If internal rotation is restricted, the little finger presses toward the vertex as the patient breaths deeply into exhalation.

7. The sphenoid is returned to neutral, recapturing the palatines by the pterygoid processes.

8. Reassess.

Note: Palatine dysfunction is a common restrictor of the anterior quadrant.

Figure 12.17.
Palatine.

Facial Balance

1. Operator sits at head of supine patient and places palm of both hands over the frontal and facial bones (Fig. 12.18).

2. Operator follows internal and external rotation motion of the facial bones and the frontal during inhalation and exhalation.

3. If asymmetric, operator exaggerates desired motion as patient deeply inhales and exhales.

4. Sometimes shearing motion is added to the internal and external rotational motions for enhanced mobility.

5. If still not symmetric, each facial bone needs to be assessed and treated as appropriate. Since the facial mechanics respond to the sphenoid, and are all suspended beneath the frontal, restoration of balance to the sphenobasilar symphysis and normal motion to the frontal usually restore mobility to the face. Most commonly, dysfunction of the zygoma is present.

Figure 12.18.
Facial balance.

Zygoma

1. Operator stands at the right side of the supine patient and with a gloved right hand slides the tip of the little finger inside of the cheek to contact the inferior margin of the zygoma and the thumb is placed on the outside of the cheek grasping the zygoma.

2. The operator's left hand stabilizes the head and monitors the attachments of the zygoma to the frontal and the great wing of the sphenoid (Fig. 12.19).

3. Operator's right hand internally and externally rotates the zygoma and the left hand monitors motion at the zygomaticofrontal and zygomaticosphenoid articulations.

4. If restricted, the longest diameter is established by dorsiflexing the right foot, and using inhalation to enhance external rotation and exhalation to enhance internal rotation as the zygoma is distracted from the frontal or sphenoid.

5. The zygoma can be mobilized from the maxilla by distracting the zygoma using the same thumb and little finger hold and stabilizing the maxilla by its frontal process attachment to the frontal, again using an appropriate respiratory assist.

6. Reassess.

Figure 12.19.
Zygoma.

Two-Person Decompression

1. Patient is supine and one operator sits at the head of the table with the occiput in the palms of the hands and the thumbs in front of the mastoid processes.

2. The second operator spans the front of the skull and contacts the two great wings of the sphenoid (Fig. 12.20).

3. The second operator directly engages the restrictive barrier of the sphenobasilar strain patterns of torsion, lateral strain, and vertical strain and puts anterior distraction on the sphenoid as the other operator stabilizes the occiput and temporals posteriorly.

4. Two or three applications of anterior distraction and flexion movement of the sphenoid are frequently necessary to restore mobility to the compressed head and reduce the restrictions of the strain patterns.

   Note: This is powerful technique and requires accurate direct engagement of the strain patterns before distraction is applied. It has been found most effective in the compressed skull associated with closed head injuries when indirect decompression is inadequate.

CONCLUSION

Craniosacral technique is a valuable addition to the armamentarium of the manual medicine practitioner. Craniosacral technique requires extensive study and practice. It should be performed within the context of total patient evaluation because of its powerful systemic effects. It influences, and is influenced by, the rest of the musculoskeletal system. This chapter includes basic and preliminary information about the craniosacral system. Students should pursue additional study from the standard texts in the field and structured courses of instruction.

SUGGESTED READINGS

Gehin A. *Atlas of manipulative techniques for the cranium and face.* Seattle: Eastland Press, 1985.

Greenman PE. Craniosacral manipulation. *Phys Med Rehab Clin N Am.* 1996;7:877–896.

Hruby RJ. *Craniosacral osteopathic technique: a manual,* second ed. Institute for Osteopathic Studies, Okemos, Michigan.

Magoun HI. *Osteopathy in the cranial field,* 2nd ed. Kirksville, MO: Journal Printing Co., 1966.

Retzlaff EW, Mitchell FL Jr. *The cranium and its sutures.* Berlin: Spinger-Verlag, 1987.

Upledger JE, Vredevoogd JD. *Craniosacral therapy.* Seattle, Eastland Press, 1983.

Figure 12.20.
Two-person sphenobasilar decompression.

13

CERVICAL SPINE TECHNIQUE

The cervical spine is an important region of the vertebral column in the field of manual medicine. It receives a great deal of attention by manual medicine practitioners. It functions as the support of the skull and biomechanically provides mobility for a number of activities of daily living. A myriad of head, neck, and upper extremity symptoms have been observed when the cervical spine is dysfunctional. Symptomatic conditions in the area can be categorized as cervicocephalic syndrome, cervical syndrome, and cervicobrachial syndrome. The cervicocephalic syndrome includes pain and restriction of motion of the upper cervical spine and associated superficial and deep pain in the head. This syndrome frequently demonstrates functional alteration in vision, vertigo, dizziness, and nystagmus. The cervical syndrome includes painful stiffness of the neck of varying severity from mild to an acute spastic torticollis. The cervicobrachial syndrome couples painful stiffness of the cervical spine with symptoms in the shoulder girdle and upper extremity. The upper extremity symptoms result from alteration of the functional capacity in the brachial plexus or altered vascular function through the arterial, venous, and lymphatic symptoms. Associated dysfunctions of the thoracic inlet, particularly the first and second ribs, and in the thoracic spine and rib cage as far as T5 or T6, contribute to the cervicobrachial syndrome.

The cervical spine is subjected to acute injuries, such as the flexion–extension "whiplash" injury and chronic, repetitive injury from improper posture and abnormal positions of the head and neck. It is seldom that the whiplash injury is a true flexion–extension injury. Most commonly, there is a rotary torque included in the trauma which gives rise to a number of motion restriction possibilities and different vectors of soft-tissue injury. It is common in our society to have patients with forward head carriage as a component of poor posture. Forward head posture results in an increase in the upper cervical lordosis and a flattening in the lower cervical spine. The balance of the head on the neck is altered, resulting in muscle imbalance with resulting tightness of the neck extensors and weakness of the deep neck flexors.

The cervical spine is the area of the musculoskeletal system in which most of the reported complications of manual medicine treatment have occurred. Traumatic insult to the vertebrobasilar artery system is a rare but catastrophic event. Congenital, inflammatory, and traumatic alterations in the upper cervical region, place the cervical spinal cord at risk from improper diagnostic and manual medicine treatment methods. Down syndrome, rheumatoid arthritis, agenesis of the odontoid process, and fracture of the odontoid base are but a few of these conditions. The student and practitioner must understand the anatomy, physiology, and biomechanics of the region to understand the therapeutic role of manual medicine and avoid potential complications.

FUNCTIONAL ANATOMY AND BIOMECHANICS

The cervical spine can be divided into the atypical segments of the upper cervical complex and the typical cervical vertebra from C3 through C7. The upper cervical complex, consisting of the Occipitoatlantal (C0-C1), atlantoaxial (C1-C2), and the superior aspect of C2, functions as an integrated unit. The biomechanics of this region are complex and are under intense research and study. Although the C0 through C3 region functions as an integrated unit, it is useful to assess each level individually to identify its contribution to the overall function of the complex.

Occipitoatlantal Articulation

The Occipitoatlantal junction (C0-C1) consists of two articulations formed by the occipital condyles and the superior articular facets of the atlas. The occipital condyles are convex from front to back and from side to side. The superior articular facets of the atlas are concave from the front to the back and from side to side. The two articulations are divergent from before backward bending. The primary movements are forward bending and backward bending (nutation and counternutation). There is a small amount of coupled side bending and rotation to opposite sides that becomes highly clinically significant when lost. During side bending, one occipital condyle slides upward on one side of the atlas and downward on the other. This side-bending component is approximately 5 degrees in each direction. Rotation couples to the opposite side of side bending and is in the range of 5 degrees to each side. The coupling of rotation to the opposite side appears to be a function of the ligamentous attachments of the occiput to the atlas and axis, the relationship of the slope of the size of the superior facets of the atlas, and the divergence posteriorly.

Atlantoaxial Articulation

There are four articulations at the atlantoaxial junction (C1-C2). The right and left zygapophysial joints are formed by the inferior facet of the atlas articulating with the convex superior facet of the axis. The inferior facet of the atlas is covered by an articular cartilage that is convex anteroposteriorly and from side to side. This relationship results in a unique convex to convex apposition of joint surfaces. The superior articular facets of the axis are convex anteroposteriorly, and from side to side, and face superiorly and laterally giving the appearance of a pair of shoulders. The other two articulations at the atlantoaxial junction involve the odontoid process. The anterior surface of the odontoid articulates with a small facet on the posterior aspect of the anterior arch of the atlas. On the posterior aspect of the odontoid process is an articulation with the transaxial ligament. The integrated functions of these four articulations, modified by ligamentous and muscular attachments, result in a small amount of forward bending, backward bending, and side bending, with the primary motion being rotation to the right and left. There is a small amount of cephalic-to-caudad translatory movement that accompanies rotation. This is a result of the unique convex-to-convex articular apposition of the zygapophysial joints. As the atlas turns right on the axis, the right facet of the atlas slides downward on the posterior aspect of the right facet of the axis, and the left inferior facet of the atlas slides downward on the anterior aspect of the left facet of the axis, resulting in caudad translation. On returning to neutral, the inferior facets of the atlas ascend on the articular shoulders of the facets of the axis resulting in a cephalic translatory movement.

C2 functions as a transitional segment with its atypical superior surface articulating with the atlas and to the occiput through ligamentous and muscular attachments. The inferior surface is the same as the remaining typical cervical segments below.

Typical Cervical Articulations

The typical cervical segments from C3 to C7 articulate at the vertebral bodies with an intervening intervertebral disc. The superior surface of the vertebral body is convex from before backward and concave from side to side while the inferior surface is convex from side to side and concave from before backward. This joint configuration, with the intervening intervertebral disc, allows it to move in all directions. The uncovertebral joints of Luschka are found at the posterolateral corner of the vertebral bodies and appear to function in the gliding movements during forward and backward bending. They also seem to protect the intervertebral disk from herniation in a posterolateral direction. These joints are subject to degenerative productive change resulting in lipping, which occasionally encroaches on the anterior aspect of the lateral intervertebral canal. The zygapophysial joints of the typical cervical vertebra face backward and upward at an angle of approximately 45 degrees. The greatest load bearing is through the posterior arches instead of the vertebral bodies as in the thoracic and lumbar spines. This loading, plus the facing of the zygapophysial joints and the characteristics of the vertebral bodies and intervening intervertebral disc, results in the motions available being forward bending, backward bending, and coupled side bending and rotation movements to the same side. This results in the typical cervical segments having only nonneutral somatic dysfunction. There are no group dysfunctions in the typical cervical segments, although several segments can become dysfunctional one on top of the other.

Vertebral Artery

The course of the vertebral artery is of major significance in the field of manual medicine. The vertebral artery begins its relationship with the cervical spine at the level of C6-C7 where it enters between the transverse processes, immediately turns cephalad, runs through the intertransverse foramen, and exits from the superior side of the transverse process of C1. Here it turns acutely posteriorly over the posterior arch of the atlas and penetrates the posterior occipitoatlantal membrane before entering the foramen magnum. It joins the vertebral artery of the opposite side to form the basilar artery. The vertebral artery is at risk at the acute angulation at C6-C7, by productive change in and around the intertransverse foramen from C7-C1, and at the occipitoatlantal junction. Normal vertebral arteries can narrow as much as 90% of their luminal size on the contralateral side during cervical rotation. This normal phenomenon is exacerbated when performed in backward bending of the head on the neck. Congenital asymmetry, and even atresia, of the vertebral arteries is not uncommon, and they are subject to degenerative vessel disease. A commonly used provocative diagnostic test for the integrity of the vertebral artery is the hanging (De Kleyn) test (Fig. 13.1). The examiner backward bends the head and neck over the end of the table (Fig. 13.2) and introduces rotation to the right (Fig. 13.3) and to the left (Fig. 13.4), holding the head in each rotated position looking for the development of nystagmus. This author does not advocate this test as it unnecessarily puts normal vertebral arteries at risk. It also has a high false-positive rate. A less aggressive test that provides equally valid information is the following: Have the sitting patient look up at the ceiling (Fig. 13.5), then turn the head to both the left (Fig. 13.6) and to the right (Fig. 13.7) while the operator observes for the initiation of nystagmus and adverse symptoms such as dizziness. This is a hands-off test by the practitioner and asks only that the patient introduce normal ranges of active movement. Probably the best sign of impending cerebral anoxia is the symptom of acute anxiety and panic. If this occurs during a structural diagnostic or manual medicine procedure in the cervical spine, the operator should stop and immediately institute evaluation and treatment for potential vascular complications.

Mechanoreceptors and Nociceptors

The articular and periarticular structures of the cervical spine, particularly the upper cervical complex, are heavily invested by mechanoreceptors and nociceptors.

Figure 13.3.

Figure 13.1.

Figure 13.4.

Figure 13.2.

Figure 13.5.

Cervical spine dysfunction can result in altered afferent stimulation by these mechanoreceptors and nociceptors and influence the integrated function of the musculoskeletal system, as well as contribute to local and regional symptoms. The suboccipital cervical muscles have a large number of spindles per unit mass. The proprioceptive function of these muscles must have a high level of significance. Recent magnetic resonance imaging (MRI) research in this region has demonstrated fatty replacement of the rectus capitis posterior major and minor muscles in some patients with posttraumatic cervicocranial syndromes (see Chapter 21).

Autonomic Nervous System Relationships

Sympathetic autonomic nervous system control of cerebral blood flow emanates from the superior cervical ganglion. This structure is intimately related to the longus colli muscle and the anterior surface of C2 to which it is intimately bound by deep connective fascia. Somatic dysfunction of C2 is frequently found in patients with cervicocephalic syndromes and in those with internal visceral disease. A small branch of the second cervical nerve connects with the vagus as it descends through the trunk. Hypothetically, this neural connection may account for the clinical observation of somatic dysfunction of C2 in the presence of visceral disease.

STRUCTURAL DIAGNOSIS

The anatomy and biomechanics of the cervical spine result in five somatic dysfunctions. The typical cervical segments have nonneutral dysfunction with either forward-bending or backward-bending restriction together with coupled side-bending and rotation restriction to the same side. At the atlantoaxial (C1-C2) junction, the primary somatic dysfunction is that of restriction of rotation to one side or the other. While there may be minor forward-bending, backward-bending, and side-bending components to the rotational restriction, adequate treatment to the rotational restriction restores the minor movement motion simultaneously. At the occipitoatlantal (C0-C1) junction, there are two dysfunctions possible. There will be either forward-bending or backward-bending restriction with coupled side-bending and rotation restrictions to opposite sides.

The structural diagnostic process begins by identifying levels of palpable deep-muscle hypertonicity. This identifies segments that need motion testing. The diagnostic and therapeutic processes seem to be most satisfactory by beginning from below and moving cephalad.

The bony landmark of most value in the typical cervical segments is the articular pillar. They are palpated in the deep fascial groove between the semispinalis medially and the cervical longissimus laterally. The paired examiner fingers can localize to the right and left articular pillars of any given cervical segment and introduce motion testing. The typical cervical segment articular pillar is the size of the examiner's finger pad. The identification of the articular pillars begins by first identifying the spinous process of C2 and C7. The C2 spinous process is the first bony prominence in the midline caudad to the external occipital protuberance (inion). The spinous process of C7 (vertebra prominens) is the spinous process that remains palpable during cervical backward bending. The articular pillars of C2 and C7 are at the same level of the spinous processes. Placing the examiner's fingers between the pillars of C2 and C7 puts the finger pads in contact with C3, C4, C5, and C6. This provides the ability to localize to any specific cervical segment. The structural diagnostic process can be performed in both the patient sitting and supine positions.

Figure 13.6.

Figure 13.7.

CERVICAL SPINE DIAGNOSIS

Typical Cervical Sitting

1. Patient sitting on table or treatment stool.

2. Operator stands behind with thumb and index finger contacting zygapophysial joints bilaterally and with left hand on vertex of head to control motion (Fig. 13.8).

3. Operator's left hand introduces forward bending; right-side bending, and right rotation with the left hand while monitoring left zygapophysial joint for opening movement (Fig. 13.9).

4. Operator introduces forward bending, left-side bending, and left rotation, palpating for opening of the right zygapophysial joint by the operator's right index finger (Fig. 13.10).

5. Operator's left hand introduces backward bending, right-side bending, and right rotation with the right index finger monitoring the right zygapophysial joint's capacity to close (Fig. 13.11).

6. Operator introduces backward bending, left-side bending, and left rotation with the left hand while monitoring the left zygapophysial joint's capacity to close with the right thumb (Fig. 13.12)

Figure 13.10.

Figure 13.8.

Figure 13.11.

Figure 13.9.

Figure 13.12.

Cervical Spine Diagnosis

Atlantoaxial (C1-C2) Sitting

1. Patient sitting on table with operator behind.

2. Operator's two hands grasp the patient's head and introduce forward bending (Fig. 13.13) to reduce rotation in lower typical cervical vertebra.

3. Operator introduces right rotation sensing for resistance to movement (Fig. 13.14).

4. Operator introduces left rotation sensing for resistance to left rotation (Fig. 13.15).

Figure 13.14.

Figure 13.13.

Figure 13.15.

Cervical Spine Diagnosis

Occipitoatlantal (C0-C1) Sitting

1. Patient sitting on table.

2. Operator stands behind with thumb and index finger of the right hand grasping the posterior arch of the atlas and the left hand on top of the head to introduce movement.

3. Operator's left hand introduces backward bending, left-side bending, and right rotation of the head sensing for prominent fullness under the right thumb indicating posterior rotation of the atlas on the left (Fig. 13.16).

4. Operator's left hand introduces backward bending, right-side bending, left rotation of the head and monitors for prominence of the right posterior arch of the atlas under the right index finger, indicative of right rotation of the atlas (Fig. 13.17).

5. Operator introduces forward bending, right-side bending, and left rotation with the left hand while monitoring for prominence of the right posterior arch of the atlas under the right index finger, indicating atlas right rotation (Fig. 13.18).

6. Operator introduces forward bending, left-side bending, and right rotation of the head with the left hand while monitoring for prominence of the left posterior arch of the atlas under the right thumb, indicating left rotation of the atlas (Fig. 13.19).

Note: The right thumb and index finger assess the rotation of the atlas in relation to the induced rotation of the occiput and not in relation to the coronal plane.

Figure 13.16.

Figure 13.18.

Figure 13.17.

Figure 13.19.

Cervical Spine Diagnosis

Typical Cervical Segments (C3-C7) Supine for Flexed, Rotated, and Side-Bent Dysfunction

1. Patient supine on table with operator sitting at head of table.

2. Operator's index and middle fingers of each hand contact the pillar of the superior vertebra of the motion segment being tested (Fig. 13.20).

3. Operator's palms and thenar eminences control the patient's head and upper cervical spine (Fig. 13.21).

Figure 13.20.

Figure 13.21.

4. Operator's finger contacts translate the vertebra anteriorly to the backward-bending barrier (lift the fingers toward the ceiling) (Fig. 13.22).

5. The operator introduces translation from right to left, sensing for resistance to movement (Fig. 13.23). If resistance is encountered, the motion restriction is backward bending, right-side bending, and right rotation [flexed, rotated, and side bent left (FRS$_{left}$)]. Something interfered with the capacity of the right facet to close.

6. Operator introduces translatory movement from left to right sensing for resistance (Fig. 13.24). If resistance is encountered, the motion restriction is backward bending, left-side bending, and left rotation (FRS$_{right}$). Something interfered with the left facet to close.

Figure 13.23.

Figure 13.22.

Figure 13.24.

Cervical Spine Diagnosis

Typical Cervical Segment (C3-C7) Supine for Extended, Rotated, and Side-bent Dysfunction

1. Patient supine on table with operator sitting at head of table.

2. Operator's index and middle fingers of each hand contact the pillar of the superior vertebra of the motion segment being tested (Fig. 13.20).

3. Operator's palms and thenar eminences control the patient's head and upper cervical spine (Fig. 13.21).

4. Operator flexes the head and neck down to the segment under examination (Fig. 13.25).

5. Operator introduces translation from right to left, sensing for resistance (Fig. 13.26). If resistance is felt, the motion restriction is forward bending, right-side bending, right rotation [extended, rotated, and side bent left (ERS_{left})]. Something has interfered with the capacity of the left facet to open.

6. Operator introduces translation from left to right sensing for resistance (Fig. 13.27). If resistance is encountered, the motion restriction is forward bending, left-side bending, and left rotation (ERS_{right}). Something interfered with the capacity of the right facet to open.

Figure 13.26.

Figure 13.25.

Figure 13.27.

Cervical Spine Diagnosis

Atlantoaxial (C1-C2) Supine

1. Patient supine on table with operator standing (or sitting) at the head of the table.

2. Operator's two hands hold each side of the patient's head with index fingers monitoring the posterior arch of the atlas. Operator flexes the patient's head and neck to provide restriction of typical cervical segment rotation through ligamentous locking (Fig. 13.28).

3. Operator's hands introduce right rotation sensing for resistance (Fig. 13.29). If resistance is encountered, the motion restriction is right rotation (atlas rotated left).

4. Operator rotates head to the left sensing for resistance (Fig. 13.30). If resistance is encountered, the motion restriction is left rotation (atlas rotated right).

Note: Neck flexion must be maintained throughout the procedure. Do not allow the head and neck to go into backward bending during the rotation effort.

Figure 13.29.

Figure 13.28.

Figure 13.30.

Cervical Spine Diagnosis

Occipitoatlantal (C0-C1) Supine Extension Restriction

1. Patient supine on table with operator sitting at the head of the table.

2. Operator's two hands grasp sides of patient's head with index fingers monitoring the posterior arch of the atlas.

3. Operator introduces backward bending to the first barrier by rolling the head posteriorly around an axis of rotation through the external auditory meati (Fig. 13.31).

4. Operator introduces translation of the head from right to left, maintaining the eyes parallel to the head of the table sensing for resistance (Fig. 13.32). If resistance is felt, motion restriction is backward bending, right-side bending, left rotation [C0 flexed (F), side bent left (S_{left}), rotated right (R_{right})]. Something interfered with the right condyle gliding forward.

5. Operator introduces translation from left to right sensing for resistance (Fig. 13.33). If resistance is encountered, the motion restriction is backward bending, left-side bending, right rotation ($FS_{right}R_{left}$). Something interfered with the left condyle to glide forward.

Figure 13.32.

Figure 13.31.

Figure 13.33.

Cervical Spine Diagnosis

Occipitoatlantal (C0-C1) Supine for Flexion Restriction

1. Patient supine on table with operator sitting at head of table.

2. Operator's hands grasp the side of the patient's head with the index fingers monitoring the posterior arch of the atlas.

3. Operator forward bends the patient's head by rotation around an axis through the external auditory meati while monitoring for first movement of the atlas (Fig. 13.34).

4. Operator introduces translation from right to left sensing for resistance (Fig 13.35). If resistance is felt, the motion restriction is forward bending, right-side bending, left rotation ($ES_{left}R_{right}$). Something interfered with the left condyle's glide posteriorly.

5. Operator introduces translation from left to right sensing for resistance (Fig. 13.36). If resistance is encountered, the motion restriction is of forward bending, left-side bending, and right rotation ($ES_{right}R_{left}$). Something interfered with the right condyle's glide posteriorly.

Figure 13.35.

Figure 13.34.

Figure 13.36.

Cervical Spine Diagnosis

Occipitoatlantal (C0-C1) Supine Condylar Glide

1. Patient supine on table with operator sitting at head of table.
2. Operator grasps the sides of the head with each hand and rotates the head 30 degrees to the right (Fig. 13.37).

3. Operator introduces anterior translation gliding the right condyle anteriorly sensing for resistance (Fig. 13.38).
4. Operator translates the head posteriorly requiring the right condyle to glide posteriorly (Fig. 13.39).
5. Operator rotates head 30 degrees to the left (Fig. 13.40).

Figure 13.37.

Figure 13.39.

Figure 13.38.

Figure 13.40.

6. Operator introduces anterior translatory movement of the head, forcing the left condyle to glide forward (Fig. 13.41).

7. Operator introduces posterior translation of the head asking the left condyle to glide posteriorly sensing for resistance to movement (Fig. 13.42).

Note: This tests for the forward-bending and backward-bending capacity of each condyle. If resistance is encountered, there will be restriction of the side-bending and rotational motion coupled to opposite sides (the minor movements).

Figure 13.41.

Figure 13.42.

CERVICAL SPINE DIAGNOSIS

Stress Tests of the Upper Cervical Complex

The upper cervical complex is subject to fracture, dislocation, and ligamentous damage after trauma. Concern for fracture and dislocation is uncommon in the practice of manual medicine. Ligamentous damage may well be of concern to the manual medicine practitioner. The preceding diagnostic tests are most valuable for determining hypomobility as the result of somatic dysfunction. Early hypermobility is much more difficult to assess. Stress testing of the craniocervical junction is difficult to interpret. If the preceding diagnostic tests for the occipitoatlantal and atlantoaxial joints have full range and asymmetric loose end feel, the index of suspicion should go up for hypermobility due to ligamentous laxity.

This author uses two stress tests of the many available. The first is an anteroposterior stress of upper cervical complex: In the supine position, the operator holds the occiput (Fig. 13.43) and anteriorly translates the atlas and axis, sensing for mobility (Fig. 13.44). The thumbs are then placed on the anterior aspect of the transverse processes of the atlas, axis and a posterior translatory force is applied (Fig. 13.45). Abnormal anterior to posterior translatory movement may indicate some laxity of the transaxial ligament. The second test is to monitor the spinous process of C2 of the flexed head (Fig. 13.46) and introduce side bending of the head on the neck (Fig. 13.47). Left-side bending of the occiput should result in immediate left rotation of C2. Then, right-side bending is introduced and right rotation elicited. Should this side bending be asymmetric or delayed, the possibility of alar ligament damage should be suspected.

A major problem in motion testing for hypermobility in this region is that it may be compensatory for restricted motion in other areas of the upper cervical

Figure 13.43.

Figure 13.45.

Figure 13.44.

Figure 13.46.

Figure 13.47.

complex. Is the side of restriction hypomobile or is the hypermobility truly due to ligamentous damage?

If there is any question of significant ligamentous damage, it can be further evaluated by rotational stress films of the upper cervical complex using either computed tomography (CT) or MRI technology. Axial views in the right and left rotated positions provide the opportunity to assess segmental mobility and its symmetry. The MRI technology is somewhat more valuable for identifying the status of individual ligaments.

MANUAL MEDICINE THERAPEUTIC PROCEDURES

The following procedures are all direct action as they directly engage the restrictive barrier. The two activating forces will be muscle energy technique, an intrinsic activating force, and mobilization with impulse technique with an extrinsic activating force. The muscle energy techniques are performed ini-tially because most of the somatic dysfunctions found within the cervical spine respond well. It is in those patients for whom muscle energy is not effective in maximizing motion that consideration should be given to the use of the mobilization with impulse technique. When the diagnostic process identifies what seems to be a deep articular or periarticular re-striction, the mobilization with impulse techniques appear to be most effective.

It is recommended that the treatment sequence begin in the lower cervical spine and move upward to-ward the craniocervical junction. One reason is that this provides easier and more accurate diagnosis of the superior segment on the inferior throughout the diagnostic process. It is not uncommon for several typical cervical segments to demonstrate stacked non-neutral dysfunction that need to be addressed indi-vidually. The goal of any manual medicine interven-tion is to balance the occiput on the vertebral column. This use of the biomechanical model would suggest that the craniooccipital junction be the last treated af-ter balancing the system below. One major exception to this rule is to approach the most restricted segment first in order to influence the system to the maximum. However, if the most restricted area is also the most acute, the practitioner might wish to work around the acute area to remove related restrictors and decongest the acute inflammatory process. In acute conditions of the cervical spine, functional (indirect) technique is the treatment of choice (see Chapter 10).

When the diagnostic procedure reveals that sev-eral of the typical cervical segments resist translation in the same direction, the probability is high that there is asymmetric hypertonicity of the scalene mus-cles resulting in a long restrictor to cervical motion. Unilateral scalene tightness is quite common. The tight scalenes should be manually stretched before ad-ditional treatment is made to the cervical spine.

Cervical Spine Scalene Muscle Stretch

1. Operator sits at the head of the table with the patient supine and head and neck over the end of the table.

2. Operator cradles patient's head with the left hand supporting the occiput and upper cervical spine and the forehead in the axilla (Fig. 13.48). Operator's right hand stabilizes the patient's right thoracic inlet, particularly the right first and second ribs.

3. Operator translates the head posteriorly (Fig. 13.49) to the barrier and resists patient's anterior transla-

tion of the head for 5 to 6 seconds with three to five repetitions. The operator engages a new barrier between patient contractions.

4. Occasionally it is useful to use a series of right-side bending efforts as well as anterior translation.

5. Comparison is made with the other side and stretching is continued to symmetry.

Note: The head and upper cervical spines are not placed in extension by posterior rotation but by posterior translation. This protects the vertebral artery from the risk of acute extension of the upper cervical complex.

Figure 13.48.

Figure 13.49.

Cervical Spine Muscle Energy Technique

Typical Cervical Vertebra (C5-C6)

Diagnosis
   Position: Flexed, rotated left, sidebend left
   (FRS$_{left}$)
   Motion Restriction: Extension, right rotation, and
   right-side bending (ERS$_{right}$)

1. Patient supine on table with operator sitting at head.

2. Operator's fingertips of the right index and middle finger are placed on the right articular pillar of C6 to hold the segment so that C5 can be moved upon it (Fig. 13.50).

3. The operator's left hand controls the left side of the patient's head and neck (Fig. 13.51).

4. The operator's right fingers translate the segment anteriorly introducing motion to the backward bending barrier (Fig. 13.52).

Figure 13.51.

Figure 13.50.

Figure 13.52.

5. Operator's left hand introduces side bending and rotation of the head and neck to the right by right-to-left translation engaging the right rotation, right-side bending barriers (Fig. 13.53).

6. The patient exerts a small isometric effort against the operator's resisting left hand into forward bending, left-side bending, or left rotation.

7. After a 3- to 5-second muscle effort, the patient relaxes and the operator increases translatory movement in an anterior and a right-to-left direction engaging the backward-bending, right-side bending, and right-rotation barriers (Fig. 13.54). The process is repeated three to five times.

8. Retest.

Note: Eye movement can be substituted for the activating force with the patient either looking down toward the feet or to the left after each localization.

Figure 13.53.

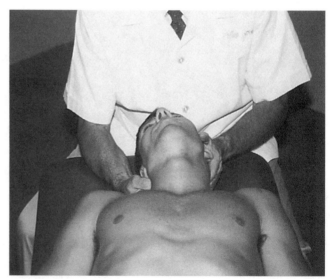

Figure 13.54.

Cervical Spine Muscle Energy Treatment

Typical Cervical Vertebra (C2-C3 Example)

Diagnosis
 Position: Extended, left side-bent, left rotated
 (ERS$_{left}$)
 Motion Restriction: Forward bending, rotation right,
 side bending right

1. Patient supine on table with operator sitting at head.

2. Operator's left hand supports the occiput with the left thumb over the left C2-C3 zygapophysial joint and the left index finger blocking the right C2-C3 zygapophysial joint (Fig. 13.55).

3. Operator's right hand is placed on the patients' right frontoparietal region to control head movement (Fig. 13.56).

4. Operator's two hands roll the head and upper neck into forward bending as far as the C2-C3 interspace (Fig. 13.57).

5. Operator introduces right-side bending and right rotation by right-to-left translation through the left index finger contact on the right zygapophysial joint of C2-C3, engaging the flexion, right-side bending, and right-rotation restriction (Fig. 13.58).

6. The patient exerts a 3 to 5 second isometric contraction into backward bending, or left-side bending, or left rotation. Following relaxation, the operator engages the new flexion, right-side bending, and right-rotational barriers and the isometric contractions are repeated three to five times.

7. Retest.

 Note: Eye movement can be substituted for the activating force with the patient either looking up toward the eyebrows or to the left after each localization.

Figure 13.55.

Figure 13.57.

Figure 13.56.

Figure 13.58.

Cervical Spine Muscle Energy Technique

Atlantoaxial (C1-C2)

Diagnosis
  Position: Atlas rotated right
  Motion Restriction: Atlas resists left rotation on axis

1. Patient supine on table with operator sitting or standing at head.

2. Operator grasps the head with the palms of the hands and flexes the head to approximately 30 to 45 degrees (Fig. 13.59).

3. Operator introduces left rotation against the restricted barrier (Fig. 13.60).

4. Patient is instructed to turn the head to the right against the operator's resisting right hand with a light isometric contraction.

5. Following a 3- to 5-second contraction and subsequent relaxation, the operator increases left rotation to the next resistant barrier.

6. Patient repeats right rotational effort against resistance three to five times.

7. Retest.

  Note: Eye movement activating force is looking to the right.

Figure 13.59.

Figure 13.60.

Cervical Spine Muscle Energy Technique

Occipitoatlantal (C0-C1)

Diagnosis
Position: $FS_{right}R_{left}$
Motion Restriction: Backward bending, left-side bending, and right rotation

1. Patient supine on table with operator sitting or standing at head.

2. Operator's left hand controls the patient's occiput with the web of the thumb and index finger along the soft tissues at the cervicocranial junction (Fig. 13.61).

3. Operator's right hand holds the patient's chin with the index finger in front and the middle finger below the tip of the ramus and with the right forearm in contact with the right side of the patient's head (Fig. 13.62).

4. The backward-bending barrier is engaged by the operator's two hands rotating the head posteriorly around a transverse axis through the external auditory meati (Fig. 13.63).

5. Left-side bending is introduced through the operator's right forearm by slight left-to-right translation (Fig.13.64). Note: rotation is not actively introduced.

6. The patient is instructed to look down at the feet or pull the chin toward the chest against resistance offered by the operator's right hand for a 3- to 5-second light isometric muscle contraction.

7. After relaxation, the new backward-bending, left-side bending, and right-rotational barriers are engaged.

8. Operator's muscle contraction is repeated three to five times with the operator relocalizing against the resisted barrier after each effort.

9. Retest.

Note: The eye movement of looking toward the feet is usually sufficient force for correction of this dysfunction.

Figure 13.61.

Figure 13.63.

Figure 13.62.

Figure 13.64.

Cervical Spine Muscle Energy Technique

Occipitoatlantal (C0-C1)

Diagnosis
  Position: $ES_{right}R_{left}$
  Motion restriction: Forward bending, left-side bending, and right rotation

1. Patient is supine on the table with the operator sitting or standing at the head.

2. Operator's left hand controls the occiput with the web of the thumb and index finger along the soft tissue of the suboccipital area (Fig. 13.61).

3. The operator's right hand cups the chin with the index finger in front and the middle finger below the tip of the ramus. The operator's right forearm is placed along the right side of the patient's head (Fig. 13.65).

4. Forward bending is introduced by rotating the head forward by the operator's two hands around a transverse axis through the external auditory meati (Fig. 13.66).

5. Left-side bending and right rotation are introduced by the operator's right forearm and with slight left-to-right translation of the patient's head to engage the restrictive barrier (Fig. 13.67). Note: Right rotation is not actively introduced.

6. Patient instruction is to push the head directly posteriorly toward the table into the hand offering resistance for 3 to 5 seconds of a mild isometric muscle contraction.

7. After relaxation, the operator engages the forward-bending, left-side bending, and right rotational barriers.

8. Patient repeats the isometric contractions three to five times.

9. Retest.

Note: An eye motion activating force is to look up toward the operator or toward the eyebrows.

Figure 13.66.

Figure 13.65.

Figure 13.67.

Cervical Spine Muscle Energy Technique

Occipitoatlantal (C0-C1)

1. Patient supine on table with operator sitting at head.

2. Operator's left thumb and index finger grasp the posterior arch of the atlas and the occiput lies in the palm of the operator's left hand (Fig. 13.68).

3. Operator's right hand spans the frontal region of the patient's head.

4. For a dysfunction that resists forward bending, left-side bending, and right rotation ($ES_{right}R_{left}$), the operator rolls the head into forward bending and with the right hand introduces left-side bending and right rotation against the resistance of the atlas held by the operator's left hand (Fig. 13.69).

5. A 3- to 5-second slight, mild isometric contraction of the head into backward bending or right-side bending that is resisted by the operator's two hands.

6. After relaxation, the new barriers are engaged and the patient repeats the isometric contraction three to five times.

7. Retest.

8. For a dysfunction showing restriction of backward bending, right-side bending, and left rotation, the operator introduces backward bending through rotation, side bending to the right, and rotation to the left with the right hand (Fig. 13.70).

9. The patient provides a mild isometric contraction in the directions of forward bending or left-side bending against resistance offered by the operator's right hand, and against the atlas stabilized by the operator's left hand.

10. After relaxation, the new backward-bending (extension), right-side bending, and left-rotation barriers is engaged and the patient repeats the isometric contraction three to five times.

11. Retest.

Figure 13.69.

Figure 13.68.

Figure 13.70.

Cervical Spine Mobilization with Impulse Technique

Typical Cervical Vertebra (C5-C6 Example)

Diagnosis
  Position: FRS$_{left}$
  Motion Restriction: Extension, right rotation, right-side bending

1. Patient supine on table with operator sitting/standing at head.

2. Operator's left hand controls left side of the patient's head and proximal neck.

3. Operator's right second metacarpophalangeal joint contacts the articular pillar of C5 (the superior vertebra of the dysfunctional vertebral motion segment) (Fig. 13.71).

4. Backward bending and right-side bending are introduced to the restricted barrier (Fig. 13.72).

   Note: Even though the head is side bent right and rotated left through the upper cervical complex, C5 is rotating right in response to the right-side bending of C5 on C6.

5. A high-velocity, low-amplitude thrust is applied in a caudad direction toward the spinous process of T1 (Fig. 13.73).

6. Retest.

   Note: Regardless of which cervical segment is dysfunctional, the thrust is always in the direction of the spinous process of T1.

Figure 13.72.

Figure 13.71.

Figure 13.73.

Cervical Spine Mobilization with Impulse Technique

C2-C3 Example

Diagnosis
   Position: ERS$_{left}$
   Motion Restriction: Forward bending, right rotation, right-side bending
   Opening facet thrust variation 1

1. Patient supine with operator standing at head of table.

2. Operator's right second metacarpophalangeal joint contacts the right zygapophysial joint of C2 through C3. The operator's left hand controls the patient's head and neck (Fig. 13.74).

3. The head is flexed and side bent right, localizing at C2-C3 (Fig. 13.75).

4. A high velocity, low amplitude thrust is applied horizontally in the plane of the involved C2-C3 joint resulting in a "gapping" opening of the left zygapophysial joint (Fig. 13.76).

5. Retest.

Figure 13.75.

Figure 13.74.

Figure 13.76.

Cervical Spine Mobilization with Impulse Technique

Typical Cervical Segments (C2-C3 Example)

Diagnosis
 Position: ERS$_{left}$
 Motion Restriction: Forward bending, right rotation, right-side bending
 Opening facet thrust variation 2

1. Patient supine with operator sitting or standing at head of table.

2. Operator controls the head through both hands with the left second metacarpophalangeal joint overlying the left pillar of C2 (Fig. 13.77). The second and third fingers of the operator's right hand contact the right zygapophysial joint of C2-C3 to serve as a blocking pivot (Fig. 13.78).

3. Using both hands the operator forward bends the head down to the flexion barrier of C2-C3 (Fig. 13.79).

4. Operator left hand rotates and right-side bends the patient's head over the fulcrum established by the right second and third fingers to the barrier (Fig. 13.80).

Figure 13.77.

Figure 13.79.

Figure 13.78.

Figure 13.80.

Note: Be sure to maintain the right-side bending component as the left hand introduces right rotation (Fig. 13.81).

5. A high-velocity, low-amplitude rotary thrust is applied through the operator's left hand by elevating the left elbow toward the ceiling (Fig. 13.82).

6. Retest.

Figure 13.81.

Figure 13.82.

Cervical Spine Mobilization with Impulse Technique

Atlantoaxial (C1-C2)

Diagnosis
  Position: Atlas rotated right
  Motion Restriction: Atlas resists left rotation on axis

1. Patient supine with operator sitting or standing at head of table.
2. Operator's right second metacarpophalangeal joint contacts the right posterior arch of the atlas. The operator's left hand controls the left side of the head and neck.

3. Patients head is flexed approximately 30 to 45 degrees to take out the flexion mobility of the typical cervical segments below (Fig. 13.83).
4. Operator's two hands rotate the atlas to the left to the restrict ional barrier and fine-tune the forward-bending, and backward-bending, and right- and left-side bending components to maximum ease (Fig. 13.84).
5. A rotary thrust is applied through both hands in a left rotational direction (Fig. 13.85).
6. Retest.

Figure 13.84.

Figure 13.83.

Figure 13.85.

Cervical Spine Mobilization with Impulse Technique

Occipitoatlantal (C0-C1)

Diagnosis
Position: $FS_{right}R_{left}$
Motion Restriction: Backward bending, left-side bending, right rotation

1. Patient supine with operator sitting at head of table.

2. Operator's left hand cradles the occiput between the web of the thumb and index finger with bony contact at suboccipital region. Do not compress the posterior occipitoatlantal membrane (Fig. 13.86).

3. Operator's right hand cradles the patient's chin with the right forearm along the right side of the patient's mandible and temporal regions (Fig. 13.87). Exten-sion is introduced through both hands by posterior rotation around a transverse axis through the external auditory meati. Left-side bending and right rotation are introduced through the operator's right forearm and with slight left-to-right translation (Fig. 13.88).

Note: Rotation is not actively introduced but follows side bending.

4. When all three barriers are engaged, a high-velocity, low-amplitude thrust is applied through operator's two hands in a cephalic, long-axis-extension direction (Fig. 13.89).

Note: The left forearm is caudad to the left hand contact on the occiput for better control of the long axis extension thrust.

5. Retest.

Figure 13.86.

Figure 13.88.

Figure 13.87.

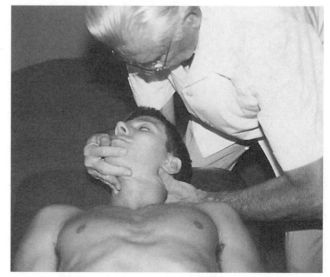

Figure 13.89.

Cervical Spine Mobilization with Impulse Technique

Occipitoatlantal (C0-C1)

Diagnosis
Position: ES$_{right}$R$_{left}$
Motion Restriction: Forward bending, left-side bending, right rotation

1. Patient supine with operator sitting or standing at head of table.
2. Operator's left hand cradles occiput with web of thumb and index finger on bone to monitor suboccipital tissue tension. Do not compress the posterior occipitoatlantal membrane (Fig. 13.86).
3. Operator's right hand cradles patient's chin with right forearm along right side of patient's face and head (Fig. 13.90).
4. Operator introduces forward bending by rotating the head anteriorly around a transverse axis through the external auditory meati.

5. Left-side bending and right rotation are introduced through the operator's right forearm and slight left-to-right translation (Fig. 13.91).

   Note: Right rotation is not actively introduced.

6. When the flexion, left-side bending, right rotational barriers are engaged, a high-velocity, low-amplitude thrust is applied in a cephalic, long-axis-extension direction simultaneously by both hands (Fig. 13.92).

   Note: The operator's left forearm to elbow is below the occipital contact giving better control of the long axis extension thrust.

7. Retest.

Figure 13.91.

Figure 13.90.

Figure 13.92.

Cervical Spine Combined Soft-tissue Inhibition and Craniosacral Condylar Decompression

Craniooccipital Junction

1. Patient supine with operator sitting at head of table.

2. Operator cradles head in both hands with finger pads along the insertion of extensor cervical muscles in the occiput.

3. Flexion of the operator's distal interphalangeal joints place inhibitory pressure against muscle insertion in the occiput (Fig. 13.93).

4. When softening of muscle hypertonicity occurs, the operator places the two middle fingers on each side of the external occipital protuberance (inion) with the heels of the hands together.

5. With the operator's forearms on the table, the middle fingers are moved anteriorly along bone as far forward as possible with contact on the condylar portion of the occipital bone (Fig. 13.94).

6. With flexion of the distal interphalangeal joints of the middle finger putting compressive force on the occipital condylar portion, the elbows are brought together resulting in a posterolateral distraction of each condylar portion of bone (Fig. 13.95).

7. Operator enhances the amount of compressive force on the condylar portion of the occiput that has less resilience until softening occurs.

8. The goal of treatment is relaxation of suboccipital muscles and symmetric resiliency of bone in the occipital condylar parts.

Figure 13.94.

Figure 13.93.

Figure 13.95.

CONCLUSION

There are a number of structural diagnostic and manual medicine therapeutic interventions for the cervical spine. Only five somatic dysfunctions occur in the cervical spine, namely, flexion or extension restriction with coupled side bending and rotation to the same side in the typical cervical segments, rotational restriction of the atlas on the axis, and either flexion or extension with side bending and rotational restriction to opposite sides at the occipitoatlantal articulation. There are many combinations of these dysfunctions. Remember that the upper cervical complex functions as an integrative unit and dysfunctions of the occipitoatlantal, atlantoaxial, and C-2 on C-3 are very common. The muscle energy and mobilization with impulse techniques described in this chapter have been most effective and safe in the hands of the author. Mastery of the diagnostic and manual medicine treatment procedures for the cervical spine is useful in managing the myriad of head, neck, and upper extremity problems presenting to the manual medicine practitioner. A thorough understanding of the functional anatomy and biomechanics of the cervical spine is essential for effective and safe manual medicine technique.

SUGGESTED READINGS

Aprill C, Dwyer A, Bogduk N. Cervical zygapophyseal joint pain patterns, II: a clinical evaluation. *Spine* 1990;15:458–461.

Dvorak J, Froelich D, Penning L, et al. Functional radiographic diagnosis of the cervical spine: flexion/extension. *Spine* 1998;13:748–755.

Dvorak J, Hayek J, Zehnder R. C-T functional diagnostics of the rotary instability of upper cervical spine, II: an evaluation on healthy adults and patients with suspected instability. *Spine* 1987;12:726–731.

Dvorak J, Orelli F. How dangerous is manipulation on the cervical spine? *Man Med* 1985;2:1–4.

Dvorak J, Panjabi MM, Gerber M, Wichmann W. C-T Functional diagnostics of the rotary instability of the upper cervical spine, I: an experimental study on cadavers. *Spine* 1987;12:197–205.

Haldeman S, ed. *Modern developments in the principles and practice of chiropractic.* New York: Appleton-Century-Crofts, 1980.

Haldeman S, Kohlbeck FJ, McGregor M. Risk factor and precipitating neck movements causing vertebrobasilar artery dissection after cervical trauma and spinal manipulation. *Spine* 1999;24:785–794.

Jull G. Management of cervical headache. *Man Ther* 1997;2:182–190.

Jull G, Bogduk N, Marsland A. The accuracy of manual diagnosis for cervical zygapophyseal joint syndromes. *Med J Austral* 1988;148:233–236.

Kleynhans AM. Complications of and contraindications to spinal manipulative therapy. In:

Patijn J. Complications in manual medicine: a review of the literature. *Man Med* 1991;6:89–92.

14

Twelve vertebrae comprise the thoracic spine and are noted for their posterior kyphosis. The thoracic spine is intimately related to the rib cage and essentially works as a single unit. Alteration in thoracic spine function influences the rib cage, and alteration in rib cage function alters the thoracic spine. Hence, from the respiratory–circulatory model of manual medicine, the thoracic spine assumes major importance in providing optimal functional capacity to the thoracic cage for respiration and circulation. The thoracic spine takes on additional importance from the neurologic perspective because of the relationship with the sympathetic division of the autonomic nervous system. All twelve segments of the thoracic spinal cord give origin to preganglionic sympathetic nerve fibers, which exit through the intervertebral canals of the thoracic vertebra and either synapse in, or traverse through, the lateral chain sympathetic ganglion lying on the anterior aspect of the costovertebral articulations. Recall that the preganglionic sympathetic nerve innervation to the soma and viscera above the diaphragm takes origin from the first four to five segments of the thoracic cord. All of the viscera and soma below the diaphragm receive their preganglionic sympathetic nerve fibers from the spinal cord below T5. Many of the tissue texture abnormalities used in the diagnosis of somatic dysfunction appear to be manifestations of altered secretomotor, pilomotor, and vasomotor functions of the skin viscera. Because the sympathetic nervous system is segmentally organized, skin viscera and internal viscera share many sympathetic nervous system reflexes. It has been clinically noted that internal viscera sharing preganglionic innervation origin in the spinal cord with somatic segments demonstrating tissue texture abnormality may be involved in dysfunctional or diseased states.

FUNCTIONAL ANATOMY

The typical thoracic vertebra has a body roughly equal in its transverse and anteroposterior diameters. The vertebral bodies have demifacets, located posterolaterally at the upper and lower margins of the body that articulate with the head of the rib. These demifacets are true arthrodial joints with a capsule and articular cartilage. The posterior arch of the thoracic vertebra has zygapophysial joints on the superior and inferior articular pillars. The superior zygapophysial joints face backward, laterally, and slightly superiorly, and the inferior zygapophysial joints face just the reverse. Theoretically this facet facing would provide a great deal of rotation to the thoracic vertebra, but rotation is restricted by the attachment of the ribs. The transverse processes are unique with the anterior surface having a small articular facet for articulation with the posterior-facing facet of the tubercle of the adjacent rib. The relationship of the costovertebral and costotransverse articulations greatly influences the type and amount of rib motion. The posterior aspects of the transverse processes are valuable anatomical landmarks for structural diagnosis of thoracic spine dysfunction. The spinous processes project backward and inferiorly and, in the midportion, are severely shingled one on the other (see rule of 3's, Chapter 5).

Atypical Thoracic Vertebrae

The atypical thoracic vertebrae are those that are transitional between the cervical and thoracic spines, and the thoracic and lumbar spines. T1 has the broadest transverse processes in the thoracic spine and they progressively become narrower from above downward. The lateral portion of the vertebral body of T1 has a unifacet for articulation with the head of the first rib. While the inferior zygapophysial joint facing is typically thoracic, the superior zygapophysial joint facing is transitional from the cervical spine and may have typical cervical characteristics. T1 is also the junction of the change in anteroposterior curve between the cervical and thoracic spines. Dysfunction of T1 profoundly affects the functional capacity of the thoracic inlet and related structures.

T12 is the location of transition to the lumbar spine. The superior zygapophysial joint facing is usually typically thoracic, whereas the inferior zygapophysial joint facing tends toward lumbar characteristics. There is a uni-facet on the lateral side of the body for articulation with the twelfth rib. The transverse processes are quite short and rudimentary and are difficult to palpate with certainty. T12 is the location for the change in the anteroposterior curve between the thoracic kyphosis and the lumbar lordosis, a location of change in mobility of two areas of the spine, and a point of frequent dysfunction.

Thoracic Kyphosis

The thoracic kyphosis is normally a smooth posterior convexity without severe areas of increased convexity or "flattening." The observation of "flat spots" within the thoracic kyphosis should alert the diagnostician to evaluate this area carefully for nonneutral, type II, vertebral somatic dysfunction. The thoracic kyphosis changes at its upper and lower extremities (at the transitional zones) to flow into the cervical and lumbar lordoses. Because of this, frequently the upper segments of the thoracic spine are viewed from the perspective of the cervical spine, while the lower thoracic segments are viewed as an extension of the lumbar spine. Many techniques for cervical dysfunction are highly appropriate and effective in the upper thoracic spine, and many lumbar techniques are effective in the lower thoracic spine.

THORACIC SPINE MOTION

Attachment of the ribs through the costovertebral, and cost-transverse articulations reduces the amount of mobility within the thoracic spine. Thoracic segments have forward-bending and backward-bending movement, as well as coupled movements of side bending and rotation to the same side and to opposite sides. The coupling of side bending and rotation in the thoracic spine is complex. Vertebral coupling depends on many factors, including whether the segments involved are above or below the apex of the thoracic kyphosis and whether you introduce side bending or rotation first. As a rule, if you introduce side bending with the thoracic spine in a neutral kyphosis, rotation occurs to the opposite side following neutral (type I) vertebral motion. If rotation is introduced first in the presence of a normal thoracic kyphosis, side bending and rotation occur to the same side following the rule of nonneutral (type II) vertebral mechanics. T1 through T3 most commonly follow nonneutral vertebral mechanics as a carry over from the lower cervical spine.

Despite the complexity of thoracic spine motion, clinical evaluation identifies that the thoracic spine can become dysfunctional with nonneutral single-segment (type II) dysfunctions and neutral (type I) group dysfunction. The screening and scanning examinations can lead the examiner to pursue specific segmental diagnosis in the thoracic spine. Identification of the dysfunctional segment begins by palpating soft-tissue change of hypertonicity in the fourth layer

of the erector spinae muscle mass in the medial groove between the spinous process and the longissimus. Palpable muscle hypertonicity of the deepest muscle layers including the multifidi and levator costales is pathognomonic of vertebral motion segment dysfunction at that level (Fig. 14.1).

Tissue texture changes of the skin and deeper layers of the posterior thoracic cage reflect the function of the sympathetic division of the autonomic nervous system. The changes include "skin drag" in areas of increased skin hydration, a "red response" following stroking of the skin from above downward reflecting change in vasomotor control, coldness or heat, bogginess, and change in thickness. Changes are seen in patients with musculoskeletal dysfunction and those with visceral disease primarily of the respiratory, cardiac, and gastrointestinal systems. It has been shown by studies of skin hydration, water evaporation loss rate, and temperature change that these palpable changes are different from those of a healthy asymptomatic population and differ between those with visceral disease or musculoskeletal disease or dysfunction. Much can be learned from judicious palpation of the soft tissues in addition to active and passive motion testing. Nonneutral dysfunctions within the thoracic spine appear to have an effect on muscle tone of segmentally related muscles, perhaps through an arthrokinetic reflex mechanism. Extended, rotated, and side-bent (ERS) dysfunctions of the midscapular region, particularly several segments stacked one on top of another, appear commonly with weakness of the serratus anterior and rhomboid muscles. Flexed, rotated, and side-bent (FRS) dysfunctions of the lower thoracic spine around T8 are associated with weakness of the lower

Figure 14.1.
Palpation of hypertonic fourth-layer muscle.

trapezius muscle, which is essential for normal scapular control.

MOTION TESTING

Vertebral motion testing and the diagnosis of restriction of vertebral motion have been described in Chapter 6. The most useful test is to monitor change in the relationship of pairs of transverse processes through an arc of forward bending to backward bending. In the upper thoracic spine from T1 to T5, the operator monitors the behavior of a pair of transverse processes during the introduction of active forward and backward bending of the head on the neck with the patient sitting. With nonneutral (type II) ERS dysfunction, the transverse process on one side will become more prominent during forward bending and the transverse processes become symmetric during backward bending. In nonneutral (type II) FRS dysfunction, one transverse process becomes more prominent during backward bending and the transverse processes become symmetric during forward bending. In the presence of a neutral group (type I) dysfunction, three or more vertebrae, the transverse processes are prominent on one side. During the forward- to backward-bending arc, the posterior transverse processes may change a little, but they never become symmetric.

In the mid and lower thoracic spine the evaluation is performed in the sitting position with the patient assuming the three positions of forward bending, neutral, and backward bending, or in the three static positions of being fully forward bent, prone in neutral on the table, and in backward bending in the prone prop position.

The examiner always relates one pair of transverse processes to the segment below, asking is it the same or different? As an example, if T8 has restriction of backward bending, left rotation, and left-side bending (FRS$_{right}$), the superior surface of T8 is unlevel with side bending to the right. When the patient is in the neutral position, the segments above T8 should form a neutral curve with side bending left and rotation right as an adaptive response to maintain the body erect. In the backward-bent body position, and in the absence of dysfunction above T8, all of the superior segments should follow the right rotation of T8 with their respective transverse processes being prominent on the right side. When the patient is in the forward-bent position, T8 becomes level in the coronal plane and all of the nondysfunctional segments above should follow and be straight in the coronal plane.

Structural diagnosis in the presence of a primary structural scoliosis of the thoracic spine becomes quite difficult. The segments involved in a primary scoliosis behave as a neutral, group (type I) dysfunction. Patients with a primary structural scoliosis of the thoracic spine have few symptoms of back pain until a relatively minor traumatic episode occurs. Pain and restriction of motion become quite evident. A nonneutral (type II) dysfunction within the primary scoliotic curve is frequently found in this situation. The diagnosis of these nonneutral (type II) dysfunctions can be quite difficult, but if the examiner is diligent in searching from one segment to the other, he or she frequently observes a nonneutral single-segment vertebral somatic dysfunction within the curve. The usual observation is a single vertebral motion segment with rotation into the concavity. Single-segment fourth-layer muscle hypertonicity is a valuable finding in making a diagnosis of the presence and location of a nonneutral dysfunction within the primary curve. The difficulty is to identify a segment that is rotated in the opposite direction of the primary curve. The principle of relating the superior segment to the one below still holds. Also, recall that by convention we speak of the scoliotic curve as being side bent and rotated to opposite sides. This is true for the entire curve in three-dimensional space. When evaluated segment by segment, the rule of side bending and rotation to opposite sides holds below the apex of the curve, but in the segments above the apex, the rotation is to the same side as the curve gradually returns to the midline.

Thoracic Spine Diagnosis

Upper Thoracic Spine (T1-T5)

1. Patient is sitting on table with operator standing behind.

2. Operator's thumbs palpate the posterior aspect of the transverse processes of the segment under diagnosis (Fig. 14.2).

3. The operator follows the pair of transverse processes during the backward-bending arc as the patient is asked to look up toward the ceiling (Fig. 14.3).

4. The operator follows the pair of transverse processes through a forward-bending arc while asking the patient to look down at the floor (Fig. 14.4).

   Note: It is easier to follow a pair of transverse processes during backward bending than forward bending.

5. Based on the behavior of the transverse processes during the forward-bending, neutral, and backward-bending arcs, an appropriate single-segment vertebral motion somatic dysfunction diagnosis is made.

Figure 14.3.

Figure 14.2.

Figure 14.4.

Thoracic Spine Diagnosis

Mid to Lower Thoracic Spine

Dynamic Process

1. The patient is sitting on table with operator standing behind.

2. The operator palpates the posterior aspect of a pair of transverse processes at the segment under evaluation (Fig. 14.5).

3. Patient is asked to look up at the ceiling and arch the back by pushing the abdomen anteriorly as the operator follows the transverse processes into backward bending (Fig. 14.6).

4. Patient is asked to slump the back and forward bend the trunk as the operator follows the transverse processes into flexion (Fig. 14.7).

5. Operator evaluates the behavior of the transverse processes through the forward- and backward-bending arcs, making a diagnosis of a single-segment vertebral somatic dysfunction of the ERS or FRS type.

Figure 14.6.

Figure 14.5.

Figure 14.7.

Thoracic Spine Diagnosis

Mid to Lower Thoracic Spine Static Three Positions

1. Patient prone on the table with the operator standing at the side with thumbs palpating a pair of transverse processes (Fig. 14.8).

2. Operator monitors the posterior aspect of the paired transverse processes in the backward-bent (prone prop) position (Fig. 14.9).

3. Operator evaluates the pair of transverse processes in the static forward-bent position (Fig. 14.7).

4. Evaluation of a single-segment nonneutral vertebral dysfunction is identified by comparing the behavior of the paired transverse processes through the three static positions of neutral, backward bent, and forward bent.

Figure 14.8.

Figure 14.9.

MANUAL MEDICINE TECHNIQUE FOR THORACIC SPINE DYSFUNCTION

In the treatment sequence of a patient presenting with multiple areas of somatic dysfunction, the thoracic spine is treated before the treatment of dysfunction of the ribs. This fundamental rule is broken only if the resolution of restriction from rib cage dysfunction assists in the treatment process of the thoracic spine dysfunction. Most muscle energy procedures for thoracic spine somatic dysfunctions are performed with the patient sitting but all can be modified for a patient in the horizontal position, either supine, lateral recumbent, or prone. As in the cervical spine, muscle energy technique is usually performed as the initial intervention. If the muscle energy procedure is ineffective and the structural diagnostic process has identified the presence of a chronic, deep motion restrictor in the articular and periarticular structures, a mobilization with impulse technique becomes indicated.

Thoracic Spine

Muscle Energy Technique
T1-T5
Sitting (Example: T4-T5)
Diagnosis
    Position: Extended, rotated left, side-bent left (ERS$_{left}$)
    Motion Restriction: Forward bending, right rotation, right-side bending

1. Patient sitting on the table with the operator behind.

2. Operator's left hand monitors the T4 to T5 segment with the left index finger in the interspinous space and the left middle finger overlying the posterior left transverse process of T4 (Fig. 14.10).

3. Operator's right hand is on the top of the patient's head, and the operator's trunk is against the posterior aspect of the patient's body.

4. Operator introduces forward bending to the T4 to T5 segment by anterior-to-posterior translation of the patient's body localized at the T4 to T5 level (Fig. 14.11).

Figure 14.10.

Figure 14.11.

5. Operator engages the right-side bending and right rotational barriers by introducing right-to-left translation through the trunk with localization at the T4 to T5 level (Fig. 14.12).

6. Operator resists a backward bending, left-side bending, or left rotational effort of the patient's head and neck by giving resistance with the right hand (Fig. 14.13). A 3- to 5-second isometric muscle contraction is requested.

7. After relaxation the operator engages the new forward-bending, right-side bending, and right rotational barriers and the patient performs three to five repetitions of the isometric muscle contraction (Fig. 14.14).

8. Retest.

Figure 14.13.

Figure 14.12.

Figure 14.14.

Thoracic Spine

Muscle Energy Technique
T1-T5
Sitting (Example T2-T3)
Diagnosis
 Position: Flexed, rotated left, side-bent left(FRS$_{left}$)
 Motion Restriction: Backward bending, right rotation, and right-side bending

1. Patient is sitting with the operator behind.

2. Operator's right index finger palpates the interspinous space between T2 to T3 and the right middle finger palpates over the right transverse process of T2 (Fig. 14.15).

3. Operator's left hand and forearm control the patient's head and neck with the operator's trunk against the posterior aspect of the left trunk of the patient (Fig. 14.16). Operator's left hand introduces a small amount of right rotation to gap the right zygapophysial joint at T2 to T3.

4. Operator translates the trunk forward with the thumb over the mid to lower scapular region. The patient is asked to tuck the chin in and carry the head into posterior translation localizing extension at the T2 to T3 segment (Fig. 14.17).

5. The patient is instructed to perform a mild isometric contraction of forward bending, left-side bending, or left rotation of the head and neck against the resisting left hand and forearm of the operator for a 3- to 5-second contraction.

6. After relaxation, a new backward-bending, right-side bending, and right rotational barrier is engaged, and the patient is instructed to repeat the isometric contraction three to five times (Fig. 14.18).

7. Retest.

Figure 14.15.

Figure 14.17.

Figure 14.16.

Figure 14.18.

Thoracic Spine

Muscle Energy Technique
T1-T5
Sitting
Diagnosis
 Dysfunction: Neutral, side-bent right, rotated left
 (NS$_{right}$/R$_{left}$), Easy normal, left convexity (EN$_{left}$)
 Motion Restriction: Side-bending left, rotation right

1. Patient sits erect with operator standing behind.

2. Operator's left thumb is localized to the apex of the
   left convexity (Fig. 14.19).

3. Operator's right hand controls the patient's head
   and stabilizes the cervical spine (Fig. 14.20).

4. Left-side bending and right rotation are introduced
   by translation from left to right localized by the
   thumb (Fig. 14.21).

5. Patient is instructed to side bend the head to the
   right against the resistance offered by the operator's
   right hand and forearm (Fig. 14.22).

6. Following relaxation, the left-side bending and right
   rotational barriers are again engaged, and the patient repeats the isometric muscle contraction of
   right-side bending.

7. Three to five repetitions are made of a 3- to second isometric contraction.

8. Retest.

Figure 14.19.

Figure 14.21.

Figure 14.20.

Figure 14.22.

Thoracic Spine

Muscle Energy Technique
- T5-T12
- Sitting (Example, T8 to T9)
- Diagnosis
  - Position: Extended (backward bent), right rotated, right side-bent (ERS_{right})
  - Motion Restriction: Flexion (forward bending), left rotation, left-side bending

1. Patient sitting with operator behind.

2. Patient's left hand holds the right shoulder. Operator's left arm controls the patient's trunk with the left hand grasping the right shoulder and the patient's left shoulder resting in the operator's left axilla (Fig. 14.23).

3. Operator's right index finger monitors the interspinous space at T8 to T9 and right middle finger monitors the right transverse process of T8 (Fig. 14.24).

4. The forward-bending (flexion) barrier is engaged by an anterior-to-posterior translation of the trunk at the T8 to T9 level (Fig. 14.25).

Figure 14.24.

Figure 14.23.

Figure 14.25.

5. The left-side bending and left rotational barriers are engaged by translation of the patient's trunk from left to right at the T8 to T9 level (Fig. 14.26).

6. Patient is instructed to perform a right-side bending isometric contraction against resistance offered by the operator's left hand and arm for 3 to 5 seconds (Fig. 14.27).

7. Following relaxation, all three barriers are reengaged and the patient performs three to five repetitions of a 3- to 5-second isometric contraction.

8. Retest.

Note: This technique can be adapted into the upper lumbar spine.

Figure 14.26.

Figure 14.27.

Thoracic Spine

Muscle Energy Technique
T5-T12 (Example, T8-T9)
Diagnosis
    Position: Flexed (forward bent), rotated right, side-bent right (FRS$_{right}$)
    Motion Restriction: Extension (backward bending), rotation left, side bending left

1. Patient sitting with operator behind.

2. Operator's left hand controls the patient's trunk through a contact on the left shoulder. Operator's right index finger monitors the interspinous space of T8 to T9 and the middle finger monitors the right transverse process of T8 (Fig. 14.28).

3. With the spine in the erect neutral position, rotation left of T8 is introduced by right-to-left translation of T8 to T9 with the patient dropping the right shoulder and shifting the weight to the left buttock (Fig. 14.29).

4. Patient is instructed to perform a left-side bending isometric contraction against resistance offered by the operator's left hand. This is repeated two to three times to enhance left rotation of T8.

5. Left-side bending and extension barriers are engaged by the operator depressing the patient's left shoulder and the patient shifting the body weight to the right buttock following the operator's instruction of projecting the abdomen over the right knee (Fig. 14.30).

6. The patient is instructed to lift the left shoulder toward the ceiling (right-side bending effort) or pull the left shoulder forward (right rotational effort) for 3 to 5 seconds and three to five repetitions.

7. After each effort, extension, left-side bending, and left rotational barriers are reengaged by projecting the abdomen over the right knee and translating the trunk from left to right at T8 to T9.

Figure 14.29.

Figure 14.28.

Figure 14.30.

8. Patient's trunk is now returned to midline with operator's right hand blocking the T9 segment (Fig. 14.31).

9. Operator resists trunk forward bending by the patient's shoulders with the resisting left arm (Fig. 14.32).

10. Retest.

Figure 14.31.

Figure 14.32.

Thoracic Spine

Muscle Energy Technique
T5-T12
Group Dysfunction
Diagnosis
    Position: NS$_{left}$R$_{right}$) or (EN$_{right}$)
    Motion Restriction: Neutral, side bending right, rotation left.

1. Patient sitting erect in neutral with operator behind.
2. Operator's right thumb is localized at the apex of the right convexity with an anteromedial vector of force (Fig. 14.33).

3. Patient's left hand grasps the right shoulder and the operator places the left arm through the patient's left axilla and grasps the right shoulder (Fig. 14.34).
4. Side-bending right and rotation left barriers are engaged by a right-to-left translatory movement at the apex of the convexity (Fig. 14.35).
5. Operator's left arm resists a 3- to 5-second isometric contraction of left-side bending by the patient (Fig. 14.36).
6. Following each isometric effort a new right-side bending and left rotational barrier is engaged and the patient repeats the left-side bending isometric contraction with three to five repetitions.
7. Retest.

Figure 14.33.

Figure 14.35.

Figure 14.34.

Figure 14.36.

Thoracic Spine

Mobilization with Impulse Technique
T1-T5
Sitting (Example: T3-T4)
Diagnosis
  Position: Extended (backward bent), left rotated, left side bent (ERS_{left})
  Motion Restriction: Flexion (forward bending), right rotation, right-side bending

1. Patient sitting with operator standing behind.

2. Operator's left hand and forearm control the patient's head and left-side of the neck. Operator's right hand is over the right shawl area with the thumb contacting the right side of the spinous process of T3 (the superior segment of the dysfunctional vertebral motion unit) (Fig. 14.37).

3. Operator's left hand introduces flexion, right-side bending, and right rotation of the patient's head and neck through translation from before backward and from right-to-left localizing at the T3-T4 level (Fig. 14.38).

4. When all barriers are engaged, a high-velocity, low-amplitude thrust is introduced through the operator's right thumb against the spinous process in a right-to-left translatory movement (Fig. 14.39).

5. Retest.

Figure 14.38.

Figure 14.37.

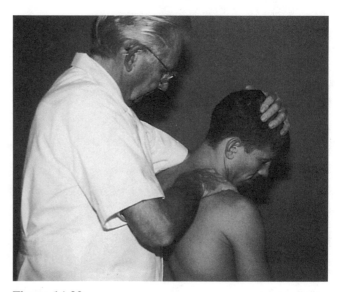

Figure 14.39.

Thoracic Spine

Mobilization with Impulse Technique
T1-T5
Sitting
Diagnosis (Example: T3-T4)
  Position: FRS$_{left}$
  Motion Restriction: Extension (backward bending), right rotation, right-side bending.

1. Patient sitting with operator standing behind. Patient's left arm may be draped over the operator's left thigh with the left foot on the table.

2. Patient's head and left side of the neck are controlled by the operator's left hand and forearm. Operator's right hand overlies the patient's right shawl area with the thumb in contact with the right side of the spinous process of T-3 (the superior segment of the dysfunctional vertebral motor unit) (Fig. 14.40).

3. Operator's left forearm and hand introduce extension (backward bending), right-side bending, and right rotation of the patient's head and neck to T3-T4 by translation from behind forward and from right to left (Fig. 14.41).

4. With the extension, right-side bending, and right rotational barriers engaged, a high-velocity, low-amplitude thrust is introduced from right to left through the thumb contact with the spinous process of T-3 (Fig. 14.42).

5. Retest.

Figure 14.41.

Figure 14.40.

Figure 14.42.

Thoracic Spine

Mobilization with Impulse Technique
T1-T5
Sitting
Diagnosis
    Group Dysfunction (type I) (Example:T1-T4)
    Position: $NS_{right}R_{left}$) or EN_{left}
    Motion Restriction: Side bending left, rotation right

1. Patient sitting with operator behind. Patient's right arm is draped over the operator's right leg with the right foot on the table.

2. Operator's right hand and forearm control the patient's head and right side of the neck. Operator's left hand is placed over the patient's left shawl area with the left thumb at the intertransverse space between T2 and T3 (Fig. 14.43).

3. Operator's right hand and forearm introduce left-side bending and right rotation with localization at the apex of the left convexity through the left thumb with an anteromedial vector of force (Fig. 14.44).

4. The left-side bending and right rotational barriers are engaged by a left-to-right translatory movement of the operator's left hand and forearm (Fig. 14.45).

5. A high-velocity, low-amplitude thrust is introduced through the operator's left hand and thumb in an anteromedial direction from left to right (Fig. 14.46).

6. Retest.

Figure 14.43.

Figure 14.45.

Figure 14.44.

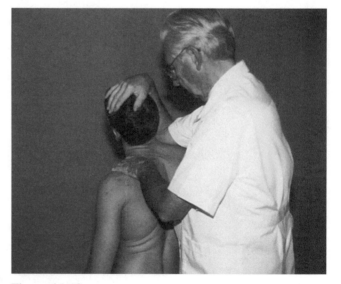

Figure 14.46.

Thoracic Spine

Mobilization with Impulse Technique
T1-T5
Prone (Example: T3-T4)
Diagnosis
  Position: FRS$_{left}$
  Motion Restriction: Extension (backward bending) right rotation, right-side bending

1. Patient prone with operator standing at head (Fig. 14.47).

2. Operator's hands move patient's chin to the right (introducing right-side bending) and rotating the face to the right (Fig. 14.48).

3. Operator's right pisiform is placed on the right transverse process of T4 (inferior segment of the dysfunctional vertebral motor unit) (Fig. 14.49).

4. A high-velocity, low-amplitude thrust is applied through the pisiform of the right hand with the operator's left hand stabilizing the head and neck in right-side bending and right rotation. The thrust direction is ventral, rotating T4 to the left with extension, resulting in closure of the right zygapophysial joint at T3-T4.

5. Retest.

Figure 14.48.

Figure 14.47.

Figure 14.49.

Thoracic Spine

Mobilization with Impulse Technique
T1-T5
Prone (Example: group dysfunction T1-T4)
Diagnosis

Position: Neutral, side-bent right, rotated left
(NS$_{right}$R$_{left}$) or (EN$_{left}$)
Motion Restriction: Side bending left, rotation right

1. Patient prone with operator standing with hand controlling patient's head (Fig. 14.50).

2. With chin staying at the midline operator's left hand introduces left-side bending and right rotation to the apex of the group dysfunction (Fig. 14.51).

3. With the thumb at the intertransverse space of T2-T3, a high-velocity, low-amplitude thrust is performed with an anteromedial thrust of the thumb with the left hand holding the patient's head and neck stable, or an exaggeration of the left-side bending and right rotation of the head and neck through the operator's left hand against a stable fulcrum of the right thumb.

4. An alternative contact is with the operator's right pisiform bone at the intertransverse space of T2 to T3 on the left with similar thrusting force anteromedially with the right hand or exaggeration of the left-side bending right rotation of the head and neck against the fulcrum of the right pisiform (Fig. 14.52).

5. Retest.

Figure 14.51.

Figure 14.50.

Figure 14.52.

Thoracic Spine

Mobilization with Impulse Technique
T5-T10
Prone (Example: T6-T7)
Diagnosis
    Position: FRS$_{right}$
    Motion Restriction: Extension (backward bent), left rotation, left-side bending

1. Patient prone with operator standing on patient's left side.
2. Operator's left pisiform contacts the superior aspect of the left transverse process of T6 with the fingers pointing in a caudad direction (Fig. 14.53).

3. Operator's right pisiform contacts the right transverse process of T6 with anterior compression introducing left rotation of T6 (Fig. 14.54).
4. The restrictive barrier is engaged by a caudad movement with the operator's left pisiform and an anterior movement of the operator's right pisiform.
5. A high-velocity, low-amplitude thrust is made through both hands in a ventral direction introducing extension, left-side bending, and left rotation of T6 (Fig. 14.55).
6. Retest.

Figure 14.54.

Figure 14.53.

Figure 14.55.

Thoracic Spine

Mobilization with Impulse Technique
T3-T12
Supine
Principles of the Technique

Principle 1. Establish Lever Arm

1. Patient supine with operator standing at side.

2. Patient crosses arms over chest and holds the opposite shoulder. The arm opposite the operator is the superior (Fig. 14.56).

3. Alternative arm position two has the patient clasp the two hands together behind the cervical spine (not the head). This arm position is particular useful in the lower thoracic region (Fig. 14.57).

4. Alternative arm position three is unilateral using the arm opposite the operator grasping the patient's opposite shoulder (Fig. 14.58).

5. Alternative arm position four has patient grasp the right shoulder with the left hand and the left elbow with the right hand (Fig. 14.59).

Principle 2. Establish Fulcrum

1. The hand is placed to control the inferior segment of the dysfunctional vertebral motion segment with the spinous processes placed in the palm of the hand and with the thumb along the side of the spinous processes (Fig. 14.60).

2. Alternative hand position two is the use of the flexed second, third, fourth, and fifth fingers on one side of the spinous process and the thenar and hy-

Figure 14.56.

Figure 14.58.

Figure 14.57.

Figure 14.59.

pothenar eminence on the other side of the spinous process (Fig. 14.61). This hand position may be uncomfortable both to the patient and operator.

3. A third alternative hand position uses flexion of the proximal and distal interphalangeal joints of the index finger against one transverse process of the inferior segment and the metacarpophalangeal joint of the thumb on the opposite transverse process (Fig. 14.62). This hand position is preferred as it provides for a contact of the thenar eminence against the rib shaft of a dysfunctional rib associated with nonneutral (ERS) dysfunctions of the thoracic spine.

Principle 3. Localization of the Lever Arm to the Fulcrum

1. The patient is rolled toward the operator to place the fulcrum on the inferior vertebra of the dysfunctional vertebral motor motion segment.

2. The patient is returned to the neutral position and a body contact is made with the crossed arm lever arm. This preferably is the epigastrium. Care should be taken not to put compressive force against the operator's rib cage, or in a female operator against breast tissue. A folded towel or small pillow can be used to cushion the patient's elbows against the operator's trunk (Fig. 14.63).

Principle 4. Localization of Thrust

1. The fulcrum holds the inferior segment so that the superior vertebra can be moved in the appropriate direction to engage the restrictive barrier.

2. The thrusting force is directed at the superior aspect of the fulcrum.

Figure 14.60.

Figure 14.62.

Figure 14.61.

Figure 14.63.

Thoracic Spine

Mobilization with Impulse Technique
T3-T12
Supine
Diagnosis
   Position: Bilaterally extended (both facets in the closed position)
   Motion Restriction: Sagittal plane flexion

1. Patient supine with operator standing at side.

2. The lever arm is established by crossing both arms over the chest (or one of the alternative lever arm positions).

3. Operator places the fulcrum hand under the patient's torso localized to the inferior segment of the dysfunctional vertebral unit.

4. Patient returned to neutral midline position with localization of lever arm to fulcrum. Operator's cephalic hand controls patient's head and neck to introduce flexion (Fig. 14.64).

5. Operator flexes thoracic spine down to the superior vertebra of the dysfunctional vertebral motion unit (Fig. 14.65).

6. A high-velocity, low-amplitude thrust is performed by dropping the operator's body weight through the lever arm to the fulcrum with slight exaggeration of the patient's flexed position.

7. Retest.

Figure 14.64.

Figure 14.65.

Thoracic Spine

Mobilization with Impulse Technique
T3-T12
Supine
Diagnosis
    Position: Bilaterally flexed (both facets in the open position)
    Motion Restriction: Sagittal plane extension

1. Patient supine with operator standing at side.

2. Lever arm is established by crossing the arms across the patient's chest holding each shoulder.

3. Operator's hand is placed as the fulcrum on the lower segment of the dysfunctional vertebral motion unit.

4. Patient returned to midline with operator controlling the patient's upper trunk, neck, and head.

5. Patient flexes upper trunk just past the fulcrum (Fig. 14.66).

6. Operator drops patient's head, neck, and upper trunk into extension just over the fulcrum.

7. A high-velocity, low-amplitude thrust through the operator's trunk against the lever arm takes the superior segment into extension over the fulcrum (Fig. 14.67).

8. Retest.

Figure 14.66.

Figure 14.67.

Thoracic Spine

Mobilization with Impulse Technique
T3-T12
Supine
Diagnosis: Example, T4-T5
Position: Extended (backward bent), rotated left, side bent left (ERS$_{left}$)
Motion Restriction: Flexion (forward bending), right rotation and right-side bending

1. Patient supine with operator standing on patient's right side.

2. Patient established lever arm by crossing hands over chest.

3. Operator's right hand establishes a fulcrum on both transverse processes of T5.

4. Patient is returned to neutral position and lever arm is localized to the fulcrum.

5. Operator's left hand introduces flexion, right-side bending, and right rotation of the neck and upper thoracic spine down to T4 (Fig. 14.68).

6. A high-velocity, low-amplitude thrust is made by the operator's body weight on the lever arm to the fulcrum resulting in flexion, right-side bending, right rotation of T4, and opening of the left zygapophysial joint (Fig. 14.69).

7. Retest.

Figure 14.68.

Figure 14.69.

Thoracic Spine

Mobilization with Impulse Technique
T3-T12
Supine
Diagnosis (Example: Group dysfunction T3 to T6)
  Position: $NS_{right}R_{left}$ or EN_{left}
  Motion Restriction: Side bending left, rotation right

1. Patient supine on table with operator standing on right side.

2. Patient establishes the lever arm by crossing the arms over the chest.

3. Operator's right hand establishes the fulcrum with the metacarpophalangeal joint localized to the left intertransverse space of T4 to T5 using the hand position shown in Fig. 14.60.

4. Operator localizes lever arm to fulcrum and with the left hand flexes and extends the head and upper trunk to ensure neutral mechanics at the dysfunctional segments (Fig. 14.70).

5. Operator's left hand introduces left-side bending and right rotation down to the dysfunctional segments (Fig. 14.71).

6. Operator's torso provides a thrusting force through the lever arm to the fulcrum resulting in left-side bending and right rotation of the dysfunctional segments.

7. Retest.

Figure 14.70.

Figure 14.71.

Thoracic Spine

Mobilization with Impulse Technique
T5-T12
Sitting

Principle 1. Establish a Lever Arm

1. Patient sitting on a stepladder treatment stool and clasps both hands together against the cervical spine (not occiput) (Fig. 14.72).

2. Operator threads both hands under the patient's axilla and grasps each forearm providing control of the patient's trunk (Fig. 14.73).

Principle 2. Establish a Fulcrum

1. Operator places the knee on the inferior vertebra of the dysfunctional vertebral motion unit, against the spinous process or a transverse process (Fig. 14.74).

2. Operator places foot on appropriate step of the stepladder treatment stool to localize the knee at the dysfunctional vertebral motion unit.

Figure 14.73.

Figure 14.72.

Figure 14.74.

3. Alternatively, a rolled towel can be used as the fulcrum with the edge against the inferior segment of the dysfunctional vertebral motion unit (Fig. 14.75).

4. The operator's trunk is placed against the towel fulcrum to control the inferior vertebra (Fig. 14.76).

Principle 3. Thrust Through the Lever Arm to the Fulcrum

1. Operator's two arms pull the patient's trunk toward the fulcrum or lift the trunk over the fulcrum depending on whether a flexion or an extension thrust is necessary.

2. The thrusting procedure occurs with operator's both arms controlling the patient's trunk through the operator's hand contact on the forearms.

Figure 14.75.

Figure 14.76.

Thoracic Spine

Mobilization with Impulse Technique
T5-T12
Sitting
Diagnosis
   Position: Bilateral extended
   Motion Restriction: Bilateral flexion

1. Operator seated on stool with hands grasped behind neck.

2. Operator places the knee or towel fulcrum on the spinous process of the inferior vertebra of the dysfunctional vertebral motion unit.

3. Operator threads both hands through the axilla and grasps each forearm of the patient.

4. Flexion is introduced until localized at the dysfunctional segment (Fig. 14.77).

5. Operator applies a high-velocity, low-amplitude thrust by pulling directly posteriorly toward the fulcrum enhancing flexion from above against the fixed lower vertebra.

6. Retest.

Thoracic Spine

Mobilization with Impulse Technique
T5-T12
Sitting
Diagnosis
   Position: Bilateral flexed
   Motion Restriction: Bilateral extension

1. Patient sitting with hands clasped behind neck.

2. Operator stands behind patient with knee or rolled towel as fulcrum on spinous process of inferior vertebra of dysfunctional vertebral motion unit.

3. Operator threads both hands under patient's axilla grasping patient's forearms.

4. Operator localizes to the dysfunctional segment by extending the patient's trunk over the fulcrum (Fig. 14.78).

5. Operator applies a high-velocity, low-amplitude thrust by a lifting motion extending the patient's upper trunk over the fulcrum.

6. Retest.

Figure 14.77.

Figure 14.78.

Thoracic Spine

Mobilization with Impulse Technique
  T5-T12
  Sitting
  Diagnosis (Example: T8-T9)
    Position: Extended, rotated left, side-bent left (ERS_{left})
    Motion Restriction: Flexion (forward bending), right rotation, right-side bending

1. Patient sitting with hands clasped behind neck.

2. Operator stands behind patient and establishes the fulcrum against the right transverse process of T9 (the inferior vertebra).

3. Operator threads arms through patient's axillae and grasps each forearm.

4. Operator localizes patient's upper trunk to the barrier of flexion, right-side bending, and right rotation (Fig. 14.79).

5. Operator applies a flexion high-velocity, low-amplitude thrust by the operator pulling the patient's upper trunk toward the fulcrum.

6. Retest.

Thoracic Spine

Mobilization with Impulse Technique
  T5-T12
  Sitting
  Diagnosis (Example: T8-T9)
    Position: Flexed, rotated left, side–bent left (FRS_{left})
    Motion Restriction: Extension (backward bending), right rotation, right-side bending

1. Patient sitting with hands clasped behind neck.

2. Operator establishes fulcrum against the right transverse process of T-9 (the inferior segment).

3. Operator threads arms through patient's axillae and grasps patient's forearms.

4. Operator engages extension, right-side bending, and right rotational barrier at the dysfunctional segment (Fig. 14.80).

5. Operator applies a high-velocity, low-amplitude thrust by lifting and posteriorly translating the patient's trunk over the fulcrum.

6. Retest.

Figure 14.79.

Figure 14.80.

Thoracic Spine

Mobilization with Impulse Technique
T5-T12
Sitting
Diagnosis (Example: Group dysfunction T7 to T10
    Position: Neutral, sidebent left, rotated right
    ($NS_{left}R_{right}$) or (EN_{right})
    Motion Restriction: Right-side bending, left rotation

1. Patient sitting with hands clasped behind neck.

2. Operator establishes the fulcrum at the intertransverse space on the right of T8 to T9.

3. Operator threads arms through patient's axillae and grasps patient's forearms.

4. Operator flexes and extends to neutral, then introduces right-side bending and left rotation to localize at the apex of the dysfunctional segments (Fig. 14.81).

5. Operator applies a high-velocity, low-amplitude thrust of the patient's upper trunk through the fulcrum enhancing right-side bending and left rotation of the dysfunctional vertebra.

6. Retest.

CONCLUSION

In the usual treatment sequence, the thoracic spine should be evaluated and treated before evaluation and treatment of rib function. Occasionally it is useful to treat a major rib dysfunction first to better evaluate and treat dysfunction of the thoracic spine.

In the seated mid to lower thoracic mobilization with impulse technique, this author prefers to use the knee or rolled towel as a fulcrum on the inferior vertebra of the dysfunctional vertebral motion unit. Other practitioners and authors will occasionally apply the fulcrum against the posterior transverse process of the superior vertebra of the dysfunctional vertebral motion unit and thrust forward with the knee or the trunk through the rolled up towel to derotate the dysfunctional vertebra. In either instance, it is imperative that there be good localization of the thrusting force to the fulcrum.

It should be noted that the prone mobilization with impulse technique for T5 through T12 is only used for FRS dysfunctions. This technique is contraindicated in an ERS dysfunction. While it is possible to adapt the supine mobilization with impulse techniques for T5 through T12 for FRS dysfunctions, it is difficult to perform. It is recommended that for FRS dysfunctions in this region that the prone technique be used. In the prone and sitting mobilization with impulse techniques, it is important that the localization to the transverse processes be precise and not against the adjacent rib shaft because repetitive thrusting on a rib shaft can cause hypermobility of the costovertebral and costotransverse articulations resulting in chronic structural rib dysfunction.

SUGGESTED READING

Flynn TA, ed. *The thoracic spine and rib cage: musculoskeletal evaluation and treatment.* Boston: Butterworth-Heinemann, 1996.

Figure 14.81.

15

RIB CAGE TECHNIQUE

The thoracic cage consists of the 12 thoracic vertebra, the paired 12 ribs, the sternum, and the related ligaments and muscles. The ribs maintain the contour of the thoracic cage, much like a cylinder, and house the thoracic viscera, primarily the heart and great vessels, the lungs, trachea, and esophagus. The thoracoabdominal diaphragm (Fig. 15.1) functions as the piston within the cylinder of the thoracic cage, changing the relative negative intrathoracic pressure for respiration. In addition to being the main muscle of respiration, the diaphragm is the major "pump" of the low pressure venous and lymphatic systems.

FUNCTIONAL ANATOMY

Thoracic Inlet

At the cephalic end of the thoracic cage is the thoracic inlet (Fig. 15.2), which is bounded by the body of T1, the medial margins of the right and left first ribs, the posterior aspect of the manubrium of the sternum, and the medial end of the right and left clavicles. Through the thoracic inlet, pass the esophagus, trachea, and major vessels of the neck and upper extremity.

Figure 15.1.
Diaphragm.

261

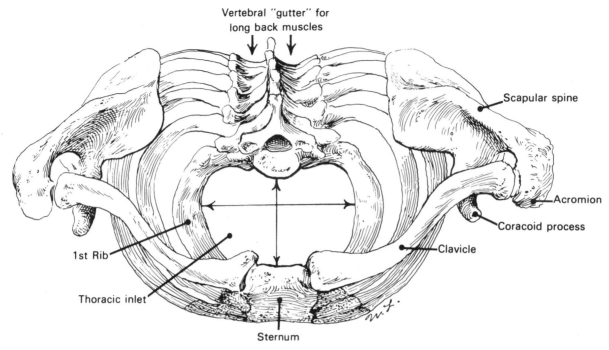

Figure 15.2.
Thoracic outlet.

Lymphatic Drainage

The thoracic inlet is of importance in lymphatic drainage because the lymphatic system for the whole body drains into the venous system immediately posterior to the medial end of the clavicle and first rib (Fig. 15.3). Altered rib cage function influences respiratory activity, circulatory activity (arterial, venous, and lymphatic), and neural activity (particularly of the intercostal nerves and the brachial plexus superior to rib one).

Sympathetic Trunk

The thoracic lateral chain ganglia of the sympathetic division of the autonomic nervous system lies anterior to the capsule of the costovertebral articulations and are tightly bound down to the posterior thoracic wall by heavy, dense fascia.

Rib cage dysfunction is frequently a major component of dysfunction in the musculoskeletal system and is frequently painless. These dysfunctions are frequently described as respiratory restrictions and contribute to the persistence and recurrence of dysfunction within the thoracic spine and can contribute as long restrictors to dysfunction of the musculoskeletal system elsewhere.

INTERCOSTAL NEURALGIA

Other rib dysfunctions are found in association with pain in the intercostal space, commonly described as intercostal neuralgia. These rib dysfunctions are de-scribed as structural rib dysfunctions. They contribute to restriction of respiratory activity of the rib cage as well, but they primarily are found as the dysfunctions associated with chest wall pain. Intercostal neuralgic symptoms in the absence of structural rib dysfunctions should alert the physician to search for organic causes of intercostal neuralgia (e.g., herpes zoster, cord tumor, and primary or secondary inflammatory or neoplastic disease of the thoracic viscera).

RIB ANATOMY

Ribs are described as typical or atypical. The atypical ribs are those with the numbers one and two, namely ribs one, two, 11, and 12. The first rib is broad, flat, and articulates with T1 by a unifacet. It is the lateral boundary of the thoracic inlet and has multiple types of dysfunction. The second rib articulates by two demifacets with T1 and T2. Anteriorly it articulates by a strong cartilaginous attachment with the manubriogladiolar junction of the sternum at the angle of Louis. Alteration in function of the second rib profoundly influences the function of the sternum and frequently contributes to pain syndromes in the upper extremity (Fig. 15.4). Ribs 11 and 12 articulate by unifacets with the eleventh and twelfth vertebra. They do not have typical costotransverse articulations. They are both associated with the muscles of the posterior abdominal wall. The quadratus lumborum muscle attaches to the inferior margin of rib 12. The twelfth rib is frequently asymmetric in length. Neither rib attaches to the costal arch.

is the posterior aspect of the rib shaft and is the attachment of the iliocostalis muscles.

DIAPHRAGM

The diaphragm (Fig. 15.1) is the primary muscle of respiration. When it contracts it descends and increases the negative intrathoracic pressure enhancing inspiration. As it relaxes, the passive recoil of the thoracic cage results in exhalation. Other inspiratory muscles include the external intercostals, the sternocostalis, and the accessory muscles of inspiration. These include the sternocleidomastoid, scalenes, pectoralis major and minor, and occasionally the serratus anterior and latissimus dorsi, serratus posterior superior, and the superior fibers of the iliocostalis. The primary exhalation muscles are the internal intercostals and the accessory exhalation muscles are the abdominals, lower fibers of the iliocostalis, serratus posterior inferior, and quadratus lumborum. The external and internal intercostal muscles are frequently viewed as respiratory muscles, but primarily their function is to maintain the integrity of the contour of the thoracic cylinder and prevent invagination during increasing negative intrathoracic pressure.

RIB MOTIONS

The primary rib motion is that of inhalation and exhalation. Inhalation and exhalation are further described as pump-handle and bucket-handle (Fig. 15.5). During inhalation the anterior extremity of a rib moves superiorly in a pump-handle fashion, and the lateral aspect of the rib goes superiorly in a bucket-handle fashion. During exhalation both the pump-handle and bucket-handle components move in a caudad direction. All ribs have both pump-handle and bucket-handle movements. The more cephalic ribs have more pump-handle motion and the more caudal ribs have more bucket-handle motion. The major determinant of this bucket-handle, pump-handle movement is the axis of motion between the costovertebral and the costotransverse articulation. In the upper ribs, this axis is transverse providing more pump-handle activity, whereas in the lower ribs, this axis is more anteroposterior providing for more bucket-handle motion. In a true bucket-handle motion, the anterior and posterior ends of the ribs should be fixed. This is not true in the normal chest wall as the anterior extremity of the rib moves laterally and somewhat superiorly during inhalation, and medially and inferiorly during exhalation. Nonetheless, the descriptors of pump-handle and bucket-handle movements are good for describing the characteristics of chest wall motion.

A third rib motion occurs at the eleventh and twelfth ribs. They have no articular attachments anteriorly and no costotransverse articulations posteriorly

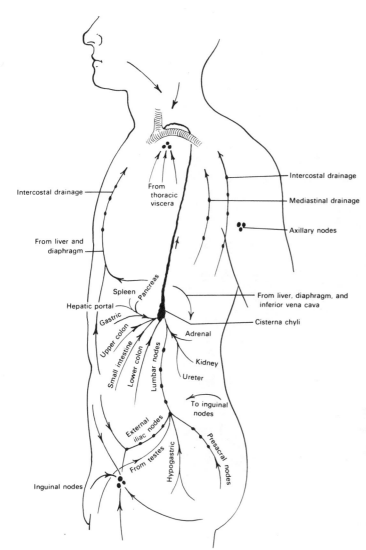

Figure 15.3.
Lymphatic drainage.

The typical ribs, ribs three through 10, have three articulations. The posterior articulations are the costovertebral, with the rib head attaching to demifacets of the thoracic vertebra above and below, and through a strong ligamentous attachment, to the annulus of the intervertebral disk. The second posterior articulation is the costotransverse. This synovial joint incorporates the anterior surface of the transverse process and the articular surface of the posterior aspect of the rib. As an example, the costovertebral articulation of rib four attaches to the inferior demifacet of T3 and the superior demifacet of T4, while the costotransverse articulation is at the T4 level. The anterior articulation is the costochondral. Each rib attaches either to the sternum directly or through the costal arch. Normal rib motion requires mobility of the thoracic vertebrae and mobility at the costovertebral, costotransverse, and costochondral articulations. The rib angle of the typical ribs

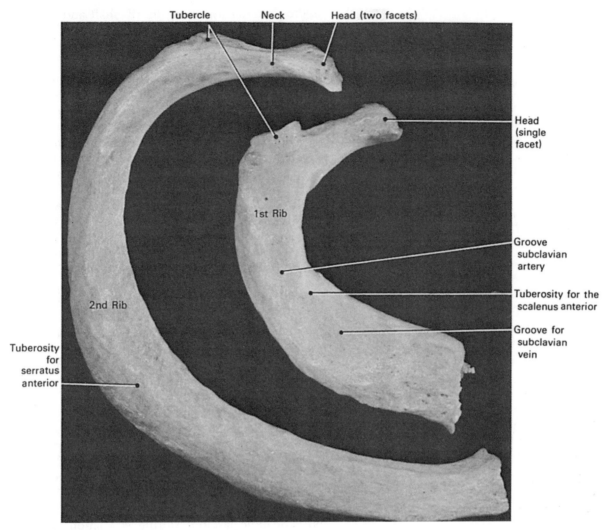

Figure 15.4.
Ribs one and two.

resulting in their motion being primarily posterior and lateral during inhalation, and anterior and medial during exhalation. This motion has been described as caliper motion simulating the action of a set of ice tongs.

A fourth rib motion is that which accompanies rotation of the thoracic spine. This motion is described as torsional movement that results when a pair of typical ribs is attached to two thoracic vertebrae involved in a rotational movement. For example, when T5 rotates to the right in relation to T6, the posterior aspect of the right sixth rib turns externally and the posterior aspect of the left sixth rib turns internally. The rib appears to twist on this long axis. This torsional movement continues around the rib cage to the sternal attachment with the anterior extremity of the right sixth rib being more flat with its inferior border sharp and the anterior extremity of the left sixth rib having its superior margin accentuated. As the thoracic spine returns to neutral, the rib torsional movement should return to bilateral symmetry.

When the rib cage is subjected to traumatic insult, abnormal rib motions can occur. Following a single traumatic episode or multiple microtraumas, one or more ribs may become subluxed anteriorly or posteriorly. These subluxations are abnormal hypermobile ribs with the rib either being carried more anteriorly or posteriorly along the axis of motion between the costovertebral and the costotransverse articulations. A third subluxation is the possibility of rib one being carried cephalad at its unifacet on the lateral side of T1 resulting in the rib shaft sitting on top of the transverse process.

Rib shafts also have a great deal of pliability and are built to sustain anteroposterior and lateral compression loads as they maintain the integrity of the chest wall cylinder. Occasionally after trauma from an anteroposterior or a lateral direction, one or more

Figure 15.5.
Pump handle–bucket handle motion.

ribs lose this plasticity and become restricted in a deformed state.

STRUCTURAL DIAGNOSIS OF THE RIB CAGE

Structural diagnosis of the rib cage assesses for the diagnostic triad of asymmetry, altered range of motion, and tissue texture abnormality. The examiner assesses the symmetry or asymmetry of the chest wall by palpation anteriorly, posteriorly, and laterally. Concurrently, the examiner can assess for tissue texture abnormality, particularly hypertonicity of the iliocostalis attachment at the rib angle and the intercostal muscles. Symmetrically palpating ribs, both in groups and singly, and following respiratory activity of inhalation and exhalation identify motion characteristics.

Rib Cage

Diagnosis
Sitting
Posterior Palpation

1. Patient sitting with operator standing behind.
2. Operator palpates the posterior convexity of the thorax in the upper region (Fig. 15.6), mid-region (Fig. 15.7), and lower region (Fig. 15.8).
3. Assessment is made of the participation of each rib angle in the posterior convexity. Is one more prominent or less prominent than another?

4. Assessment is made of the hypertonicity and tenderness of the iliocostalis muscle at the rib angle.
5. Assessment is made of the posterior contour of the rib shaft. There is a normal posterior convexity with the lower border of the rib being somewhat more easily palpable than that of the superior.
6. Assessment is made of the width of the intercostal space and the intercostal muscle hypertonicity and tenderness. Each interspace should be symmetric with its fellow on the opposite side and with the ones above and below.

Figure 15.7.

Figure 15.6.

Figure 15.8.

Rib Cage

Diagnosis
Sitting
Anterior Palpation

1. Patient sitting on table with operator standing in front.

2. Operator palpates the anterior contour of the chest wall and its anterior convexity beginning at the upper region (Fig. 15.9) with the longest finger palpating the costal cartilage of rib one under the medial extremity of the clavicle. The middle ribs (Fig. 15.10) and lower ribs (Fig. 15.11) are palpated.

3. Assessment is made for the participation of the anterior aspect of each rib in the normal convexity. Is one more or less prominent than the one above or below?

4. Assessment is made of the symmetry of the intercostal spaces and the tissue tension and tenderness of intercostal muscles.

5. Assessment is made of the costochondral junction (Fig. 15.12) assessing for prominence, depression, tissue reaction, and tenderness.

Figure 15.9.

Figure 15.11.

Figure 15.10.

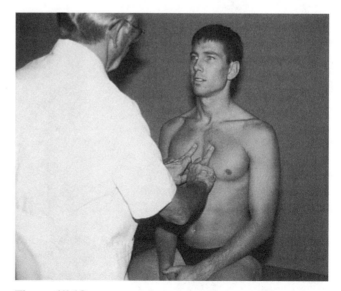

Figure 15.12.

Rib Cage

Diagnosis
Sitting
Lateral Palpation

1. Patient sitting on table with operator standing in front.
2. Operator palpates the lateral contour of the chest wall from above downward assessing for the participation of all ribs in the lateral convexity (Fig. 15.13). Is one more or less prominent than the one above or below?

Figure 15.13.

3. Operator assesses for symmetry of intercostal spaces and for tissue tension in intercostal muscles.
4. The ribs in the mid-axillary line are noted for tenderness in the presence of rib dysfunction.

Rib Cage

Diagnosis
Sitting
First Rib for Superior Subluxation

1. Patient sitting on table with operator standing behind.
2. Operator grasps anterior aspect of the superior trapezius on each side and pulls posteriorly (Fig. 15.14).
3. With posterior retraction of the upper trapezius, the long fingers are directed caudally on to the posterior shaft of the first rib.
4. Unleveling of one rib in comparison to the other by 5 mm is a positive finding (Fig. 15.15).
5. The dysfunctional rib is markedly tender on its superior aspect.
6. The dysfunctional rib has significant exhalation restriction.
7. There is usually hypertonicity of the ipsilateral scalene muscles.

Figure 15.14.

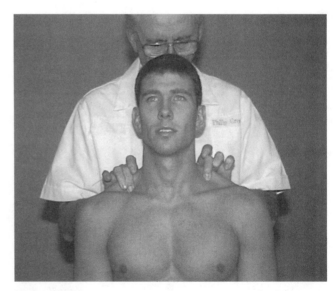

Figure 15.15.

Rib Cage

Diagnosis
Supine
Respiratory Motion Restriction

1. Patient supine with operator standing at side with dominant eye over the midline.
2. Operator symmetrically places hands over lateral aspect of lower rib cage with fingers in interspaces (Fig.15.16).

3. Operator follows inhalation and exhalation effort looking for symmetry or asymmetry of full inhalation and exhalation excursion. Identifying which side stops moving first during the inhalation or exhalation effort makes the diagnosis of either inhalation or exhalation restriction.
4. Palpation is performed on the anterior extremity of the lower ribs (Fig. 15.17) assessing pump-handle motion.

Figure 15.16.

Figure 15.17.

5. Similar assessment of bucket-handle movement (Fig. 15.18) and pump-handle movement (Fig.15.19) is made of the middle ribs.

6. Similar assessment of the bucket-handle movement (Fig. 15.20) and pump-handle movement (Fig. 15.21) of the upper ribs is made. Note that the long finger is in contact with the anterior extremity of the first rib.

Note: It is important to challenge the end range of inhalation and exhalation for accurate diagnosis.

Figure 15.18.

Figure 15.20.

Figure 15.19.

Figure 15.21.

Rib Cage

Diagnosis
Supine
Identification of "key rib"

1. Patient supine with operator standing at side with dominant eye over the midline.
2. Operator symmetrically places a finger on the superior aspect of a pair of ribs and follows inhalation and exhalation effort (Fig. 15.22).
3. A rib that stops first during inhalation effort has inhalation restriction.
4. A rib that stops first during exhalation effort has exhalation restriction.

   Note: The "key" rib designation denotes the rib that seems to prevent the ribs below (in inhalation restriction) and the ribs above (in exhalation restriction) from moving in their normal fashion.

Rib Cage

Diagnosis
Prone
Respiratory Movement of the 11th and 12th Ribs

1. Patient prone on table with operator standing at side and dominant eye over the midline.
2. Operator identifies the tip of the 11th rib usually found in the mid-axillary line just superior to the iliac crest.
3. Operator follows the contour of the eleventh rib medially and places the thumbs and thenar eminences over the posterior shaft of the 11th and 12th ribs (Fig. 15.23).
4. Operator follows inhalation and exhalation effort of the patient.
5. The 11th and 12th ribs that do not move posteriorly during inhalation have inhalation restriction.
6. The 11th and 12th ribs that do not move anteriorly during exhalation have exhalation restriction.
7. The 12th rib is notoriously asymmetric but always follows the 11th rib.

Figure 15.22.

Figure 15.23.

RIB CAGE SOMATIC DYSFUNCTION

Rib dysfunctions are classified as structural and respiratory. The structural rib dysfunctions include:

1. Anterior and posterior subluxation,
2. Superior subluxation of the first rib,
3. Anteroposterior compression,
4. Lateral compression.

The subluxations and compressions follow acute or chronic recurrent trauma. They are frequently related to motor vehicle and sports injuries. In many instances, their presentation suggests that a rib is fractured but imaging studies fail to demonstrate a fracture. They frequently present as intercostal neuralgia. If a patient presents with intercostal neuralgia symptoms and no structural rib dysfunctions are identified, the practitioner should consider organic neurologic disease as the cause of the symptoms.

Another rib dysfunction that some classify as structural is rib torsion usually accompanying a nonneutral dysfunction of the thoracic spine, particularly of the extended, rotated, and side-bent (ERS) variety. Rib torsional dysfunctions frequently resolve when the non-neutral thoracic spine dysfunction has been successfully treated. In other instances, particularly if the torsion has been present for a long time, the rib undergoes torsional deformity that persists and is a leading cause of recurrence of the thoracic spine dysfunction. This chronic torsion alters the bony architecture and is why some call it a structural rib dysfunction.

Another rib dysfunction classified by some as structural is observed at rib two and is described as being "laterally flexed." Another term used is "bucket-bail." In this dysfunction, the rib behaves as though the anterior and posterior ends of the first rib were fixed in a true bucket-handle fashion and the traumatic episode results in the rib being laterally flexed. This usually occurs in a superior direction. Some authors describe this as a major bucket-handle exhalation restriction but they do not respond to the usual respiratory rib techniques. Other authors suggest that there is a subluxation of the rib shaft on top of the transverse process of the associated vertebra. While radiographs have demonstrated this phenomenon in the superior subluxation of rib one, it has not been demonstrated in the laterally flexed rib. They usually result from acute side-bending injuries to the cervical thoracic junction. Shortening and hypertonicity of the posterior scalene muscles is an important associated finding.

The diagnostic criteria for structural rib dysfunctions are as follows:

1. Anterior Subluxation:
    *   Rib angle less prominent in posterior rib cage contour.
    *   Rib angle tender with tension of iliocostalis muscle.
    *   Prominence of anterior extremity of the rib in the anterior rib cage contour.
    *   Marked motion restriction of inhalation and exhalation.
    *   Frequently present with complaint of "intercostal neuralgia" in adjacent interspace.

2. Posterior Subluxation:
    *   Rib angle more prominent in posterior rib cage contour.
    *   Rib angle tender with tension of iliocostalis muscle.
    *   Anterior extremity of the rib less prominent in anterior rib cage contour.
    *   Marked restriction of rib in inhalation and exhalation movement.
    *   Frequent complaint of "intercostal neuralgia" in adjacent interspace.

3. Superior First Rib Subluxation:
    *   Palpation of superior aspect of first rib anterior to the upper trapezius muscle shows dysfunctional rib to be 5 to 6 mm cephalic in relation to contralateral side.
    *   Marked tenderness of superior aspect of first rib.
    *   Restriction of respiratory motion primarily exhalation.
    *   Hypertonicity of scalene muscles on ipsilateral side.

4. Anteroposterior rib compression:
    *   Less prominence of the rib shaft in the anterior and posterior convexities of the thoracic cage.
    *   Prominence of the rib shaft in the mid-axillary line.
    *   Tenderness and tension of the intercostal space above and below dysfunctional rib.
    *   Frequent complaint of chest wall pain of the "intercostal neuralgia" type.
    *   Motion restriction of respiratory activity.

5. Lateral Rib Compression:
    *   Prominence of the rib shaft in the anterior and posterior convexities of the rib cage.
    *   Dysfunctional rib shaft less prominent in the mid-axillary line.
    *   Tenderness and tension of the intercostal space above and below dysfunctional rib.
    *   Complaint of chest wall pain consistent with "intercostal neuralgia."
    *   Respiratory motion restriction.

Note: Both anteroposterior and lateral rib compressions simulate rib fracture.

6. External Rib Torsion:
    *   Superior border of dysfunctional rib more prominent posteriorly.

- Inferior border of dysfunctional rib less prominent posteriorly.
- Tension and tenderness at iliocostalis muscle attachment at rib angle.
- Widened intercostal space above and narrowed intercostal space below dysfunctional rib with tension of the intercostal muscles on the inferior interspace.
- Respiratory motion restriction primarily of exhalation.
- These dysfunctions are frequently the key rib in exhalation group rib restrictions.

Note: External torsional dysfunctions are commonly associated with ERS dysfunction to the ipsilateral side. Internal torsional dysfunction has the reverse findings and is usually found on the contralateral side. Rib torsion dysfunctions are seldom found associated with flexed, rotated, and side-bent (FRS) dysfunctions.

7. Lateral Flexed Rib:
- Prominence of the rib shaft in the mid-axillary line.
- Marked respiratory rib restriction usually exhalation.
- Asymmetry of interspace above and below dysfunctional rib with the superior usually narrow and the inferior wider.
- Marked tenderness of the interspace usually the one above.
- Most commonly seen in rib two, being dysfunctional in a superior position (laterally flexed superiorly).
- Marked tenderness of the superior intercostal space of rib two at its lateral aspect just beneath the lateral extremity of the clavicle.
- Frequently associated with brachalgia-type symptoms in the upper extremity.

RESPIRATORY RIB DYSFUNCTIONS

A single rib, or a group of ribs, can demonstrate restriction of either inhalation or exhalation movement. When a group of ribs has restriction of inhalation or exhalation function, we look for the *key rib*. The key rib is the major restrictor of the group's ability to move into either inhalation or exhalation. The key rib is found at the upper or lower end of the group. In exhalation group rib dysfunction, the key rib is at the bottom of the dysfunctional group. In inhalation group rib dysfunction, the key rib is at the upper end of the group. The key rib is frequently one of the structural rib dysfunctions. If a structural rib dysfunction is identified, it should be appropriately treated before dealing with the respiratory rib dysfunctions. In treating group respiratory rib restrictions of the inhalation and exhalation type, the key rib is the rib usually addressed in the treatment procedure. Caution must be advised for the be-

ginning student when assessing for respiratory restrictions. The diagnostic criterion is based on the rib group that stops first during inhalation or exhalation. It is not the rib group that has the alteration in the excursion of range. For example, a group of ribs that has exhalation restriction stops first during the exhalation phase of respiration. Because the ribs are already held in a position of inhalation, they have a reduced range of inhalation. These rib dysfunctions are frequently misdiagnosed as inhalation restrictions because the range is reduced. However, they are really exhalation restrictions because they have reduced range of exhalation when compared to the opposite side. The converse is true of inhalation restrictions. Because they are already held in a position of exhalation, they have a reduced range of exhalation, but their major restriction is in the direction of inhalation.

Diagnostic criteria for respiratory rib dysfunctions are:

Exhalation Restriction:
1. A rib or group of ribs that ceases movement first during exhalation effort.
2. The key rib is at the bottom of the group.
3. Assessment is made as to which of the pump-handle and bucket-handle components is the most restricted.

Inhalation Restriction:
1. A rib or group of ribs that ceases moving first during inhalation effort.
2. The key rib is at the top of the group.
3. Assessment is made as to whether the pump-handle or bucket-handle component is most restricted.

In group rib respiratory restrictions, there may be more than one key rib. Each rib must be assessed for its compliance in the overall inhalation and exhalation effort of that group of ribs.

TREATMENT OF RIB CAGE DYSFUNCTION

There are general principles of treatment sequence that should be followed for the successful treatment of rib cage dysfunction. As a general rule, treatment of the thoracic spine should precede treatment of the ribs, either individual or in groups. Torsional rib dysfunction frequently responds simultaneously with the treatment of the associated non-neutral thoracic dysfunction. The unique anatomy at the thoracic inlet requires that T1 be adequately evaluated and treated before addressing dysfunction of ribs one and two. The unifacet for the first rib on the lateral side of T1 allows a great deal of variable motion of the first rib.

The second principle of treating rib dysfunctions is to address the structural rib dysfunctions prior to treatment of respiratory rib restriction. The key rib of a group of respiratory rib dysfunction is usually a structural rib at the top or bottom of the group. Appropriate treatment to the structural rib dysfunction frequently restores normal movement to the group of ribs and their respiratory capacity. Following treatment of structural rib dysfunction, the respiratory rib dysfunctions are addressed with the goal of restoration of maximal, symmetric, inhalation/exhalation movement.

Technique of rib cage dysfunction is usually direct action with combined activating forces of muscle energy, respiratory effort, and operator guiding.

Rib Cage

Structural Rib Dysfunction
Diagnosis
Superior Subluxation First Rib (left-side example)

1. Patient sitting with operator standing behind.

2. Patient's right arm is draped over the operator's right thigh with foot on the table.

3. Operator's right hand and forearm control the patient's head and neck with the fingers of the left hand overlying the upper trapezius muscle that is pulled posteriorly (Fig. 15.24).

4. Operator's left thumb contacts the posterior shaft of rib one through the trapezius muscle (Fig. 15.25).

5. Operator's right hand introduces left-side bending and rotation of the patient's neck to unload the left scalene muscles and with the tips of the forefingers continuing to maintain the trapezius posteriorly; a caudal force is placed upon the shaft of the first rib (Fig. 15.26).

6. Simultaneously the operator's left thumb maintains an anterior force on the posterior aspect of the shaft of the first rib to slide it forward in relation to the left transverse process of T1 (Fig. 15.27).

7. Patient performs a right-side-bending effort of the head and neck against operator's resistance through the right hand activating the right scalene muscles and resulting in inhibition of the left scalenes.

8. Two to three efforts may be necessary before release is felt of the superior subluxation restoring symmetry with the opposite side.

9. Retest.

Figure 15.24.

Figure 15.26.

Figure 15.25.

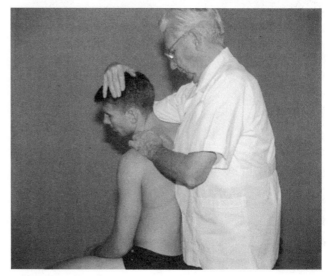

Figure 15.27.

Rib Cage

Structural Rib Dysfunction
Diagnosis
Anterior Subluxation (Example: right fifth rib)

1. Patient sitting on table with right hand holding left shoulder.

2. Operator stands behind the patient with the right thumb on the shaft of the fifth rib medial to the rib angle (Fig. 15.28) and with the left hand controlling the patient's right elbow (Fig. 15.29).

3. Operator applies and maintains a posterolateral "pull" force on the rib shaft (Fig. 15.30).

Figure 15.29.

Figure 15.28.

Figure 15.30.

4. Patient is instructed to "pull" the right elbow laterally or caudally (Fig. 15.31). Three to five repetitions are made of a 3- to 5-second muscle contraction of the patient with operator monitoring rib motion.

5. Patient's left fist can be applied to the anterior extremity of the dysfunctional rib so that when the cau-

dad pulling motion is performed there is anterior-to-posterior force directed at the dysfunctional rib (Fig. 15.32).

6. Retest.

Figure 15.31.

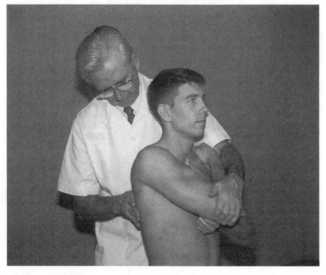

Figure 15.32.

Rib Cage

Structural Rib Dysfunction
Diagnosis
Posterior Subluxation (Example: right fifth rib)

1. Patient sitting on table with right hand grasping left shoulder.

2. Operator stands behind patient with thumb placed on shaft of right fifth rib lateral to the angle (Fig. 15.33), and with left hand holding the patient's right elbow (Fig. 15.34).

3. Operator maintains an anteromedial "push" force on the rib shaft and resists the patient's instructed "push" of the elbow to the left (Fig. 15.35), or a "push" of the right elbow toward the ceiling (Fig. 15.36).

4. Three to five repetitions of a 3- to 5-second muscle effort are usually necessary to restore symmetry.

5. Retest.

   Note: Rib subluxations are frequently hypermobile and following treatment stabilization of the rib cage by strapping or a rib belt is frequently useful.

Figure 15.33.

Figure 15.35.

Figure 15.34.

Figure 15.36.

Rib Cage

Structural Rib Dysfunction
Diagnosis
Rib Torsion (Example: right fifth rib)

1. Patient sitting on table with right hand holding left shoulder.
2. Operator stands behind with thumb contacting the rib angle of the right fifth rib in a vertical fashion (Fig. 15.37).
3. With external torsional restriction, the thumb applies an anterior force on the superior border of the dysfunctional rib.
4. For internal torsional restriction, the operator's thumb applies an anterior force on the inferior margin of the dysfunctional rib.

5. Patient is instructed to alternately pull the elbow to the lap (Fig. 15.38) and push toward the ceiling (Fig. 15.39) with the operator maintaining the appropriate compressive force on the superior or inferior aspect of the rib shaft.
6. Pulling toward the lap introduces internal torsional movement, and pushing toward the ceiling introduces external torsional movement. Operator resists the rib motion during the appropriate muscle effort and takes up the slack to the new barrier during each relaxation.
7. Three to five repetitions of 3- to 5-second contractions are made.
8. Retest.

Figure 15.38.

Figure 15.37.

Figure 15.39.

Rib Cage

Structural Rib Dysfunction
Diagnosis
External Torsion (Example: right fifth rib)

1. Patient sitting on table with right hand grasping left shoulder.

2. Operator stands behind with the left arm controlling the patient's trunk with the left axilla over the patient's left shoulder and the left hand grasping the right shoulder. Operator's right hand identifies dysfunctional rib angle and shaft (Fig. 15.40).

3. Operator introduces small amount of flexion, left-side bending, and left rotation of the trunk and right hand follows the right fifth rib anteriorly (Fig. 15.41).

4. Operator's thumb and thenar eminence contact the anterior shaft of the right fifth rib exerting an internal rotary force over the prominent inferior margin of the shaft (Fig. 15.42).

Figure 15.41.

Figure 15.40.

Figure 15.42.

5. Operator increases the forward bending, left-side bending, and left rotation of the trunk (Fig. 15.43).

6. Operator resists a right rotation, right-side bending, and extension effort of the patient while maintaining a compressive force on the inferior margin of the anterior shaft of the fifth rib (Fig. 15.44).

7. Three to five repetitions of a 3- to 5-second effort are made with the operator engaging a new barrier after each effort.

8. Retest.

Figure 15.43.

Figure 15.44.

Rib Cage

Structural Rib Dysfunction
Diagnosis
Anteroposterior Compression (Example: right sixth rib)

1. Patient sits on end of table with operator standing on the side opposite of the dysfunction and patient's arm is draped over the operator's shoulder (Fig. 15.45).

2. Operator's middle finger of both hands contacts the prominent rib shaft in the mid-axillary line (Fig. 15.46).

3. Operator side bends patient to the right while applying a medial compressive force on the shaft of the dysfunctional rib (Fig. 15.47).

4. Patient is instructed to deeply inhale, hold the breath, and perform a left-side bending effort of the trunk against operator resistance while the operator maintains a medial compressive force on the dysfunctional rib (Fig. 15.48).

5. Three to five repetitions are made.

6. Retest.

Figure 15.45.

Figure 15.47.

Figure 15.46.

Figure 15.48.

Rib Cage

Structural Rib Dysfunction
Diagnosis
Lateral Compression (example, left fifth rib)

1. Patient sitting on end of table with operator standing on the side of dysfunction with patient's left arm draped over the operator's right shoulder (Fig. 15.49).

2. Operator places the thenar eminence of each hand over the prominent posterior and anterior shaft of the dysfunctional fifth rib (Fig. 15.50).

3. Operator side bends the patient to the right while maintaining anteroposterior compression on the dysfunctional rib (Fig. 15.51).

4. Patient takes a deep breath in, holds the breath, and performs a left-side bending effort against the resistance to the operator's shoulder (Fig. 15.52).

5. Three to five repetitions of a 3- to 5-second effort are performed with the operator engaging a new barrier after each effort.

6. Retest.

Figure 15.49.

Figure 15.51.

Figure 15.50.

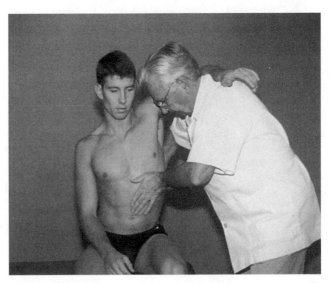

Figure 15.52.

Rib Cage

Structural Rib Dysfunction
Diagnosis
Laterally Flexed Superior (Example: left second rib)

1. Patient supine on table with operator standing on side of dysfunction facing cephalad with the right hand against the mid-axillary line of the patient's thorax (Fig. 15.53).

2. Operator slides right hand cephalically along the lateral rib shaft with the left hand holding the patient's left arm inferiorly (Fig. 15.54).

3. Operator's left hand introduces left-side bending of the head and neck and the patient is instructed to fully exhale and reach toward the left knee to increase left-side bending (Fig. 15.55).

4. After several respiratory efforts with increased left-side bending, operator's right hand grasps the su-

Figure 15.54.

Figure 15.53.

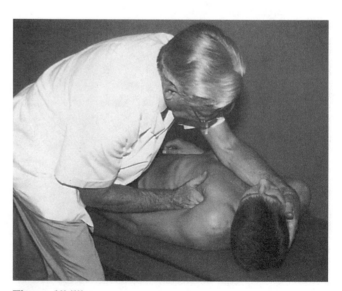

Figure 15.55.

perior aspect of the shaft of the second rib and the left hand is switched to the opposite side of the patient's head (Fig. 15.56).

5. While holding the superior aspect of the dysfunctional rib, operator's left hand introduces acute right-side bending of the head and neck, stretching the left scalene muscles (Fig. 15.57).

6. Retest.

   Note: This dysfunction is exquisitely tender to the patient and the treatment procedure is significantly painful. The patient should be appropriately informed.

Figure 15.56.

Figure 15.57.

Rib Cage

Structural Rib Dysfunction
Laterally Flexed Rib (Example: left second rib)

1. Patient supine on the table with operator sitting at head.

2. Operator's right hand contacts the superior aspect of the left second rib as far laterally as possible and maintains a caudad pressure (Fig. 15.58).

3. Operator's left hand stabilizes the thoracic inlet and the lower cervical spine.

4. Patient abducts, externally rotates left arm, dorsiflexes the left hand and provides an on-and-off dural mobilization of the left upper extremity with a median nerve bias (Fig. 15.59). The operator frequently feels a release of the restricted rib during the mobilization by the patient.

5. Retest.

Note: This technique uses operator guiding and dural mobilization as the activating forces. It is much more comfortable for the patient than the previous technique. If ineffective, the previous direct action technique can be used.

Figure 15.58.

Figure 15.59.

RESPIRATORY RIB RESTRICTIONS

Following the treatment of structural rib dysfunctions, respiratory rib restrictions are addressed. The respiratory rib restrictions are more myofascial problems than the bone and joint restrictions of the structural rib dysfunctions. The practitioner needs to be able to deal with both inhalation and exhalation rib restriction.

PRINCIPLES OF TREATMENT OF INHALATION RESTRICTION

1. Operator distracts the rib angle laterally and caudad to disengage the rib head at the costovertebral articulation.
2. Patient applies respiratory activating force by deep inhalation.
3. Patient's muscle activating force uses scalenes for ribs one and two, pectoralis minor for ribs three through five, and serratus anterior for ribs six through nine.

PRINCIPLES OF TREATMENT OF EXHALATION RESTRICTION

1. Operator positions patient in combined side bending and flexion to the side of dysfunction.
2. Operator contacts superior shaft and costochondral junction of the dysfunctional rib.
3. Patient provides a maximum exhalation effort while operator follows and holds the dysfunctional rib in an exhalation position.
4. Following a series of patient exhalations, operator returns patient to a neutral trunk position while holding the rib in an exhalation position and slowly releases pressure on the rib shaft.

Rib Cage

Respiratory Restriction
Ribs 1 and 2
Diagnosis
   Inhalation Restriction (Example: right side)

1. Patient supine with operator standing on left side of table.
2. The fingers of operator's left hand contact the medial aspect of the first and second ribs as close to the transverse process as possible (Fig. 15.60).
3. Patient's trunk is returned to the table with the operator's elbow on the table and operator's hand providing a lateral and inferior pull on the first and second ribs.

4. Operator's right hand introduces left-side bending and rotation of the head and neck putting the right scalenes on tension (Fig. 15.61).
5. Patient is instructed to deeply inhale and lift the head off the table for pump-handle restriction or to side bend the head to the right for bucket-handle restriction, against the resistance of the operator's right hand (Fig. 15.62).
6. Three to five repetitions are made of a 3- to 5-second effort.
7. This can be done in the presence of pathology of the right shoulder. If the right shoulder is healthy, an alternate hand position has the patient's forearm resting against the head (Fig. 15.63) reducing the caudad traction on the first and second ribs by the fascia of the right upper extremity.
8. Retest.

Figure 15.60.

Figure 15.62.

Figure 15.61.

Figure 15.63.

Rib Cage

Respiratory Restriction
Ribs 3 to 5
Diagnosis
   Inhalation Restriction (Example: right side)

1. Patient supine on table with operator standing on left side and with the left hand grasps the shafts of ribs three, four, and five medial to the angle (Fig. 15.64).

2. Operator returns the patient to neutral on the table and with the left forearm on the table applies a lateral and caudad distraction on the dysfunctional ribs.

3. Patient's right arm is elevated and abducted putting the pectoralis minor muscle on stretch.

4. Patient is instructed to take and hold a deep breath.

5. Patient performs a muscle effort of adduction against the operator's resistance for bucket-handle restriction (Fig. 15.65) or a flexion effort against operator resistance for a pump-handle restriction (Fig. 15.66).

6. Patient performs three to five repetitions of a 3- to 5-second contraction.

7. In the presence of right shoulder pathology the alternative procedure finds the operator's thumb medial to the right coracoid process to resist an anterior motion of the right shoulder girdle (Fig. 15.67).

8. Retest.

Figure 15.64.

Figure 15.66.

Figure 15.65.

Figure 15.67.

Rib Cage

Respiratory Restriction
Ribs 6, 7, 8, and 9
Diagnosis
  Inhalation Restriction (Example: right side)

1. Patient supine on table with operator standing on left side.

2. The fingers of the operator's left hand contact the sixth, seventh, eighth, and ninth ribs medial to the angle (Fig. 15.68).

3. Operator returns patient to neutral position and with the left elbow on the table puts a lateral and caudad distractive force on the four ribs.

4. Operator's right hand controls the patient's right upper extremity.

5. Patient is instructed to take and hold a deep breath, and for a pump-handle restriction flexes the upper extremity against operator resistance (Fig. 15.69), or in a lateral direction for bucket-handle restriction (Fig. 15.70).

6. Patient performs three to five repetitions of a 3- to 5-second muscle effort.

7. In the presence of shoulder dysfunction, operator resists a protraction action of the right scapula at the inferior scapular angle (Fig. 15.71).

8. Retest.

Figure 15.68.

Figure 15.70.

Figure 15.69.

Figure 15.71.

Rib Cage

Respiratory Restriction
Lower ribs
Diagnosis
    Exhalation Restriction (Example: left side)

1. Patient supine on table with operator standing at the left side of the head of the table.

2. Operator's left thumb and thenar eminence contacts the superior aspect of the dysfunctional key rib, including the costochondral junction (Fig. 15.72).

3. Operator's right hand supports head, neck, and upper thorax to control patient body position (Fig. 15.73).

4. Operator introduces left-side bending and flexion of the trunk down to the key rib (Fig. 15.74).

5. Patient is instructed to exhale completely.

6. Operator follows exhalation movement of the rib and holds it in that position.

7. Operator resists patient's inhalation respiratory effort. During patient's next exhalation a new barrier is engaged by trunk flexion and side bending (Fig. 15.75).

8. After three to five repetitions of maximum exhalation, patient's head, neck, and upper trunk are returned to neutral while the operator holds the key rib in an exhalation position.

9. Operator slowly releases the left thumb from the key rib.

10. Retest.

Figure 15.72.

Figure 15.74.

Figure 15.73.

Figure 15.75.

Rib Cage

Respiratory Restriction
Upper Ribs
Diagnosis
  Exhalation Restriction (Example: left side)

1. Patient supine on table with operator standing at left side of head of table.
2. Operator's left thumb and thenar eminence contact the superior aspect of the shaft of the dysfunctional rib spanning the costochondral junction. Note that the more cephalic the rib the more medial is the costochondral junction (Fig. 15.76).
3. Operator's right hand controls patient's head, neck, and upper thorax and introduces flexion and side bending to the side of dysfunction (Fig. 15.77).
4. Operator introduces more flexion for pump-handle component and side bending for the bucket-handle component (Fig. 15.78).

Figure 15.77.

Figure 15.76.

Figure 15.78.

5. Patient is instructed to exhale completely while operator follows the rib in exhalation with increasing flexion and side bending (Fig. 15.79).

6. Three to five repetitions are performed. When maximum exhalation movement has been achieved, patient's head and neck are returned to neutral while

operator holds dysfunctional rib in exhalation position (Fig. 15.80).

7. Operator slowly releases compressive left thumb.

8. Retest.

Figure 15.79.

Figure 15.80.

Rib Cage

Respiratory Restriction
Upper Ribs
Diagnosis
   Exhalation Restriction (Example: left side)

1. Patient supine with operator standing at head of table.

2. Operator's left hand controls the patient's head and neck while the right thumb and thenar eminence contacts the shaft and costochondral articulation of the dysfunction rib (Fig. 15.81).

3. Operator introduces flexion and side bending toward the side of dysfunction.

4. Patient is instructed to fully exhale and the operator follows the dysfunctional rib into an exhalation position and holds it there (Fig. 15.82).

5. Following several respiratory efforts with increasing flexion and side bending, operator returns the head to neutral and slowly releases the compressive force on the dysfunctional rib.

6. Retest.

   Note: This alternative position avoids compressive force on breast tissue particularly in females. It is also particularly valuable for the pump-handle component of upper rib restrictions.

Figure 15.81.

Figure 15.82.

Rib Cage

Respiratory Restriction
First Rib
Diagnosis
    Exhalation Restriction: pump-handle component
    (Example: left side)

1. Patient supine on table with operator sitting at head.

2. Operator's right hand controls the patient's head while the left thumb contacts the superior aspect of the anterior extremity of the first rib, either lateral to or between the heads of the sternocleidomastoid muscle (Fig. 15.83).

3. Operator introduces flexion with some left-side bending (Fig. 15.84).

4. Patient fully exhales while the operator increases flexion and left-side bending following the left first rib into exhalation (Fig. 15.85).

5. Operator resists inhalation movement of the first rib and during patient's next exhalation follows the first rib into the exhalation position.

6. Three to five efforts are performed and when maximum exhalation has been achieved, operator returns the head to neutral and slowly releases the contact on the first rib.

7. Retest.

Figure 15.84.

Figure 15.83.

Figure 15.85.

Rib Cage

Respiratory Restriction
First Rib
Diagnosis
Exhalation Restriction: bucket-handle component
(Example: left side)

1. Patient supine with operator sitting at head of table.

2. Operator's right hand grasps patient's head and neck while left thumb contacts the superior aspect of the lateral shaft of the first rib just anterior to the trapezius and posterior to the clavicle (Fig. 15.86).

3. Patient performs a forced exhalation while operator side bends the head to the left with a small amount of flexion and follows the lateral shaft of the rib into exhalation (Fig. 15.87).

4. Operator continues holding the first rib in exhalation and patient repeats the maximal exhalation effort with increasing left-side bending of the head and neck by the operator's right hand (Fig. 15.88).

5. When maximal exhalation effort has been achieved, operator holds first rib in exhalation position and returns head to neutral.

6. Operator's left thumb is released slowly.

7. Retest.

Figure 15.87.

Figure 15.86.

Figure 15.88.

Rib Cage

Respiratory Restriction
Ribs 11 and 12
Diagnosis
   Exhalation Restriction (Example: right side)

1. Patient prone on table with operator standing on left side of patient.
2. Operator's heel of left hand contacts the medial side of the shafts of the eleventh and twelvth ribs (Fig. 15.89).
3. Patient's right arm is placed on the table and reaches toward the feet with trunk side bending toward the right.

4. Operator's right hand grasps the patient's right anterior superior iliac spine (Fig. 15.90).
5. Patient is instructed to maximally exhale.
6. Operator's left hand carries the eleventh and twelvth ribs in a lateral and caudad direction.
7. At the end of full exhalation patient pulls the right anterior superior iliac spine toward the table for 3 to 5 seconds (Fig. 15.91).
8. After each effort operator engages a new barrier. Three to five repetitions are made.
9. Retest.

Figure 15.90.

Figure 15.89.

Figure 15.91.

Rib Cage

Respiratory Restriction
Ribs 11 and 12
Diagnosis
   Inhalation Restriction (Example: right side)

1. Patient prone on table with operator standing on the left side.

2. Operator's heel of left hand contacts the medial aspect of the patient's eleventh and twelvth ribs (Fig 15.92) and exerts a lateral and cephalic force.

3. Patient's right hand is placed over the head and the feet to the left introducing left-side bending (Fig. 15.93).

4. Operator's right hand grasps the right anterior superior iliac spine.

5. Patient is instructed to take and hold a maximal inhalation effort.

6. Operator lifts patient's right pelvis off table and resists the patient's effort to pull the right anterior superior iliac spine down to the table (Fig. 15.94).

7. Three to five repetitions are made with a new barrier being engaged after each effort.

8. Retest.

Figure 15.93.

Figure 15.92.

Figure 15.94.

MOBILIZATION WITH IMPULSE (HIGH-VELOCITY THRUST) DIRECT ACTION TECHNIQUE FOR RIB DYSFUNCTION

The major restrictors of rib cage dysfunction are primarily myofascial. Occasionally a rib will become dysfunctional with palpable characteristics of deep articular and periarticular tissue reaction. Mobilization with impulse technique would then be of assistance in the management of the rib cage. Mobilization with impulse technique can be used to treat single rib and group rib dysfunctions of both the structural and respiratory type. Mobilizations with impulse techniques are contraindicated in the presence of rib subluxations. The treatment sequence is the same as previously described.

The structural rib dysfunction most frequently treated with mobilization with impulse technique is external rib torsional dysfunction associated with a nonneutral ERS dysfunction of the thoracic spine.

Rib Cage

Respiratory Restriction
Mobilization with Impulse Technique
Supine
Diagnosis
  External Torsion Dysfunction (Example: left fifth rib)

1. The patient and operator positions are the same as for the thoracic spine, mobilization with impulse technique for an ERS left dysfunction at T4 to T5 (Figs. 14.68 and 14.69).

2. Operator establishes lever arm.

3. Operator's right hand establishes a fulcrum to stabilize both transverse processes of T5 and with the thenar eminence on the inferior aspect of the left 5th rib.

4. Following return of patient to neutral position and the establishment of the lever arm to the fulcrum, operator's left hand introduces flexion, right-side bending, and right rotation of the neck and upper thoracic spine down to the left fifth rib.

5. The force through the lever arm to the fulcrum is somewhat more to the left side than midline as for the thoracic dysfunction, and a high-velocity, low-amplitude thrust is made by the body weight of the operator on the lever arm to the fulcrum resulting in flexion, right-side bending, and right rotation of T4 on T5, the opening of the left zygapophysial joint, and the mobilization of the left fifth rib. The thenar eminence of the operator's right hand maintains a cephalic pressure on the inferior aspect of the 5th rib at the time of the thrust.

6. Commonly, two cavitation pop sounds occur in rapid sequence when the thrust is applied.

7. Retest.

Rib Cage

Respiratory Restriction
Mobilization with Impulse Technique
Rib 1
Diagnosis
  Inhalation or Exhalation Restriction (Example: left first rib)

1. Patient supine on table with operator standing on right side and slides arm under patient with fingers of the right hand grasping the superior aspect of the left first rib (Fig. 15.95).

2. With exhalation restriction, operator depresses anterior aspect of the rib shaft. With inhalation restriction, operator depresses posterior aspect of first rib.

3. Operator's left hand side bends patient's head and neck to the left, rotates to the right, localizing to T1 (Fig. 15.96).

4. A mobilization with impulse thrust is performed by the operator with either an acute exaggeration of the head and neck position into left-side bending, or stabilizing the head and neck with the left hand and performing an acute caudad thrust through the right hand in the axis of the right forearm.

5. Retest.

Figure 15.95.

Figure 15.96.

Rib Cage

Respiratory Restriction
Mobilization with Impulse Technique
Rib 1
Diagnosis
   Exhalation Restriction (Example: left first rib)

1. Patient sitting on the table with operator standing behind.
2. Operator's right foot is placed on the table and the patient's right upper extremity is draped over the operator's right thigh.
3. Operator's right hand contacts the right side of the head and neck of the patient, while the left hand contacts the left first rib over its anterior and posterior extremity (Fig. 15.97).
4. Operator's left forearm is angled from above downward against the hand contact on the first rib (Fig. 15.98).
5. Operator introduces left-side bending and right rotation of the patient's head and neck localized at T1 (Fig. 15.99).
6. A mobilization with impulse thrust is performed through the operator's left forearm in a caudad and medial direction (Fig. 15.100).
7. Retest.

Figure 15.97.

Figure 15.99.

Figure 15.98.

Figure 15.100.

Rib Cage

Respiratory Restriction
Mobilization with Impulse Technique
Rib 2
Diagnosis
  Exhalation restriction (Example: left second rib)

1. Patient sitting on table with operator standing behind with right foot on the table and patient's right arm draped over the operator's right thigh.

2. Operator's right hand controls the right side of the patient's head and neck and the left hand is over the patient's left shoulder (Fig. 15.101).

3. Operator's left thumb is on the posterior shaft of rib two (Fig. 15.102).

4. Operator introduces left-side bending, right rotation of the head and neck, with translation of the trunk from left to right localizing to T1 to T2 and the left second rib (Fig. 15.103).

5. When the barrier is engaged, a mobilization with impulse technique is performed through the left forearm with an anterior and medial thrust against the resistance of the stabilizing right arm (Fig. 15.104).

6. Retest.

Figure 15.101.

Figure 15.103.

Figure 15.102.

Figure 15.104.

Rib Cage

Respiratory Restriction
Mobilization with Impulse Technique
Typical Ribs (3 to10)
Diagnosis
  Inhalation or Exhalation Restriction (Example: left ribs)

1. Operator's thumb and thenar eminence function as the fulcrum. The thumb contacts either the superior or the inferior aspect of the dysfunctional rib (Fig. 15.105).

2. For inhalation restriction, the thumb and thenar contact is on the superior aspect of the rib shaft with the rib being carried caudad (Fig. 15.106).

3. For exhalation restriction the thumb is placed below the rib shaft and exerts a superior force (Fig. 15.107).

4. Patient's left hand grasps the right shoulder establishing the lever arm (Fig. 15.108).

Figure 15.105.

Figure 15.107.

Figure 15.106.

Figure 15.108.

5. Operator places the fulcrum on the dysfunctional rib as appropriate for the respiratory restriction (Fig. 15.109).

6. Patient's trunk is returned to midline and operator's body (either chest wall or abdomen) localizes to fulcrum through the lever arm (Fig. 15.110).

7. A mobilization with impulse thrust is made by the operator's body dropped through the lever arm to the fulcrum with the right thumb and thenar eminence exerting a cephalic-directed force for exhalation restriction and a caudad-direction force for inhalation restriction.

8. A respiratory assist of inhalation or exhalation can be made, but usually exhalation for relaxation of the patient is more helpful.

9. Retest.

Figure 15.109.

Figure 15.110.

Rib Cage

Respiratory Restriction
Mobilization with Impulse Technique
Lower Typical Ribs and ribs 11 and 12
Diagnosis
Inhalation or exhalation restriction (Example: left side)

1. Patient in lateral recumbent position with the dysfunctional side up.

2. Operator stands in front of patient with the pisiform of the right hand in contact with the posterior aspect of the dysfunctional rib (Fig. 15.111).

3. Operator's left hand contacts the anterior aspect of the patient's left shoulder.

4. For exhalation restriction, the pisiform contact is on the inferior aspect of the rib shaft and operator's right forearm directs the rib in an anterior and superior direction (Fig. 15.112).

5. For inhalation restriction, the pisiform contact is on the superior aspect of the rib shaft and operator's right arm carries it caudally (Fig. 15.113).

6. A mobilization with impulse thrust is performed by a body drop of the operator directing force through the right forearm in the appropriate direction for inhalation or exhalation restriction.

7. Retest.

Figure 15.112.

Figure 15.111.

Figure 15.113.

Rib Cage

Respiratory Restriction
Mobilization with Impulse Technique
Diagnosis
    Ribs 11 and 12 (Example: right side)

1. Patient prone on table with operator standing on left side with left hand medial to the shafts of ribs 11 and 12 and the right hand grasping the patient's right anterior superior iliac spine.

2. For exhalation restriction, the patient is side bent to the right with the right arm reaching toward the right knee (Fig. 15.114).

3. For inhalation restriction, the patient is left-side bent with the right hand over the head (Fig. 15.115).

4. The barrier is engaged by lifting the anterosuperior iliac spine from the table.

5. A mobilization with impulse thrust is performed through the operator's left hand in a lateral and inferior direction for exhalation restriction and in a lateral and superior direction for inhalation restriction.

6. Retest.

Figure 15.114.

Figure 15.115.

CONCLUSION

Dysfunction of the rib cage is highly significant in many problems of the musculoskeletal system. The structural rib dysfunctions can be major pain generators. Respiratory rib restriction compromises the patient's capacity for respiration and efficient circulation of the low pressure venous and lymphatic systems. There are extensive muscle attachments to the rib cage that can serve as restrictors of the cervical spine, the upper extremities, the lumbar spine, and even into the pelvis and lower extremities. Restoration of symmetric thoracic cage function for respiration and circulation is as important as restoring symmetric mobility of the lumbar spine, pelvis, and lower extremities in the walking cycle.

SUGGESTED READINGS

Andriacchi T, Schultz A, Belytschko T, et al. A model for studies of mechanical interactions between the human spine and rib cage. *J Biomech* 1974;7:497–507.

Bourdillon J. Treatment of respiratory rib dysfunctions. *J Orthop Med* 1990;12:63–68.

Bourdillon J. Treatment of structural rib dysfunctions. *J Orthop Med* 1991;13:20–22.

Lee R, Farquharson T, Domelo S. Subluxation and locking of the first rib: a cause of thoracic outlet syndrome. *Aust Assoc Man Med Bull* 1988;6:50–51.

Lindgren KA, Leino E. Subluxation of the first rib: a possible thoracic outlet syndrome mechanism. *Arch Phys Med Rehabil* 1988;68:692–695.

Lindgren KA, Mannimen H, Rytkonen H. Thoracic outlet syndrome: a functional disturbance of the upper thoracic aperture? *Muscle Nerve* 1995;5:526–530.

16

LUMBAR SPINE TECHNIQUE

The lumbar spine and pelvic girdle (see Chapter 17) contain many of the structures incriminated in the complaint of "low back pain." The classic report of Mixter and Barr in 1934 brought the lumbar intervertebral disc to the attention of physicians in many disciplines. The differential diagnosis of low back pain continues to be a dilemma for the examining physician. 60% to 80% of cases of low back pain are still classified as idiopathic. After the exclusion of organic and pathologic conditions by orthodox orthopedic and neurologic testing, the examiner is left with the difficulty of determining if any other treatable source for the back pain can be identified. It is in these patients that the ability to identify and treat functional abnormalities of the musculoskeletal system has been found to be clinically effective. It is strongly recommended that the structural diagnostic procedures identified here and in Chapter 17, be used concurrently with orthopedic and neurologic testing of the lower trunk and lower extremities. Including functional diagnosis in these patients greatly reduces the number that need to be classified as idiopathic. More clinical research is needed into the origin of pain in dysfunctions of the lumbar spine and pelvis, the efficacy, and the mechanisms of manual medicine therapeutic applications.

FUNCTIONAL ANATOMY

The five lumbar vertebrae are the most massive in the vertebral column. The vertebral bodies are kidney shaped and are solidly constructed to participate in weight bearing of the superincumbent vertebral column. The posterior arches are strongly developed with large spinous processes projecting directly posterior from the vertebral bodies. The transverse processes are quite large and those at L3 are usually the most broad. The lumbar lordosis has an anterior convexity with L3, usually the most anterior segment. L4 and L5 have limited motion because of the strong attachments of the iliolumbar ligaments to the osseous pelvis; therefore, L3 becomes the first lumbar segment that is freely movable.

The articular pillar has a superior zygapophysial joint that faces posteriorly and medially, and an inferior zygapophysial joint that faces laterally and anteriorly. The superior facet is somewhat concave and the inferior facet somewhat convex. The facing of the lumbar zygapophysial joint is variable and asymmetry is quite common. Because of the shape of the zygapophysial joints, only a small amount of axial rotation movement is present. When the plane of the zygapophysial joints is more sagittal, there appears to be increased stability of the lumbar spine. The more coronal facing the lumbar zygapophysial joints are, the more mobility and potential hypermobility appear to be present. The presence of asymmetry, with one zygapophysial joint being sagittal and the other being coronal, appears to increase the risk of disc degeneration and herniation, with a tendency toward herniation on the side of the coronal facing facet. Asymmetric zygapophysial joints also appear to influence the motion characteristics of the segment and are frequently found in patients with recurrent and refractory dysfunctional problems in the lumbar spine. Between the superior and inferior zygapophysial joints lies the structure called the pars interarticularis. Disruption through the pars without separation is called spondylolysis. With separation at this level, the body, pedicle, and superior articular pillar slide anteriorly while the spinous process, laminae, and inferior articular pillar are held posteriorly, resulting in spondylolisthesis.

The lower lumbar region is frequently the site of developmental variations. In addition to asymmetric development of the zygapophysial joints, other variations in the posterior arch occur resulting in unilateral and bilateral changes in size and shape of the transverse process, culminating in a transitional lumbosacral vertebra that may have lumbar or sacral characteristics, (previously referred to as lumbarization and sacralization). Failure of closure of the posterior arch is not infrequently seen and occasionally the spinous process of L5 is missing. Absence of these structures must result in alteration of the usual ligamentous and muscular attachments in the region.

LUMBAR MOTION

The motions available in the lumbar spine are primarily flexion and extension. There is a small amount of right- and left-side bending and a minimal amount of rotation. The coupled movements of side bending and rotation available in the lumbar spine are both neutral (type I) and nonneutral (type II). In the absence of dysfunction, when in the neutral and the backward-bending positions, side bending and rotation are coupled to opposite sides. In the forward-bent position, side bending and rotation couple to the same side (nonneutral mechanics). Neutral coupling is the lumbar motion that occurs during normal gait. The lumbar lordosis is present and the lumbar spine side bends and rotates to opposite sides with each step. The nonneutral behavior of the lumbar spine, when it is forward bent, places the lumbar spine at risk for injury of the zygapophysial joints for dysfunction, the paravertebral muscles for strain, the posterior ligaments for sprain, and the intervertebral disc for torsional injury and potentially herniation. The L4 and L5 segments have less mobility than the upper three due to the attachment of the iliolumbar ligaments with the osseous pelvis.

MOTION AT THE LUMBOSACRAL JUNCTION

During neutral vertebral mechanics, and in the absence of dysfunction, the lumbar spine and the sacrum move in opposite directions. As the sacrum moves into anterior nutation (sacral flexion), the lumbar spine moves into backward bending (extension) in relation to the sacrum. With the sacrum moving into posterior nutation (sacral extension), the lumbar moves into forward bending (flexion) in relation to the sacrum. With side bending right and rotation left of the sacrum between the hip bones, the lumbar spine adapts by side bending left and rotating right in three-dimensional space. Sometimes this lumbar to sacral coupling occurs at the lumbosacral junction (L5 on S1) and occasionally it occurs at L4-L5. The reason for the difference may be in the location of the lower lumbar segments in relation to the hip bones. Previous studies have shown that if L5 is located deep within the pelvis, the L4-L5 disc is more likely to herniate. If L5 is high and above the level of the hip bones, the L5 to S1 disc is more likely to herniate. This may be due to the different orientation of the iliolumbar ligaments. The obvious conclusion is that the torsional load on the disc is different. This anatomy may also explain the different coupling seen at the lumbosacral junction. Suffice it to say, the lumbar spine and sacrum, as units, should move in opposite directions during neutral mechanics.

In the absence of dysfunction all lumbar segments should follow the segment below during the forward-bending/backward-bending arc. The paired transverse processes of each segment should remain in the same relevant plane as the segment below. Loss of the normal, neutral, relationship of the lumbar spine to the sacrum is of great clinical significance and is termed "nonadaptive lumbar response" to sacral function. Restoration of this normal relationship at the lumbosacral junction (whether at L4-L5 or L5-S1) is one of the major reasons for diagnosing and treating lumbar spine dysfunctions before addressing the two sacroiliac joints. Many of the techniques to be described in Chapter 17 require the normal, neutral, relationship of L5 to the sacrum.

STRUCTURAL DIAGNOSIS OF LUMBAR SPINE DYSFUNCTION

The lumbar spine has the capacity for three dysfunctions. There can be the two nonneutral (type II) dysfunctions of either the extended, rotated, and side-bent (ERS) type or the flexed, rotated, and side-bent (FRS) type or can have a neutral (group) dysfunction. Group dysfunctions frequently occur in the upper lumbar spine and carry over into the lower thoracic spine segments. In the presence of flattening of the lumbar lordosis, the probability of FRS dysfunction with extension restriction is high. If the lumbar lordosis is increased, the probability of ERS dysfunction with flexion restriction is high. The diagnosis of lumbar segmental dysfunction combines tissue texture changes of the deeper layers of paravertebral muscles, particularly hypertonicity of the multifidi, rotatores, and intertransversarii, and alteration in motion characteristics. Evaluation of lumbar segmental motion can be done in a variety of ways. For the reasons described in Chapter 6, the recommended process is to evaluate the location of the posterior aspect of the transverse processes in three positions. This process requires the assessment of the superior segment in relation to the inferior. In the lumbar spine, this requires that L5 be assessed in relation to the sacrum. Therefore, assessment of the lumbar spine begins by identifying the sacral base, the posterior aspect of the transverse processes of S1. Because of the anatomy of the lumbosacral junction, it is not possible to palpate the transverse processes of L5. Instead, the examiner identifies the symmetric portions of the posterior arch of L5, as far laterally as possible, to assess rotation of L5 in relation to S1.

The diagnostic procedure requires the assessment of the paired transverse processes in neutral, forward-bent, and backward positions. A sequence that is the easiest for the beginning student is to first assess in the prone (neutral) position on the table (Fig. 16.1). Beginning at the sacral base, each lumbar vertebra is assessed for its relationship to the one below up to the thoracolumbar junction. Assessment is now made in the backward bent (extended) prone prop position on the table (sphinx position) (Fig. 16.2). Despite the mass size of the lumbar musculature, the transverse processes are quite easily palpated in this position. Assessment is then made in the fully forward-bent position with the patient seated with the feet on the floor or a stool. Assessment is made from below upward in a similar fashion. It is more difficult to palpate transverse processes in this position because of the tension through the lumbar muscles and the lumbodorsal fascia (Fig. 16.3). If one transverse process is more pos-

terior in the fully forward-bent position and become symmetric in the prone prop (sphinx position), a nonneutral (type II) ERS dysfunction is present at this level. If one transverse process is more prominent in the prone prop (sphinx position) and becomes symmetric in the forward-bent position, a nonneutral (type II) FRS restriction is present. If three or more transverse processes remain prominent throughout all three positions, a neutral (type I) dysfunction is present. It is difficult to evaluate the functional capacity of the upper lumbar segments until those identified as dysfunctional in the lower region are successfully treated. Nonneutral dysfunctions are common at L4 and L5, as well as at the thoracolumbar junction. Nonneutral dysfunctions at L4 and L5 are frequently seen in association with dysfunction of the sacroiliac joints.

The lumbar spine also has the capacity for bilateral dysfunction at the same vertebral motion segment. The most common is bilateral flexed or bilateral extended dysfunction. These are seen more frequently at the lumbosacral and thoracolumbar junctions. These dysfunctions are more difficult to diagnose since there is no rotational asymmetry. The major clue to their existence is bilateral tissue texture abnormality at a given segment and some overall motion loss. The diagnosis is made by finding no change in the interspinous space between two segments during the forward bending–backward bending arc. The segment is either bilaterally flexed or bilaterally extended. These dysfunctions are classified as sagittal plane dysfunction.

In the presence of unleveling of the sacrum, in the absence of dysfunction of the lumbar spine, there will

Figure 16.1.
Transverse process, palpation-neutral position.

Figure 16.2.
Transverse process, palpation backward bent (extended) position (prone prop).

Figure 16.3.
Transverse process palpation, forward-bent position.

be a side bending and rotation to opposite sides of the lumbar vertebra in order to compensate and maintain the trunk erect. This adaptive response is only found in neutral. The longer this is present, the more likely it is to develop a neutral (group) dysfunction.

MANUAL MEDICINE PROCEDURES FOR DYSFUNCTIONS OF LUMBAR SPINE

The treating clinician needs to have manual medicine techniques to treat group (type I) dysfunctions and the nonneutral (type II) ERS and FRS dysfunctions. In the treatment sequence, it is recommended that nonneutral dysfunctions be treated first and group dysfunctions last. Usually one begins by treating the lower segments first and sequentially from below upward. Exceptions to this below upward rule are those cases in which the major restrictor is higher in the lumbar spine or in which the lowest segment is so acute that it is difficult to directly address it. One should be able to treat a patient in the erect sitting posture or recumbent on the table. It is frequently valuable to treat a large patient in the sitting position so that gravity can be used as an assisting activating force.

Lumbar Spine

Muscle Energy Technique
Sitting
Nonneutral Dysfunction (Example: L4 ERS_left)
Position: Backward bent (extended), rotated left, sidebent left (ER_left S_left)
Motion Restriction: Forward bending (flexion), right-side bending, right rotation

1. Patient sitting on stool with left hand holding the right shoulder and right arm dropped at the side.

2. Operator stands at left side of patient straddling the patient's left knee with the left hand grasping patient's right shoulder and controlling the left shoulder with the left axilla (Fig. 16.4). Operator's right middle finger monitors the L4-L5 interspinous space and the right index finger monitors the left transverse process of L4.

3. The forward-bending (flexion) barrier is engaged by an anterior-to-posterior translatory movement at L4-L5 (Fig. 16.5).

4. Right-side bending and right rotation are introduced at L4-L5 by the operator's left arm and asking the patient to reach to the floor with the right hand (Fig. 16.6) with a controlled concentric isotonic contraction.

5. Patient is instructed to side bend to the left against equal resistance for 3 to 5 seconds using an isometric contraction. Following relaxation, a new forward-bending, right-side bending, and right rotational barrier is engaged and three to five repetitions are made of the left-side bending isometric effort.

Figure 16.5.

Figure 16.4.

Figure 16.6.

6. When all right rotation and right-side bending restrictions are removed, operator forward bends the patient while maintaining right rotation (Fig. 16.7).

7. Operator's left hand resists a patient trunk extension effort, fully forward bending the segment and opening both zygapophysial joints at L4 to L5 (Fig. 16.8).

8. Retest.

Figure 16.7.

Figure 16.8.

Lumbar Spine

Muscle Energy Technique
Sitting
Nonneutral Dysfunction (Example: L3 FRS$_{left}$)
  Position: Forward bent$_{(F)}$, rotated$_{(left)}$, sidebent$_{(left)}$
  Motion Restriction: Backward bending (extension),
  right-side bending, right rotation

1. Patient sitting on stool with operator sitting behind controlling patient's trunk with the right hand and monitoring the interspinous space of L3 to L4 with the left index finger and the left transverse process of L3 with the left middle finger.

2. Operator introduces side bending left and rotation right in neutral mechanics by the patient dropping the left shoulder and shifting the weight to the right buttock.

3. Three to four repetitions of a right-side bending effort by the patient pushing the right shoulder into the operator's right hand introducing right rotation at L3 on L4 (Fig. 16.9).

4. Operator introduces extension and right-side bending while right rotated by pressing inferiorly on the right shoulder while the patient shifts the weight to the left buttock and projects the abdomen over the left knee (Fig. 16.10).

5. Operator resists a series of three to five isometric contractions of 3 to 5 seconds with the patient either pulling the right shoulder forward against resistance or lifting the right shoulder toward the ceiling against resistance (Fig. 16.11). After each repetition, a new barrier is engaged.

6. When all right-side bending and right rotation restriction is removed, operator maintains extension and straightens patient's shoulders, while blocking the L4 segment bilaterally with the left hand (Fig. 16.12). Operator's right hand resists flexion effort by the patient's trunk to fully extend L3 on L4, closing both zygapophysial joints.

7. Retest.

Figure 16.9.

Figure 16.11.

Figure 16.10.

Figure 16.12.

Lumbar Spine

Muscle Energy Technique
Sitting
Neutral (group dysfunction)
Variation 1
    Position: Neutral, side-bent right, rotated left
    ($NS_{right}R_{left}$ or EN_{left})
    Motion Restriction: Side bending left, rotation right

1. Patient sitting on table with right hand grasping the left shoulder. Operator standing behind with right arm under patient's right axilla and grasping patient's left shoulder to control upper trunk (Fig. 16.13).

2. Operator's left thumb is placed at the apex of the left lumbar convexity for localization (Fig. 16.14).

3. Operator introduces left-side bending and right rotation by left-to-right translation localized by the left thumb contact at the apex of the left lumbar convexity (Fig. 16.15).

4. Operator resists a series of 3- to 5-second right-side bending efforts against operator's resistance through the right hand (Fig. 16.16). The localizing thumb maintains a force anteromedially against the left lumbar curve.

5. Retest.

Figure 16.13.

Figure 16.15.

Figure 16.14.

Figure 16.16.

Lumbar Spine

Muscle Energy Technique
Sitting
Neutral (group dysfunction)
Variation 2
    Position: $NS_{right}R_{left}$ or EN_{left}
    Motion Restriction: Side bending left, rotation right

1. Patient sitting on table with left hand holding the right shoulder. Operator stands behind with the left hand grasping patient's right shoulder and with left axilla over patient's left shoulder. Operator's right thumb is at the apex of the left lumbar convexity pressing anteromedially (Fig. 16.17).

2. Operator introduces left-side bending and right rotation through the left arm contact with translation from left to right at the apex of the curve localized by the right thumb (Fig. 16.18).

3. Operator resists patient's right-side bending effort of 3 to 5 seconds repeated three to five times (Fig. 16.19).

4. Following each effort the operator engages the new left-side bending right rotational barrier with left-to-right translation localized at the apex.

5. Retest.

Figure 16.18.

Figure 16.17.

Figure 16.19.

Lumbar Spine

Muscle Energy Technique
Sitting
Bilateral Extension Restriction (Example: L1-L2)
    Position: Bilaterally flexed
    Motion Restriction: Bilateral extension

1. Patient sitting on table with hands holding opposite shoulder. Operator stands behind with left hand holding both elbows to control patient's trunk (Fig. 16.20).
2. The heel of the operator's hand blocks the L2 segment in the midline (Fig. 16.21).

3. Operator engages extension barrier by backward bending the trunk while translating from posterior to anterior through the right hand (Fig. 16.22). Note the blocking of the right elbow against the operator's trunk.
4. Operator's left arm resists a forward bending effort by the patient with a 3- to 5-second contraction repeated three to five times (Fig. 16.23).
5. The extension barrier is engaged after each patient effort.
6. Retest.

Figure 16.20.

Figure 16.22.

Figure 16.21.

Figure 16.23.

Lumbar Spine

Muscle Energy Technique
Lateral Recumbent (Sims Position) (Example: L4 ERS$_{right}$)
    Position: Backward bent (ERS$_{right}$)
    Motion Restriction: Forward bending (flexion), rotation left, side bending left

1. Patient prone on table with operator standing at right side. Operator flexes patient's knees; rolls lower extremity onto left hip into the Sims position (Fig. 16.24).

2. Operator's left middle finger palpates the L4 to L5 interspace with the index finger over the right transverse process of L4. Operator's right hand introduces left rotation of the trunk down to L4. Patient assists by reaching toward the floor (Fig. 16.25).

3. Operator switches hands with right hand monitoring the L4 to L5 level as the left arm and left thigh flex the patient's knees up to L5, engaging the flexion barrier (Fig. 16.26).

Figure 16.25.

Figure 16.24.

Figure 16.26.

4. While continuing to monitor the L4 to L5 level, operator drops both feet to the floor introducing left-side bending to the barrier (Fig. 16.27). Note that the patient's knees are resting on the operator's left thigh.

5. Operator resists a muscle effort by the patient to lift the feet to the ceiling attempting to introduce a right-side bending effort against resistance (Fig. 16.28). Operator's right hand monitors over the L4 to L5 level ensuring localization of muscle contraction at that level.

6. Three to five repetitions of a 3- to 5-second muscle contraction are performed by the patient with the

operator engaging a new flexion, left rotation, and left-side bending barrier after each effort.

7. Retest.

Note: Caution must be used to protect the lateral aspect of the patient's left thigh against the edge of the table. If the operator is unable to stabilize the patient's legs against the left thigh, a rolled towel or small pillow can be placed between the patient's thighs and the edge of the table. Another option is for the operator to sit on the end of the table with the left hand monitoring the L4-L5 level, controlling the lower extremities with the right hand, with the patient's left knee over the operator's left thigh.

Figure 16.27.

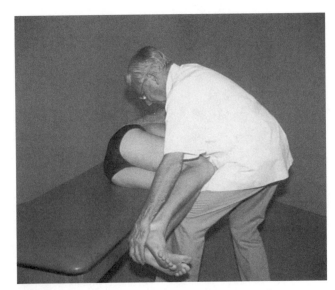

Figure 16.28.

Lumbar Spine

Muscle Energy Technique
Lateral Recumbent
Nonneutral Dysfunction (Example: L4 ERS$_{left}$)
    Position: Backward bent (ERS$_{left}$)
    Motion Restriction: Forward bending (flexion), rotation right, side bending right

1. Patient lying in the left lateral recumbent position with neck supported by a pillow, the feet and knees together, and shoulders and hips perpendicular to the table. Operator stands in front of patient and with right hand flexes patient's trunk down to L4 from above maintaining the shoulders perpendicular to the table for right-side bending (Fig. 16.29).

2. Operator flexes the lower extremities up to L5 while monitoring at the L4-L5 level with the right hand (Fig. 16.30).

3. Operator introduces right rotation through the right forearm rotating the patient's right shoulder posteriorly while monitoring at the L4-L5 level with the right hand.

4. Operator introduces right-side bending by lifting both feet toward the ceiling (Fig. 16.31) engaging the combined right rotation, right-side bending barrier.

5. Operator resists patient effort to pull the feet back toward the table (a left-side bending effort) while monitoring for contraction of the erector spinae muscles at the L4-L5 level.

6. Patient performs three to five repetitions of a 3- to 5-second contraction. During each relaxation phase the operator reengages the forward bending, right rotation, right-side bending barrier.

7. Retest.

Figure 16.30.

Figure 16.29.

Figure 16.31.

Lumbar Spine

Muscle Energy Technique
Lateral Recumbent (Example: L4 FRS$_{left}$)
  Position: Forward bent (FRS$_{left}$)
  Motion Restriction: Backward bending (extension), right rotation, right-side bending

1. Patient in the left lateral recumbent position with the knees and feet together and with shoulders and pelvic perpendicular to the table (begins right-side bending by position).
2. Operator stands in front of the patient and with two hands contacts the L4-L5 level (Fig. 16.32).

3. Operator engages first backward bending (extension) barrier by translating the L4-L5 level from posterior to anterior (Fig. 16.33).

   Note: Patient is lying on a sheet or towel to facilitate sliding on the table.

4. Operator fine-tunes backward bending (extension) barrier from above by translating the left shoulder posteriorly, maintaining both shoulders perpendicular to the table, and monitoring with the left hand for motion down to L4 (Fig. 16.34).
5. Operator fine-tunes backward bending (extension) barrier from below by extending the lower extremities and monitoring with the right hand for movement up to L5 (Fig. 16.35).

Figure 16.32.

Figure 16.34.

Figure 16.33.

Figure 16.35.

6. Operator engages right rotation barrier by rotating the right shoulder posteriorly with the right hand monitoring for rotation to L4 with the left hand (Fig. 16.36). Patient grasps the edge of the table to maintain the right rotation and to introduce more extension.

7. Operator's left hand lifts the right leg to engage the right-side bending barrier while monitoring with the right hand at the L4-L5 level (Fig. 16.37).

8. Patient pulls right knee down toward the left knee for three to five repetitions of a 3 to 5 second muscle contraction against resistance provided by the operator's left hand. After each effort, the operator engages a new right-side bending barrier by lifting the knee toward the ceiling, and a new backward

bending barrier by translating L4-L5 anteriorly by the right hand.

9. Operator returns patient's right knee to the table and places right forearm against the patient's right shoulder maintaining right rotation. Operator's right hand monitors at the L4-L5 level. Operator's left hand on patient's right buttock engages right-side bending barrier by cephalic translation (Fig. 16.38). Operator resists with the right forearm a left rotation effort of the patient's trunk by pushing the right shoulder into the operator's right forearm or a left-side bending effort by pushing the right buttock caudad. Again, three to five repetitions are performed.

10. Retest.

Figure 16.37.

Figure 16.36.

Figure 16.38.

Lumbar Spine

Lateral Recumbent Position
Neutral (group dysfunction) (Example: L1-L4 convex left)

Position: $NS_{right}R_{left}$ or EN_{left}
Motion Restriction: Left-side bending, right rotation

1. Patient in right lateral recumbent position with shoulders and pelvis perpendicular to the table and with knees and feet together. Operator stands in front.
2. Operator flexes and extends the lower extremities to ensure the point of maximum ease of the forward bending/backward bending movement of the L1 to L4 lumbar neutral curve. Operator monitors with the left hand (Fig. 16.39).
3. Operator lifts both feet toward the ceiling, introducing a left-side bending, right rotational movement to the lumbar spine (Fig. 16.40).
4. Operator's right hand resists patient's effort of pulling the feet back to the table for 3 to 5 seconds and three to five repetitions (a right-side bending effort).
5. Operator's left hand monitors the muscle contraction and postcontraction stretch of the right paravertebral muscles (the concavity).
6. Retest.

Figure 16.39.

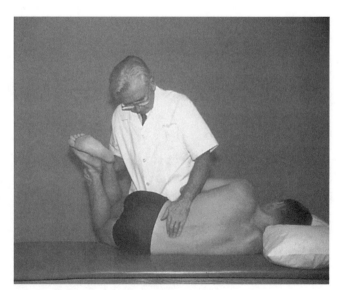

Figure 16.40.

Lumbar Spine

Mobilization with Impulse Technique
Lateral Recumbent Position
Neutral (group) Dysfunction (Example: L1-L4 convex left)

Position: $NS_{right}R_{left}$ or EN_{left}
Motion Restriction: Side-bending left, rotation right

1. Patient in the left lateral recumbent position (most posterior transverse processes toward the table) with operator standing in front.

2. Patient's lower extremities are flexed and extended to the point of maximum ease of the forward bending/backward bending range of the lumbar lordosis.

3. Operator monitors dysfunctional lumbar segments with the left hand and grasps the patient's left elbow (Fig. 16.41).

4. Operator pulls patient's left elbow forward and caudad (Fig. 16.42), introducing left-side bending and right rotation from above (Fig. 16.43).

5. Operator's right forearm in contact with the patient's right axilla and pectoral region maintains right rotation from above while operator's left forearm pulls patient's pelvis into left rotation (Fig. 16.44). The transverse processes of the apex of the dysfunctional group are perpendicular to the table.

6. A mobilization with impulse thrust is made through the left forearm by the operator's body drop rotating the pelvis anteriorly into left rotation.

Figure 16.41.

Figure 16.43.

Figure 16.42.

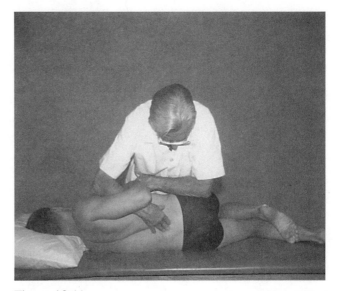

Figure 16.44.

7. An alternate arm position finds the operator's right forearm stabilizing the patient's right shoulder and pectoral region and both hands monitoring at the dysfunctional lumbar segments. Again, an anterior rotary thrust is applied through the left forearm by an operator body drop (Fig. 16.45).

8. An alternate arm position has operator's right hand stabilizing the anterior aspect of the pectoral region (not grasping the humerus) and the left forearm incorporated as part of the operator's body provides the anterior rotational thrust. Note operator's left hand monitoring dysfunctional segments (Fig. 16.46).

9. Retest.

Figure 16.45.

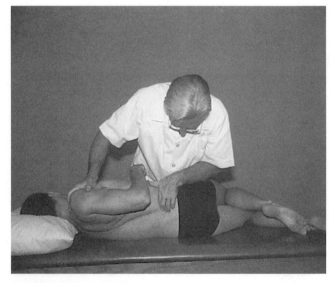

Figure 16.46.

Lumbar Spine

Mobilization with Impulse Technique
Lateral Recumbent Position
Nonneutral Dysfunction (Example: L4 ERS$_{left}$)
   Position: Backward bent (ERS$_{left}$)
   Motion Restriction: Forward bending (flexion), right rotation, right-side bending

1. Patient in the left lateral recumbent position (most posterior transverse process toward the table) with a pillow supporting the cervical spine, knees and

feet together and shoulders and pelvis perpendicular to the table (initiating beginning right-side bending). Operator stands in front monitoring L4-L5 level with the left hand (Fig. 16.47).

2. While maintaining the patient's shoulders perpendicular to the table, operator introduces forward bending down to L4 from above by curling the patient's trunk forward (Fig. 16.48).

3. Operator now monitors the L4-L5 segment with the right hand and flexes the lower extremities up to L5 (Fig. 16.49).

Figure 16.48.

Figure 16.47.

Figure 16.49.

4. Operator places the patient's right foot in the left popliteal space. Operator's right forearm introduces right rotation down to L4 (Fig. 16.50).

5. Operator's left forearm in contact with the patient's right buttock rotates the pelvis anteriorly and superiorly (Fig. 16.51).

6. Operator fine-tunes forward bending, right rotation, and right-side bending to the elastic barrier and provides an anterior and cephalad thrust through the left forearm by a body drop. The localization attempts to maintain the transverse processes of L4 perpendicular to the table.

7. Retest.

Figure 16.50.

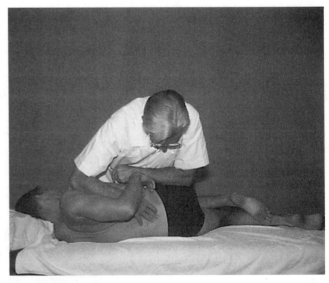

Figure 16.51.

Lumbar Spine

Mobilization with Impulse Technique
Lateral Recumbent Position
Nonneutral Dysfunction (Example: L4 FRS$_{left}$)
    Position: Forward bent rotated left, sidebent left
    (FRS$_{left}$)
    Motion Restriction: Backward bending (extension),
    right rotation, right-side bending

1. Patient lies in the left lateral recumbent position
    (most posterior transverse process toward the
    table) with a pillow under the cervical spine, knees
    and feet together, shoulders and pelvis perpendicu-
    lar to the table.

2. Operator stands in front and grasps the L4-L5 seg-
    ment level between the two hands (Fig. 16.52).

3. Operator's hands localizes to the first backward-
    bending barrier by translating the patient's trunk
    from posterior to anterior (Fig. 16.53).

4. Operator fine-tunes extension barrier from above by
    translating patient posteriorly through the operator's
    right forearm (Fig. 16.54) while monitoring with the
    left hand over the L4-L5 segment (Fig. 16.55).

Figure 16.52.

Figure 16.54.

Figure 16.53.

Figure 16.55.

5. Operator fine-tunes extension barrier from below by extending the lower extremities with the left arm for movement up to L5 being monitored by the right hand (Fig. 16.56).

6. Operator's left hand places patient's right foot in the left popliteal space while the right forearm, in contact with the patient's right pectoral region, introduces right rotation from above monitoring with the fingers of the right hand over the L4-L5 level (Fig. 16.57).

7. Operator's left forearm contacts patient's right buttock and introduces anterior and cephalad rotation of the pelvis engaging the barrier at the L4-L5 level (Fig. 16.58).

8. Operator introduces mobilizing thrust through the left forearm by a body drop in an anterior and cephalad direction.

9. Retest.

Figure 16.57.

Figure 16.56.

Figure 16.58.

Lumbar Spine

Mobilization with Impulse Technique
  Sitting
  Sagittal Plane Restriction (Example: L1 bilaterally flexed)
      Position: Bilaterally forward bent (flexed)
      Motion Restriction: Bilateral backward bending (extension)

1. Patient sitting in table with arms crossed holding the opposite shoulder. Operator stands behind grasping patient's elbows for trunk control (Fig. 16.59).
2. The heel of operator's right hand is placed in the midline over the spinous process of L2 with localization to the inferior segment (Fig. 16.60).

3. Operator applies a backward-bending (extension) thrust by lifting the patient's trunk through the elbows over the fulcrum applied by the right hand on L2 (Fig. 16.61).
4. An alternate thrust is a body drop of the operator's body through a lever arm of the right forearm in an anterior direction against the right hand contact on L2 (Fig. 16.62).
5. When using either of the thrust options, the operator tries to thrust with one hand only while the other maintains stabilization. However, both options require two-handed coordination.
6. Retest.

Figure 16.59.

Figure 16.61.

Figure 16.60.

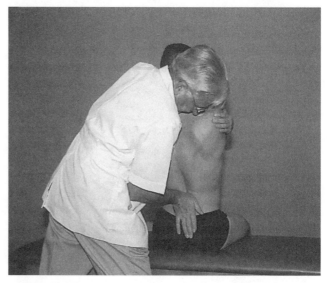

Figure 16.62.

Lumbar Spine

Mobilization with Impulse Technique
Nonneutral Dysfunction (Example: L3 ERS$_{left}$)
    Position: Backward bent (ERS$_{left}$)
    Motion restriction: Forward bending (flexion), right rotation, right-side bending

1. Patient sitting astride the table with arms crossed holding each shoulder.

2. Operator stands at right side of patient with right hand grasping patient's left shoulder and right axilla over patient's right shoulder. Operator's reinforced left thumb is in contact with the right side of the spinous process of L3 (Fig. 16.63).

3. Operator engages the forward bending, right-side bending, and right rotational barrier through move-ment of the patient's trunk by the right arm and with right-to-left pressure of the left thumb on the spinous process of L3 (Fig. 16.64).

4. The mobilizing thrust is applied by exaggerating the patient's body position by dropping the operator's weight toward the floor while simultaneously thrusting from right to left with the left thumb on the spinous process of L3.

5. An alternative localizing hand position is the use of the left pisiform through the operator's hypothenar eminence on the right side of the spinous process of L3 (Fig. 16.65). Note the blocking of the operator's left forearm against the left hip.

6. Retest.

Figure 16.64.

Figure 16.63.

Figure 16.65.

Lumbar Spine

Mobilization with Impulse Technique
Sitting
Nonneutral Dysfunction (Example: L3 FRS$_{left}$)
  Position: Forward bent (flexed), rotated left, side bent left
  Motion Restriction: Backward bending (extension), right rotation, right sidebending

1. Patient sitting astride the table with the right hand holding the left shoulder.
2. Operator stands at the right side with the right hand holding patient's left shoulder and the right axilla on top of the patient's right shoulder. Operator's reinforced left thumb is on the right side of the spinous process of L3 (Fig. 16.66).

3. Operator introduces backward bending, right-side bending, and right rotation through the right arm contact with the patient's trunk, while localizing by translation from right to left on the spinous process of L3 (Fig. 16.67).
4. The mobilizing thrust is introduced by inferior body drop of the operator on the patient's right shoulder and a right-to-left force through the left thumb.
5. An alternative hand contact is the operator's pisiform through the left hypothenar eminence on the right side of the spinous process of L3 (Fig. 16.68). Note that operator's left elbow is in contact with the left hip, providing a lever arm to the contact on L3.
6. Retest.

Figure 16.67.

Figure 16.66.

Figure 16.68.

Lumbar Spine

Mobilization with Impulse Technique
Sitting
Neutral (group dysfunction) (Example: L1 to L4 convex left)
    Position: NS$_{right}$R$_{left}$ or EN$_{left}$
    Motion Restriction: Side bending left, rotation right

1. Patient sitting astride the table with the left hand on the right shoulder.
2. Operator stands at the left side of the patient with the left hand holding the right shoulder and the left axilla on top of the patient's left shoulder and the reinforced thumb in the intertransverse space between L2 to L3 (Fig. 16.69).

3. Operator engages the left-side bending and right rotation barrier through the control of the patient's trunk with the left arm while maintaining an antero-medial-localizing fulcrum with the right thumb (Fig. 16.70).
4. The mobilizing thrust is a body drop of the operator toward the floor enhancing the left-side bending and right rotation with localization at the apex of the curve.
5. An alternate hand position is the use of the right pisiform and right hypothenar eminence at the apex of the lumbar curve (Fig. 16.71).
6. Retest.

Figure 16.70.

Figure 16.69.

Figure 16.71.

Lumbar Spine

Mobilization without Impulse (articulatory)
Technique
Activating force variations

1. All previous mobilization with impulse techniques can be modified using a mobilization without impulse activating force.

2. Patient and operator positions remain the same.

3. Follow the principles found in Chapter 7.

4. Use repetitive oscillatory operator efforts in the direction of the restrictive barrier, gradually increasing the range of movement.

5. This technique is frequently applied before the use of final mobilizing with impulse thrust.

6. Retest.

Lumbar Spine

Muscle energy activating force

1. Any of the mobilizing with impulse techniques can be modified to use a muscle intrinsic activating force.

2. Patient's activating force is in the direction opposite to the operator-localized position.

3. Three to five repetitions of a 3- to 5-second muscle contraction are used with the operator reengaging the new barrier after each patient contraction.

4. Frequently two or three muscle energy efforts are used before the application of a mobilization with impulse thrust.

5. Retest.

CONCLUSION

The lumbar spine is a frequent site of dysfunction, particularly nonneutral dysfunctions of the FRS type. These dysfunctions are frequently associated with a herniated intervertebral disc at the same level. Restoration of more normal mobility at the segment is frequently most helpful in managing the discogenic radiculopathy, if present.

The lumbar spine should be examined, and treated if dysfunctional, before addressing the pelvis, as many of the techniques for sacral dysfunction use the lumbar spine as a lever.

SUGGESTED READINGS

Bogduk N. The innervation of the lumbar spine. *Spine* 1983;8:286–293.

Bogduk N, Towmey L. *Clinical anatomy of the lumbar spine.* London: Churchill Livingstone, 1987.

Cossette JW, Farfan HF, Robertson GH, et al. The instantaneous center of rotation of the third lumbar intervertebral joint. *J Biomech* 1971;4:149–153.

Farfan HF. The effects of torsion on the intervertebral joints. *J Bone Joint Surg Am* 1970;52:468–497.

Farfan HF, Sullivan JD. The relation of facet orientation to intervertebral disc failure. *Can J Surg* 1967;10:179–185.

Mixter WJ, Barr SS. Rupture of the intervertebral disc with involvement of the spinal canal. *N Eng J Med* 1934, 211:210–215.

17

The increase in research in the past 10 to 15 years has diminished the controversy surrounding the role of the sacroiliac joint in the production of lower back pain. Several world congresses in the past decade addressed the sacroiliac joint in back pain. Sacroiliac joint motion has been reported in the medical literature since the mid 19th century. Some of the orthopedic literature in the first half of the 20th century included descriptions of pain syndromes related to the joint and various therapeutic methods for its control. Despite these publications, many authorities held the view that there was no movement at the sacroiliac joints and therefore they were not clinically significant. Based on the recent contributions from basic and clinical science, there has been a change in perception of the role of the sacroiliac joint in clinical pain syndromes. Movement within the sacroiliac joint, although small, is now generally recognized. Controversy continues as to the type of motion available and the axes of motion. Sacroiliac arthrography has demonstrated that some sacroiliac joints are painful on injection and pain relief occurs following instillation of local anesthetic. Normal sacroiliac joints do not appear to be painful on injection. Controversy continues as to the ability of a clinician to use physical assessment to identify a significant sacroiliac dysfunction. Additional basic research and clinical research are clearly needed.

It is beyond the scope of this volume to review all of the research on sacroiliac motion. The generally accepted pelvic girdle motions will be discussed and a diagnostic and therapeutic system for pelvic girdle dysfunction will be described. The system described will allow the clinician to diagnose and treat all of the physical findings of pelvic girdle dysfunctions. It builds on the current knowledge of pelvic girdle movement and dysfunction and adds a theoretic construct and terminology to describe the various physical findings encountered during examination of the pelvic girdle.

MODELS OF PELVIC GIRDLE DYSFUNCTION

The postural–structural, or biomechanical, model is the one most commonly used by the manual medicine practitioner in dealing with the pelvis because it is the key to the gait cycle on which all activities of daily living are based. The pelvis links the mobile extremities with the trunk in the highly complex mechanism of ambulation. Manual medicine management of the pelvic girdle restores functional symmetry to the three bones and joints of the pelvic girdle during the walking cycle. The superior surface of the body of the sacrum supports the vertebral column. Alteration in the sacrum has a significant effect on the vertebral function above. We owe a large debt of gratitude to Fred L. Mitchell, Sr., for his seminal work in defining the role of the pelvis in musculoskeletal function. He is acknowledged as the father of the muscle energy system of manual medicine, but his insight into the pelvic girdle could be viewed as a more significant contribution to the field. Instead of referring to his work as the muscle energy system, we could describe it as the Mitchell pelvic biomechanical model.

The pelvic girdle is also important in the respiratory–circulatory model because of its relationship to the pelvic diaphragm. Dysfunction of the osseous pelvis alters the functional capacity of the muscles of the pelvic diaphragm in a manner similar to those of thoracic spine and rib dysfunctions on the thoracoabdominal diaphragm. Many patients with pelvic girdle dysfunction have vague and persistent symptoms of the lower urinary tract, the genital system, and the rectum that resolve when pelvic girdle function is restored.

The sacral component of the pelvis is of importance within the craniosacral system. The sacrum has inherent mobility between the two hip bones (innominates) as part of craniosacral rhythm and is linked with the motion of the occiput. Altered mechanical function of the pelvic girdle can negatively influence the craniosacral mechanism and, alternatively, altered craniosacral mechanics can influence the biomechanical function of the osseous pelvis. The osseous pelvis has a significant contribution to the functional capacity of the musculoskeletal system and warrants appropriate investigation and management in all patients.

FUNCTIONAL ANATOMY

The pelvic girdle consists of three bones and three joints (Fig. 17.1). The sacrum is formed by the fused elements of the sacral vertebrae and articulates superiorly with the last lumbar vertebra and caudally with the coccyx. The sacrum should be viewed as a component part of the vertebral axis. In many ways, the sacrum functions as an atypical lumbar vertebra between the two hip bones, with the sacroiliac joints as atypical zygapophysial joints. The right and left hip bones consist of the fused elements of the ilium, ischium, and pubis. The two hip bones are joined anteriorly by the symphysis pubis joint. Each hip bone articulates cephalically with the sacrum at the ipsilateral sacroiliac joint and caudally with the femur at the hip joint. Functionally, the hip bone should be viewed as a lower extremity bone and the two sacroiliac joints as the junction of the trunk and the lower extremity.

The joints of the pelvic girdle consist of the symphysis pubis and the two sacroiliac joints. The symphysis pubis is an amphiarthrosis with strong superior and inferior ligaments and a thinner posterior ligament. The opposing surfaces can range from symmetrically flat to quite asymmetric and interlocking. The minimal amount of motion available at this joint is strongly influenced by the shape of the joint, the ligamentous integrity of the joint (particularly under the influence of hormonal changes), and the actions of the abdominal muscles from above and the adductor muscles of the lower extremity below.

The sacroiliac joints are true arthrodial joints with a joint space, synovial capsule, and articular cartilage. They are unique in that the cartilage on the sacral side is hyaline cartilage and the cartilage on the ilial side is fibrocartilage. The articular cartilage on the sacral side is much thicker than that on the ilial side. The joints are L-shaped in contour with a shorter upper arm and a longer lower arm. The joint contour usually has a depression on the sacral side at approximately S-2 and a corresponding prominence on the ilial side. The shape of the sacroiliac joint varies markedly from individual to individual and from side to side in the same individual. During the aging process, there is an increase in the grooves on the opposing surfaces of the sacrum and ilium that appear to reduce available motion and enhance stability. It is of interest to note that the age of the highest incidence of disabling back pain (range, 25 to 45 years) is the same age when the greatest amount of motion is available in the sacroiliac joints. Asymmetric dysfunction of this movement may contribute to disabling back pain. The sacroiliac joint usually has change in anteroposterior beveling at approximately the junction of the upper and lower arms. The plane of the upper portion is convergent from be-

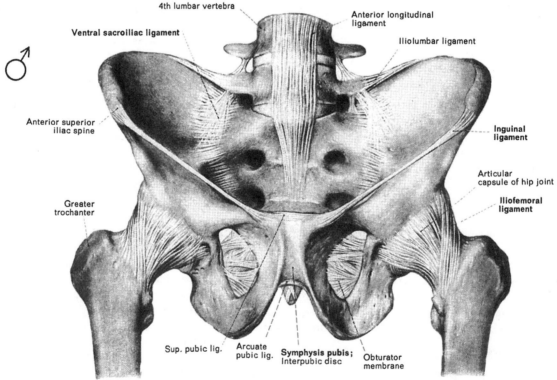

Figure 17.1.
Pelvic girdle.

hind forward whereas the lower portion is divergent from behind forward, resulting in an interlocking mechanism centering at approximately S2. This interlocking mechanism of joint beveling and the concave–convex relationship at S2 provides some of the stability of the joint and is described as form closure. Occasionally the opposing joint surfaces are quite flat and do not have the interlocking joint bevel change at S2 or the ilial prominence within the sacral depression. This type of sacroiliac joint is much less stable and the possibility of superior and inferior translatory movement, or shearing, exists. Occasionally the sacral concavity is replaced by a convexity with the ilial side being more concave. This joint structure provides increased mobility, primarily in rotation medially and laterally, around a vertical axis.

Much of the integrity of the sacroiliac joint depends on ligamentous structures (Figs. 17.1 and 17.2). The iliolumbar ligaments attach to the transverse processes of L4 and L5 and to the anterior surface of the iliac crest. The lower fibers extend inferiorly and blend with the anterior sacroiliac ligaments. The anterior sacroiliac ligaments are two relatively flat and thin bands. They can be viewed as providing a sling from the two hip bones for the anterior surface of the sacrum. They are the anterior aspect of the synovial portion of the joint. The posterior sacroiliac ligaments have three layers. The deepest layer consists of short interosseous ligaments running from the sacrum to the ilium. The intermediate layer runs from the posterior arches of the sacrum to the medial side of the ilium, occupying most of the space overlying the posterior aspect of the sacroiliac joint. The long posterior sacroiliac ligaments blend together and course vertically from the sacral crest to the ilium. Inferiorly these posterior sacroiliac ligaments blend with the accessory sacroiliac ligaments, the sacrotuberous and the sacrospinous. Of particular interest is the long dorsal sacroiliac ligament that courses from the posterior superior iliac spine inferiorly and inserts into S4. The role of this ligament is to prevent posterior sacral nutation. In sacral dysfunctions with a posterior sacral base this ligament in under tension stress and becomes painful to palpation. Tenderness of this ligament is one of the more reliable physical findings in symptomatic sacroiliac dysfunction. The sacrotuberous ligament runs from the inferior lateral angle (ILA) of the sacrum to the ischial tuberosity and has a crescent-shaped medial border. It is continuous with the fascia of the hamstring muscles and forms an im-

Figure 17.2.
Sacroiliac joint.

portant link between the lower extremity and the trunk. The sacrotuberous ligament restricts anterior nutation of the sacrum and is under tension stress in sacral dysfunctions with an anterior base and can become tender at its sacral or ischial end. The sacrospinous ligament lies under the sacrotuberous and runs from the ILA of the sacrum to the ischial spine. These two accessory ligaments contribute to the formation of the greater and lesser sciatic notches that are divided by the sacrospinous ligament.

Muscular attachment to the pelvic girdle is extensive but there are few muscles that directly influence sacroiliac motion. Movement of the sacroiliac mechanism appears to be mainly passive, in response to muscle action in the surrounding areas above and below. The abdominal muscles, including the transversus, the two obliques, and the rectus abdominus, insert on the superior aspect of the pelvic girdle and are joined posteriorly by the quadratus lumborum, the lumbodorsal fascia, and the erector spinae mass. Six groups of hip and thigh muscles attach to the pelvic girdle and lower extremities. These hip muscles strongly influence the movement of the two hip bones within the pelvic girdle. Anterior to the sacroiliac joints are two highly significant muscles, the psoas and piriformis. The psoas crosses over the anterior aspect of the sacroiliac joints in its travels from the lumbar region to insert into the lesser trochanter of the femur. The right and left piriformis muscles originate from the anterior surface of the sacrum, travel through the sciatic notch, and insert into the greater trochanter of the femur. Asymmetry of length and tone of the piriformis is frequently observed in recurrent dysfunction of the sacroiliac joints.

Two other muscles have recently been shown to be highly significant in sacroiliac motion and sacroiliac dysfunction. They are the gluteus maximus and the latissimus dorsi muscles. The gluteus maximus attaches to the posterolateral aspect of the sacrum, and the latissimus dorsi attaches to the base of the sacrum through the lumbodorsal fascia. Contraction of these muscles provides a force that helps the joint to be stable during the stance phase of gait and mobile during the swing phase. The fiber directions of these four muscles form an "X" on the dorsal aspect of the back. Gluteal function coupled with the contralateral latissimus dorsi are important in what is currently called "force closure of the sacroiliac joint." The form closure of the joints beveling, the force closure of the gluteal–latissimus mechanism, and the strength of the posterior sacroiliac ligaments provide for sacroiliac stability.

Muscle imbalance in any of these groups affects pelvic girdle function. Imbalance in piriformis length and strength strongly influences movement of the sacrum between the hip bones. Imbalance of the pelvic diaphragm is significant in patients with rectal,

gynecologic, and urologic problems. The reader is encouraged to review the anatomy of all these muscles in a standard anatomic text.

MOTION IN THE PELVIC GIRDLE

The pelvic girdle functions as an integrated unit with all three bones moving at all three joints, influenced by the lower extremities below and the vertebral column and trunk above. This integration results in torsional movement of the pelvis, both left and right, around a vertical (y) axis. In torsional movement to the left, the symphysis turns left of the midline, the right hip bone is carried forward, the left hip bone is carried backward, and the sacrum faces somewhat to the left (counterclockwise pelvic rotation). Torsion to the right (clockwise rotation) is just the reverse. A simple screening test for this global torsional movement involves the patient in the supine position with the operator placing the palm of the hands over each anterior superior iliac spine (ASIS). Alternate rocking of the osseous pelvis by pushing posteriorly on each ASIS results in a sensation of symmetry or asymmetry. If movement seems to be more restricted when pushing posteriorly on the right ASIS than with the left, one can presume that the pelvic girdle is torsioned to the left and that there is some restrictor in the mechanism that needs further evaluation.

The amount of movement present at the symphysis pubis and at both sacroiliac joints is certainly not great and more biomechanical research is needed to identify the specific motions available and to determine their axes. The descriptions that follow are based on current biomechanical information and clinical observations. Many of the clinical observations cannot be adequately explained by current biomechanical information. A theoretic construct is offered to explain some of the clinical observations and to establish a vocabulary to describe both available normal motions and dysfunctions.

MOVEMENT AT THE SYMPHYSIS PUBIS

Movement at the symphysis pubis is quite small. It occurs in one-legged standing and during the walking cycle. Strong ligaments maintain the normal integrity of the joint, primarily superiorly and inferiorly. The ligaments become more lax as a result of hormonal change in females, particularly during pregnancy and delivery, and separation occurs to widen the internal pelvic diameter during delivery. There is a normal superior shearing movement if one-legged standing is maintained for several minutes. If one-legged standing on one side is habitual, chronic recurrent pubis dysfunction appears. Muscle imbalance between the abdominal muscles above and the thigh adductors from below is secondary to prolonged one-legged standing. After standing on the opposite leg, or with prolonged standing on both legs, the shearing movement should return to normal. During normal walking, the symphysis pubis serves as the anterior axis for alternating hip bone rotation. Symphysis pubis dysfunction, either superior or inferior, alters the anterior and posterior hip bone rotation during walking.

SACROILIAC MOTION

Sacroiliac motion is the movement of the sacrum between the two hip bones and requires the participation of both sacroiliac joints. Nutation and counternutation (anterior nutation–posterior nutation) is the sacral motion about which the most is known from biomechanical and radiographic research. "Nutation" and "counternutation" are the terms used in the anatomic literature, but this author prefers the use of anterior nutation for nutation and posterior nutation for counternutation, because this terminology allows one to describe a neutral point between anterior and posterior nutation. Nutation (anterior nutation) is a forward nodding movement of the sacrum between the hip bones with the sacral base moving anteriorly and inferiorly and the sacral apex moving posteriorly and superiorly. Counternutation (posterior nutation) occurs when the sacral base moves posteriorly and superiorly and the sacral apex moves anteriorly and inferiorly. This is the sacroiliac movement that occurs in a two-legged stance with trunk forward and backward bending. Many other structures participate in trunk forward and backward bending, but the sacroiliac motion is described as nutation and counternutation. The horizontal axis around which this anteroposterior nutation occurs has been described differently by various investigators, but appears to be related to the upper and lower limbs of the sacroiliac joint and their junction somewhere around S2. This axis is the middle transverse axis in Mitchell terminology. A superior-to-inferior translatory movement accompanies the overturning of anterior and posterior nutation. During anterior nutation (nutation), there is an inferior translatory movement of the sacrum. During posterior nutation (counternutation), there is superior translatory movement. This superior-to-inferior translatory movement accompanying the overturning of anterior and posterior nutation has some authors describing it as "shear" and using the "shear" term as part of the description of unilateral dysfunction. "Shear" is not an appropriate term as it is not a true shearing motion but rather the normal translation component of the nutational movement. Bilateral symmetry of anteroposterior nutation depends on the symmetry of the two sacroiliac joints. With asymmetry of a patient's two sacroiliac joints being so common, asymmetry of this anteroposterior nutation is also quite common. This explains why it is possible for unilateral restriction to occur.

There is a craniosacral component to anterior and posterior nutational movement of the sacrum that follows the cranial rhythmic impulse. The axis for this motion is called the superior transverse axis in Mitchell terminology. Anterior nutation is called sacral flexion in the biomechanical model and sacral extension in the craniosacral model. Posterior nutation is called sacral extension in the biomechanical model and sacral flexion in the craniosacral model.

Movement of the sacrum between the two hip bones during walking is more complex and less well understood. If one palpates the right side of the sacral base with the right thumb, the right ILA with the right index finger, the left sacral base and left ILA with the left thumb and index finger, and follows movement of the sacrum during walking, the sacrum appears to have an oscillatory movement: first left, then right. The right base appears to move anteriorly while the left ILA moves posteriorly, and then the reverse occurs, with the left sacral base moving anteriorly and the right ILA moving posteriorly. This sacral motion has been described as torsion to describe the coupling of side bending and rotation to opposite sides.

Most of the studies of sacral side bending and rotational coupling have them always couple to opposite sides. In only one cadaveric study, using a unilateral preparation, the coupling of sacral side bending and rotation appeared to depend on whether side bending or rotation was introduced first. Clinical observation of the walking cycle demonstrates that sacral side bending and rotation couple to opposite sides. In left torsional movement, the anterior surface of the sacrum rotates to face left (left rotation), while the superior surface of S1 (sacral base plane) declines to the right (right-side bending). Right torsion is the exact opposite. For descriptive purposes, this complex, polyaxial, torsional movement is considered to occur around an oblique axis. By convention, and from the Mitchell terminology, the left oblique axis runs from the upper extremity of the left sacroiliac joint to the lower end of the right sacroiliac joint, and the right oblique axis runs from the upper end of the right sacroiliac joint to the lower extremity of the left sacroiliac joint. Although the biomechanics of the torsional movements of the sacrum are unknown, the hypothetic left and right oblique axes are useful for descriptive purposes.

In the normal walking cycle, the sacrum appears to move with left torsion on the left oblique axis, return to neutral, rotate in right torsion on the right oblique axis, and then return to neutral. With left torsion on the left oblique axis, the sacrum rotates left, and side bends right, with the right sacral base moving into anterior nutation. In right torsional movement on the right oblique axis, the sacrum rotates right and side bends left, with the left sacral base moving into anterior nutational movement. Because the nutational component of this normal walking movement is anterior in direction, left torsion on the left oblique axis and right torsion on the right oblique axis are described as anterior torsional movements. The nutational movement in normal walking is anterior on one side, return to neutral, anterior to the opposite side, and return to neutral. Posterior nutational movement does not appear past neutral in the normal walking cycle.

Since much of the activity of the musculoskeletal system involves the walking cycle, maintenance of normal left-on-left and right-on-right sacral movement is an important therapeutic objective. Since walking occurs with the vertebral column in the erect, neutral (neither flexed nor extended) position, the anterior torsional sacral movements are called neutral mechanics. During walking, the thoracolumbar spine side bends left and rotates right, then side bends right and rotates left with each step. This neutral movement of the vertebral column requires normal segmental mobility, and starts with the response of the lumbar spine, usually L5, at the lumbosacral junction. (See Chapter 16 for description of lumbar linkage to the sacrum.) As the sacrum side-bends right and rotates left, L5 side-bends left and rotates right. Each vertebra above L5 should appropriately respond as part of the adaptive neutral curve. A vertebra, particularly in the lower lumbar spine, with nonneutral dysfunction results in a "nonadaptive" vertebral response to the sacrum. Treatment of lumbar spine dysfunction should always precede treatment of sacroiliac dysfunction because many sacroiliac treatments require the use of the lumbar spine as a lever.

A third sacral movement occurs when the trunk is forward bent and side bent or rotated to one side. This maneuver results in the nonneutral behavior of the lumbar spine with side bending and rotation coupled to the same side. The sacrum between the hip bones participates in this maneuver by backward or posterior torsional movement. Posterior torsional movement occurs on the left or right oblique axes, and the coupling of side bending and rotation occurs to opposite sides. In posterior torsional movement, one side of the sacral base moves beyond neutral into posterior nutation. In posterior or backward torsion to the right on the left oblique axis, the sacrum rotates right, side bends left, and the right base moves into posterior nutation. In backward or posterior torsion to the left on the right oblique axis, the sacrum rotates left, side bends right, and the left base goes into posterior nutation. These posterior torsional movements are nonneutral sacroiliac mechanics and are not part of the normal walking cycle.

The sacroiliac joint is at risk for injury, as is the lumbar spine, when the trunk is forward bent and side bending/rotation are introduced. In this posture, the lumbar spine is at risk for annular tear of the disc, strain of deep lumbar muscles, and sprain of the zygapophysial joints. The posterior torsional movement of the sacrum appears to sprain the posterior sacroiliac ligaments. Nonneutral dysfunction of the lower lumbar spine and backward torsional dysfunction of the sacroiliac joint occur in the well-known syndrome of "the well man bent over and the cripple stood up."

ILIOSACRAL MOVEMENT

The sacroiliac mechanism can be viewed from the perspective of each hip bone articulating with the sacrum. The motion can be described as one hip bone moving on one side of the sacrum (iliosacral movement). Each hip bone in the walking cycle rotates anteriorly and posteriorly around the anterior axis at the symphysis pubis, and anteriorly and posteriorly with each side of the sacrum on a posterior axis (the inferior transverse axis in Mitchell terminology). In anterior hip bone rotation, the hip bone rotates forward in relation to the sacrum with the ASIS being carried anterior, inferior, and a little laterally; the posterior superior iliac spine being carried anterior and superior; and the ischial tuberosity being carried posterior and superior. In posterior hip bone rotation, the ASIS is carried superior, posterior, and a little medially; the posterior superior iliac spine is carried posterior and inferior; and, the ischial tuberosity is carried anterior and superior. Anterior and posterior hip bone rotations occur in the presence of normal sacroiliac joint contour. If the opposing surfaces of the sacrum and ilium at the sacroiliac joint are altered, atypical movements appear clinically. In approximately 10% to 15% of the population, the sacroiliac joint does not have the form closure of the bevel change and convex-to-concave relationship at S2. The opposing joint surfaces are more flat and parallel. This configuration makes the joint susceptible to a superior-to-inferior translatory movement that can become dysfunctional. This is a true "shear" motion of one joint surface on the other. In those sacra in which the sacral side is convex and the ilial concave, internal and external rotation around a vertical axis appears possible. These very rare movements can occasionally become dysfunctional and are termed "in-flare" and "out-flare," describing the medial and lateral rotation around a vertical axis observed clinically.

Somatic dysfunction can occur with any of these motions within the pelvic girdle. Each of these motions is quite small, but when lost, each has a significant clinical effect. In dysfunctions within the pelvic girdle, it is common to find restriction of several movements within the mechanism.

STRUCTURAL DIAGNOSIS OF PELVIC GIRDLE SOMATIC DYSFUNCTION

In the structural diagnosis of the pelvic girdle, the examiner looks for the diagnostic triad of asymmetry, range of motion alteration, and tissue texture abnormality. Evaluation is made of asymmetry of paired anatomic landmarks within the pelvic girdle and lower extremity; altered range of motion (by the standing and seated flexion tests, the stork test, and various springing movement tests of the sacroiliac joints); and tissue texture abnormality in the deep fascia and ligaments over the sacroiliac joints, the sacrotuberous ligament, and the gluteal and perineal muscles. A combination of findings within the asymmetry, range of motion, tissue texture abnormality (ART) diagnostic triad leads to the diagnosis of pelvic girdle dysfunction. The diagnostic process identifies dysfunction at the symphysis pubis (dysfunction between the two pubic bones), the sacroiliac joints (sacrum between the two hip bones), and the iliosacral joints (each hip bone as it articulates with its respective side of the sacrum). The diagnostic sequence is standing, sitting with feet on floor or supported on a stool, supine, prone, and supine again.

The motion tests of the standing and seated flexion test have been classically used to assess sacroiliac restriction on one side. Recent research has shown that even in a symptomatic sacroiliac dysfunction, the joint still moves, albeit somewhat less than normal. What is important is that these tests show relative asymmetry of pelvic motion and are useful in lateralizing the relative restriction to one side. The two flexion tests are very sensitive but not very specific for joint restriction. The standing flexion test is highly sensitive to restrictors influencing the pelvis from the lower extremity, and the seated flexion test takes out the influence of the lower extremities and is more sensitive to restrictors from the trunk.

Pelvic Girdle

Diagnosis: Standing

1. Patient stands with weight equally distributed on both feet acetabular distance apart.

2. Operator stands or sits behind patient with the dominant eye in the midline and on the horizontal plane where the hands are placed.

3. Operator palpates superior aspect of each iliac crest evaluating relative height (Fig. 17.3).

4. Operator palpates superior aspect of greater trochanter of each femur evaluating relative height (Fig. 17.4).

5. If one crest and greater trochanter are higher than the other, there is presumptive evidence of anatomic shortening of lower extremity.

6. Level crest height but unlevel trochanters or unlevel crests and equal trochanters are presumptive evidence of bony asymmetry of the pelvic girdle.

Figure 17.3.

Figure 17.4.

Pelvic Girdle

Diagnosis: Standing Flexion Test

1. Patient stands with weight equally distributed on both feet acetabular distance apart.

2. Operator stands or sits behind patient.

3. Operator palpates inferior slope of each posterior superior iliac spine (Fig. 17.5).

4. Patient is instructed to smoothly bend forward as far as possible without bending the knees (Fig. 17.6).

5. Examiner follows the excursion of each posterior superior iliac spine. The test is deemed positive on the side that the posterior superior iliac spine appears to move more cephalad and/or ventral.

6. The test is sensitive but not specific for restricted motion of the sacroiliac joint on the positive side. False-positives are found with asymmetric tightness of the contralateral hamstring and of the ipsilateral quadratus lumborum. The test is sensitive to the role of the long fasciae of the lower extremity on pelvic mobility.

7. Operator observes the response of the vertebral column for dysrhythmia and the presence of altered lateral curvatures.

8. The standing flexion test is used to identify the side of restricted pelvic motion for pubic and iliosacral dysfunction.

   Note: If both thumbs move symmetrically, the interpretation is that the test is negative, however, it might also be a bilaterally positive test.

Figure 17.5.

Figure 17.6.

Pelvic Girdle

Diagnosis: One-Legged Stork Test (Gillet)

1. Operator stands or sits behind the standing patient.
2. Operator's right thumb is placed on the posterior aspect of the right posterior superior iliac spine and the left thumb on the midline of the sacral promontory at the same level (Fig. 17.7).
3. Patient raises right knee toward the ceiling.

4. A normal response finds the thumb on the posterior superior iliac spine moving caudad in relation to the thumb on the sacrum (Fig.17.8).
5. A positive response finds the thumb on the posterior superior iliac spine moving cephalically (Fig. 17.9).
6. Comparison is made with the opposite side by reversing the procedure.

Figure 17.8.

Figure 17.7.

Figure 17.9.

7. Lower pole movement is tested by placing the left thumb on the sacral hiatus and the right thumb at the same level on the posterior inferior aspect of the iliac bone (Fig. 17.10).

8. Patient lifts the right knee toward the ceiling.

9. A normal response finds the right thumb moving laterally, caudally, and ventrally (Fig. 17.11).

10. A positive response finds the right thumb moving cephalad in relation to the left thumb on the sacrum (Fig. 17.12).

11. If the patient is unable to do the one-legged standing required for this test, suspect sensory motor balance dysfunction and assess accordingly (see Chapter 20).

Note: The one-legged stork test is more specific than the standing flexion test for sacroiliac joint restriction. This test is helpful in differentiating a bilateral positive standing flexion test from a negative standing flexion test.

Figure 17.11.

Figure 17.10.

Figure 17.12.

Pelvic Girdle

Diagnosis: Standing
Trunk Side Bending

1. Operator stands or sits behind patient standing with feet acetabular distance apart.

2. Operator palpates each posterior superior iliac spine with the thumbs (Fig. 17.13).

3. Patient side bends trunk to the left (Fig. 17.14) without forward bending, while operator observes behavior of the induced lumbar curve and the pelvic motion.

4. Patient side bending of trunk to the right is performed (Fig. 17.15).

5. Operator observes symmetry of induced side-bending curve. A normal response is a smooth C-curve of the spine with fullness of the side of the convexity. A positive finding is a straightening of the lumbar curve and/or fullness of the side of concavity.

6. Operator observes behavior of the pelvis during trunk side bending. The normal response is pelvic rotation opposite to the induced lumbar rotation above. A positive response is any other pelvic motion.

Figure 17.14.

Figure 17.13.

Figure 17.15.

Pelvic Girdle

Diagnosis: Sitting
Sitting Flexion Test

1. Patient sits on examining stool with feet on the floor or on the table with feet supported.

2. Operator sits or kneels behind the patient with the thumbs on the inferior aspect of the posterior superior iliac spines and the index fingers on the iliac crests (Fig. 17.16).

3. Unleveling of the crest in the seated position is strong evidence of bony asymmetry in the bony pelvis.

4. Patient is asked to smoothly forward bend as far as possible with the arms between the knees (Fig. 17.17).

5. A positive finding has the posterior superior iliac spine on one side moving more cephalad and/or more ventral than the other. A false-positive response is found in the presence of ipsilateral quadratus lumborum tightness.

6. Operator observes the behavior of the lumbar and lower thoracic spine for dysrhythmia and abnormal lateral curves. Comparison is made with that observed while standing.

7. With the patient in the fully forward-bent position, operator palpates the posterior aspect of the ILA of the sacrum, searching if they are symmetrically in the coronal plane or if one is more posterior than the other (Fig. 17.18). This finding will be used in sacroiliac diagnosis.

Note: If altered vertebral mechanics are more severe during the standing flexion test than when seated, major restriction in the lower extremities is suggested. If vertebral dysrhythmia is worse during the seated flexion test, major restriction above the pelvic girdle is suggested.

Figure 17.17.

Figure 17.16.

Figure 17.18.

Pelvic Girdle

Diagnosis: Supine
  Pubic Symphysis Height

1. Patient supine on table.
2. Operator stands at side of table with dominant eye over the midline.
3. Operator place palm of hand on abdomen and moves caudally until the heel of the hand strikes the superior aspect of the symphysis pubis (Fig. 17.19).
4. Operator places the pads of the index fingers on the superior aspect of the symphysis pubis (Fig.

17.20). (Be sure to use finger pads and not thumbs, and be above the symphysis.)

5. Operator moves index finger pads laterally approximately 2 cm palpating the superior aspect of the pubic tubercles (Fig. 17.21).
6. A positive finding is one pubic tubercle being more superior or inferior to the other and tension and tenderness of the medial attachment of the inguinal ligament.

Note: If a positive finding for dysfunction of the pubic symphysis is found, it should be appropriately treated before proceeding with the diagnostic process.

Figure 17.20.

Figure 17.19.

Figure 17.21.

Pelvic Girdle

Diagnosis: Supine and Prone
Iliac Crest Height

1. Patient supine on table with operator standing at side with dominant eye over the midline.
2. Operator palpates the superior aspect of each iliac crest in relation to the horizontal plane by symmetric placements of the index fingers (Fig. 17.22).

3. Patient prone on table with operator standing at side with dominant eye over the midline.
4. Operator palpates the superior aspect of each iliac crest in relation to the horizontal plane with the index fingers (Fig. 17.23).
5. If one crest is higher than the other, operator is highly suspicious of the presence of a hip bone shear dysfunction. If subsequently verified, it should be treated before proceeding with the remaining examination of the pelvic girdle.

Figure 17.22.

Figure 17.23.

Pelvic Girdle

Diagnosis: Prone
Leg Length at Medial Malleolus

1. Patient prone on table with dorsum of the foot free and distal tibia and fibula at edge of table.

2. Operator stands at end of table and palpates the most inferior aspect of each medial malleolus, determining if one is longer or shorter than the other (Fig. 17.24).

3. A confirmatory test is to dorsiflex the feet and sight down perpendicularly on the pads of each heel to determine which is longer or shorter.

4. Inequality may be a function of asymmetric leg length.

5. In the presence of symmetric leg length, inequality in the medial malleolus is usually a function of the adaptation of the lumbar spine to sacral base unleveling in sacroiliac dysfunction.

Figure 17.24.

Pelvic Girdle

Diagnosis: Prone
Ischial Tuberosity Level

1. Patient prone on table with operator standing at side and dominant eye over the midline.
2. Operator places the side of the thumbs in gluteal fold and presses ventrally into the posterior aspect of the hamstring fascia (Fig. 17.25).
3. Operator's thumbs move superiorly until the pad strikes the inferior aspect of the ischial tuberosity (Fig. 17.26).
4. Evaluation is made of the level of the ischial tuberosities against the horizontal plane.
5. Unleveling of the ischial tuberosity the width of the thumb (6 mm) is considered positive.

   Note: Care must be exercised to palpate the inferior aspect of the ischial tuberosity, as the structure is quite round.

Figure 17.25.

Figure 17.26.

Pelvic Girdle

Diagnosis: Prone
Sacrotuberous Ligament Tension

1. Patient prone with operator standing at side with dominant eye over the midline.
2. Operator's thumbs are placed on the inferior aspect of the ischial tuberosities (Fig. 17.26).
3. Operator's thumbs stay on bone and move medially, curl cephalad, and hook out posterolaterally on each side under each sacrotuberous ligament (Fig. 17.27).
4. Operator assesses the symmetry of tone of the sacrotuberous ligament. Laxity or increased tension with associated tenderness is a positive finding.
5. Unleveling of the ischial tuberosity and asymmetric tension of the sacrotuberous ligaments are positive findings for hip bone shear dysfunction.

Note: Tenderness of the sacrotuberous ligament is common in association with sacroiliac dysfunction.

Figure 17.27.

Pelvic Girdle

Diagnosis: Prone
Inferior Lateral Angle (ILA)

1. Patient prone on table with operator standing at side with dominant eye over the midline.
2. Operator palpates the sacral hiatus at the caudal end of the sacral crest (Fig. 17.28).
3. Operator identifies the posterior aspect of the ILA 1.5 to 2 cm lateral to the sacral hiatus (Fig. 17.29).
4. Operator places the pad of each thumb over the posterior aspect of the ILA evaluating the level against the coronal plane. A small depression of bone makes this landmark easily palpable (Fig. 17.30).

5. Operator's thumbs are turned under the inferior aspect of the ILA without lifting thumbs off bony contact for evaluation of the level against the horizontal plane (Fig. 17.31).
6. In the presence of a symmetrically shaped sacrum, a posterior ILA is always inferior, and an inferior ILA is always posterior. Occasionally, the finding is more posterior than inferior or more inferior than posterior.
7. While palpating the inferior aspect of the ILA, tension and tenderness of the superior attachment of the sacrotuberous ligament are assessed. Sacrotuberous ligament is palpably tense and usually tender in the presence of many sacroiliac dysfunctions.

Figure 17.28.

Figure 17.30.

Figure 17.29.

Figure 17.31.

Pelvic Girdle

Diagnosis: Prone
Posterior Superior Iliac Spine, Sacral base, and L5

1. Patient prone on the table with operator standing at side with dominant eye over the midline.
2. Operator places thumb pads on the inferior slope of the posterior superior iliac spine to assess level against the horizontal plane (Fig. 17.32).
3. Operator places pads of thumbs on the most posterior aspect of the posterior superior iliac spine and curls thumbs medially and caudally approximately 30 degrees. The tip of the thumb strikes the sacral base. Assessment is made of the level of the sacral base against the coronal plane (Fig. 17.33).

4. Operator's thumbs begin at the same most posterior aspect of the posterior superior iliac spine and curl medially and cephalad approximately 30 degrees to strike the posterior arch of L5 (Fig. 17.34). Assessment is made of the level of L5 against the coronal plane.
5. The level of the sacral base is frequently referred to as "depth of the sacral sulcus." If one sacral base is more anterior than the other, the sacral sulcus is said to be "deep" on that side. The term "depth of the sacral sulcus" should be reserved for a finding of depth difference from the posterior superior iliac spine to a sacral base that is level in the coronal plane.

Figure 17.33.

Figure 17.32.

Figure 17.34.

Pelvic Girdle

Diagnosis: Prone
Four-Point Sacral Motion

1. Patient prone on table with operator standing at side and dominant eye over the midline.

2. Operator's thumbs are on the posterior aspect of each ILA and the index fingers are over each side of the sacral base (Fig. 17.35). Assessment is made of the level of the ILA and the sacral base against the coronal plane.

3. Operator monitors the movement of the four-point contact on the sacrum while the patient deeply inhales and exhales several times. Normal function finds the sacral base to move dorsally and the sacral ILA to move ventrally during deep inhalation and the reverse during exhalation.

4. Patient is asked to assume trunk extension through the prone prop position with the chin in the hands (Fig. 17.36). Assessment is made as to the level of the ILA and sacral base against the coronal plane in comparison with the prone neutral position.

5. The level of the ILA during trunk forward bending has previously been assessed (Fig. 17.18).

6. The behavior of the ILA and sacral base during the three positions of neutral, backward bent (prone prop position), and forward bent (during seated flexion), is the most reliable sign of sacroiliac dysfunction.

Figure 17.35.

Figure 17.36.

Pelvic Girdle

Diagnosis: Prone
Spring Test

1. Patient prone on table with operator standing at side with dominant eye over the midline.

2. Operator places the palm of the hand over the midline of the lumbar region with the heel of the hand over the lumbosacral junction and the middle finger over the lumbar spinous processes (Figure 17.37).

3. Operator evaluates the lumbar lordosis for normal, increase, or flattening.

4. Operator provides a short quick push with the heel of the hand toward the table evaluating for yielding of the lumbar spine. This maneuver should cause lumbar spine extension and sacral nutation (anterior nutation).

5. If the operator feels no resistance, and there is yielding of the lumbar lordosis, the test is recorded as negative.

6. A lumbar spine resisting this maneuver is recorded as positive.

7. The status of the lumbar lordosis and the presence of a positive or negative spring test are useful findings in the diagnosis of sacroiliac dysfunction.

Figure 17.37.

Pelvic Girdle

Diagnosis: Prone
Sacroiliac Rocking Test

1. Patient prone on table with operator standing at side.
2. Operator places right thumb over the left ILA and the left thumb over the left sacral base (Fig. 17.38).
3. Alternate ventral pressure of each thumb tests the capacity of the left sacroiliac joint to nutate anteriorly and posteriorly across the transverse axis.
4. Operator's thumbs are placed over the right ILA and sacral base (Fig. 17.39) and the right sacroiliac joint

is similarly tested for nutation anteriorly and posteriorly across the transverse axis.

5. Operator's right thumb is over the posterior aspect of the left ILA and the left thumb over the right sacral base (Fig. 17.40).
6. Alternate ventral pressure by the thumbs tests the capacity of the sacrum's torsional movement around the left oblique axis.
7. Operator's right thumb is over the right ILA and the left thumb over the left sacral base (Fig. 17.41). A similar ventral pressure motion tests the capacity of the sacrum to move around the right oblique axis.

Figure 17.38.

Figure 17.40.

Figure 17.39.

Figure 17.41.

Pelvic Girdle

   Diagnosis: Prone
      Sacroiliac Motion Spring Test

1. Patient prone on table with operator standing at side.

2. Operator's right thenar eminence is over the left ILA and the index and middle fingers of the left hand are over the left sacral base (Fig. 17.42).

3. Ventral pressure through the right hand while monitoring movement at the left fingers tests for posterior nutation capacity of the left sacroiliac joint.

4. Operator places the right thenar eminence over the right ILA and the left fingers over the right sacral base and springs ventrally, testing posterior nutation capacity of the right sacroiliac joint.

5. Operator's places right thenar eminence over the left ILA and the monitoring left fingers are over the right sacral base (Fig. 17.43).

6. Ventral springing through the right thenar eminence with monitoring of motion of the right sacral base identifies coupled side-bending and rotational torsional movements around the left oblique axis.

7. Operator's places right thenar eminence over the right ILA and the left fingers monitor the left sacral base (Fig. 17.44). Ventral pressure through the right hand monitored at the left base identifies torsional movement around the right oblique axis.

Figure 17.43.

Figure 17.42.

Figure 17.44.

Pelvic Girdle

Diagnosis: Prone
Sacroiliac Motion Test by Gapping

1. Patient prone on table with operator standing at side.
2. Operator's fingers of the left hand overlie the posterior aspect of the left sacroiliac joint while the right hand controls the left lower extremity with contact at the ankle (Fig. 17.45).
3. With patient's knee below 90 degrees of flexion, operator introduces internal rotation of the lower extremity through the femur, hip joint, and hip bone while monitoring movement of the left sacroiliac joint.
4. The normal motion is gapping of the joint posteriorly.
5. Internal rotation of the leg with the knee below 90 degrees primarily tests the lower pole of the left sacroiliac joint.
6. Operator repeats the maneuver with the knee flexed above 90 degrees (Fig. 17.46), which primarily tests movement of the upper pole.

Figure 17.45.

Figure 17.46.

Pelvic Girdle

Diagnosis: Supine
Leg Length

1. Patient supine with operator standing at end of table.
2. Operator grasps patient's feet and ankles with the thumbs under the inferior aspect of each medial malleolus (Fig. 17.47).
3. Operator sights down perpendicular to each thumb identifying which leg appears longer or shorter.
4. In the absence of anatomic difference in leg length, inequality of leg length in the supine position is a function of hip bone rotation due to iliosacral dysfunction.

Figure 17.47.

Pelvic Girdle

Diagnosis: Supine
Anterior Superior Iliac Spine (ASIS)

1. Patient supine with operator standing at side with dominant eye over the midline.
2. Operator places the palms of the hands over each ASIS for precise localization (Fig. 17.48).
3. Operator places both thumbs on the inferior aspect of the ASIS testing against the horizontal plane for hip bone rotation (Fig. 17.49).

4. Operator places each thumb on the anterior aspect of the ASIS testing against the coronal plane to determine if one hip bone is more anterior or posterior than the other (Fig. 17.50).
5. Operator's thumbs are placed on the medial side of the ASISs, testing their relationship to the mid-sagittal plane to see if one is more medial or lateral than the other (Fig. 17.51).

Figure 17.48.

Figure 17.50.

Figure 17.49.

Figure 17.51.

PELVIC GIRDLE DYSFUNCTIONS

There are fourteen different dysfunctions possible within the pelvic girdle (Table 17.1). It is seldom that one finds a single dysfunction within the pelvis. Combinations of dysfunctions of the pubis, sacroiliac, and iliosacral mechanisms are quite common.

Diagnosis of these dysfunctions is made from a combination of physical findings of asymmetry of osseous parts, asymmetric range of motion of the right and left side of the pelvis, and tissue texture abnormalities, primarily of ligamentous tension and tenderness.

Pubic Symphysis Dysfunction

Dysfunctions of the symphysis pubis are very common and frequently overlooked. The main reason they are overlooked is because they seldom have associated local pain. The unleveling of the pubic symphysis could also be called a subluxation. It is always either superior or inferior. A unilateral anterior or posterior symphysis does not occur except in association with pelvic ring fracture. Muscle imbalances between the abdominals above and the adductors below are major contributors to the presence and persistence of this dysfunction. They frequently result from the chronic posture of one-legged standing. Pubic dysfunction restricts symmetric motion of the hip bones during the walking cycle and interferes with all other motions in the pelvis. The diagnostic criteria for pubic dysfunction are based on three diagnostic findings. The determination of the side of restriction is based on the standing flexion test and one-legged stork test as the motion test. The asymmetry finding is that one pubic tubercle is either high or low on one side against the horizontal plane. The third finding is tension and tenderness on the insertion of the inguinal ligament. The most common dysfunctions are of the right inferior pubic symphysis and left superior pubic symphysis.

Table 17.1.
Pelvic Girdle Dysfunctions

Pubis
  1. Superior
  2. Inferior
Sacroiliac
  1. Bilaterally nutated anteriorly
  2. Bilaterally nutated posteriorly
  3. Unilaterally nutated anteriorly (sacrum flexed)
  4. Unilaterally nutated posteriorly (sacrum extended)
  5. Torsioned anteriorly (left on left or right on right)
  6. Torsioned posteriorly (left on right or right on left)
Iliosacral
  1. Rotated anteriorly
  2. Rotated posteriorly
  3. Superior (cephalic) shear
  4. Inferior (caudad) shear
  5. Rotated medially (inflare)
  6. Rotated laterally (outflare)

Right Inferior Pubic Symphysis
- Positive right standing flexion test
- Right pubis inferior
- Tension and tenderness of right inguinal ligament

Left Superior Pubic Symphysis
- Positive left standing flexion test
- Left pubis superior
- Tension and tenderness of the left inguinal ligament

The less common right superior and left inferior dysfunctions differ only on the level of the pubis against the horizontal plane. If these less common dysfunctions are present, suspect a more complex musculoskeletal problem.

Sacroiliac Dysfunctions

The sacrum becomes dysfunctional between the two iliac bones either unilaterally or bilaterally (Table 17.2). The bilaterally anteriorly and bilaterally posteriorly nutated dysfunctions are rare, probably because symmetry of both sides of a sacrum is so rare. They are frequently missed because of the findings of the bilateral positive standing flexion test initially appearing negative. The one-legged stork test then becomes most valuable, as it will be bilaterally positive indicating bilateral restriction. Another reason they are missed is because the sacral base and ILAs are level against the coronal plane. They also are frequently related to bilateral dysfunction of L5 with a bilaterally extended L5 associated with a bilaterally anteriorly nutated sacrum and a bilaterally flexed L5 with the bilaterally posteriorly nutated sacrum. The rocking, springing, and gapping sacroiliac motion tests are valuable in diagnosing the bilateral sacral dysfunctions.

A difficult concept to grasp is the unilateral anteriorly or posteriorly nutated sacrum. One wonders how rigid bones can anteriorly nutate (flex) or posteriorly nutate (extend) on one side. In fact, the bone does not change its shape; the findings are the result of the unilateral restriction of both the overturning and translatory movement on one side. One-sided dysfunction is easily explained by the common asymmetry of the two sacroiliac joints. One appears to continue to function normally and the other becomes restricted, either anteriorly or posteriorly nutated. The unilaterally nutated dysfunctions have also been described as "sacral shear," either superior or inferior. The "shear" term comes from the observation of the inferior lateral angle being more inferior than posterior in its asymmetry. It is as though the sacrum "sheared" either down or up. "Shear" is a misnomer because the joint surfaces do not actually shear against each other; rather the translatory component

Table 17.2.
Sacroiliac Dysfunctions

Diagnosis	Seated Flexion Test Positive	Base of Sacrum	Inferior Lateral Angle Position	Inferior Lateral Angle Motion	Lumbar Scoliosis	Lumbar Lordosis[a]	Medial Malleolus Prone
Unilateral nutated anteriorly (flexed)	Right	Right	Anterior right	Inferior right	—	Convex right	Normal to increased	Long right
	Left	Left	Anterior left	Inferior left	—	Convex left	Normal to increased	Long left
Unilateral nutated posteriorly (extended)	Right	Right	Posterior right	Superior right	—	Convex left	Reduced	Short right
	Left	Left	Posterior left	Superior left	—	Convex right	Reduced	Short left
Anterior torsion	Left on left	Right	Anterior right	Posterior left	Left, increased on forward-bending	Convex right	Increased	Short left
	Right on right	Left	Anterior left	Posterior right	Right, increased on forward-bending	Convex left	Increased	Short right
Backward torsion	Right on left	Right	Posterior right	Posterior right	Right, increased on backward-bending	Convex left	Reduced	Short right
	Left on right	Left	Posterior left	Posterior left	Left, increased on backward-bending	Convex right	Reduced	Short left
Bilateral nutated anterior (flexed)	—	Bilateral	Anterior	Posterior	—	—	Increased	Even
Bilateral nutated posterior (extended)	—	Bilateral	Posterior	Anterior	—	—	Reduced	Even

[a]Reduced is also a positive spring test.

of the nutational motion causes the inferiority or superiority of the ILA. The incidence of the anteriorly nutated (flexed) sacrum is high and it is usually found on the left, although it does occur on the right. It is a common sacroiliac dysfunction. The incidence of posteriorly nutated sacrum is rare, but when it does occur it is usually found on the right side. Since the asymmetry of the sacral base and the ILA is the same in both dysfunctions, the differences in the motion tests and the spring test are needed for an accurate diagnosis.

The bilateral anterior and posterior nutated dysfunctions and the unilateral anteriorly and posteriorly nutated dysfunctions are all related to the transverse axis. The bilateral dysfunctions involve both joints, whereas the unilateral only involve restriction on one side. The torsional restrictions include both joints and involve the oblique axes. Remember, the oblique axis is a descriptive one and the coupled side bending and rotation to the opposite side result from a complex polyaxial system.

The diagnostic finding that identifies the torsional dysfunctions is the sacral base and ILA being posterior on the same side. A posterior base and an ILA on the same side is always torsion. The differentiation of between an anterior and posterior torsional dysfunction is primarily made by the behavior of the sacral base and ILA in the forward bending and backward bending of the trunk. Forward torsions become asymmetric in forward bending and become symmetric in backward bending. The posterior torsions are the reverse. They get more asymmetric in backward bending and symmetric in forward bending. With the torsional dysfunctions the ILA become symmetric in one position, either trunk forward or backward bent. This is not true of the unilaterally nutated sacrum, either anterior or posterior, as the ILA in these dysfunctions is never symmetric, either forward bent or backward bent. The unilaterally anteriorly nutated sacrum may seem to get a little more asymmetric in forward bending, and the unilaterally posteriorly nutated a little more asymmetric in backward bending, but they never become symmetric.

The behavior of the ILA in the forward-bent position then becomes a very valuable clue to sacroiliac dysfunction. If the ILA is symmetric in the forward-bent position while doing the seated flexion test, the examiner has ruled out four of the possible sacroiliac dysfunctions, the two unilaterally nutated restrictions, and the forward torsions. If the seated flexion test is positive on one side, the examiner has ruled out the bilaterally anteriorly or posteriorly nutated sacral dysfunctions as well. The only possibility left is one of the posterior torsion dysfunctions.

Iliosacral Dysfunctions

The diagnosis of iliosacral dysfunction follows the diagnosis and treatment of the pubic and sacroiliac dysfunctions (Table 17.3). The iliosacral dysfunctions are unilateral dysfunctions, although there may be one on each side of the pelvis. Remember that there are two different axes for motion of the ilium: the symphysis pubis is front, and with the sacrum posteriorly. The examiner primarily assesses the hip bones with the patient in the supine position. Therefore, the pelvis must be balanced and symmetrically placed on the sacrum if possible. The bony asymmetries most important for the iliosacral dysfunctions are the level of the ischial tuberosities; the anterior or posterior, inferior or superior, medial or lateral placement of the anterior iliac spines; and the level of the medial malleolus in the supine position.

The superior and inferior hip bone shear dysfunctions are true "shears" as the joint apposition is altered. They can also be classified as true subluxations. They occur in those patients who do not have good form closure of the sacroiliac joint. They are the result of a shearing force, either superior or inferior, on one sacroiliac joint. The inferior shears will frequently self-correct on loading of the involved leg, whereas the superior shears persist unless appropriately treated. The superior shear results from some trauma such as a slip and fall of the buttocks or during a motor vehicle collision when the patient has one foot firmly placed on the brake pedal when the impact occurs. Another characteristic of the shear dysfunctions is symptom severity that appears to be greater than expected from the injury described. They are common in the patient with chronic lower back pain syndrome and when present interfere with all other motions within the pelvis. The hip bone shears also have a characteristic tissue texture finding in the sacrotuberous ligament. The ligament is lax in the superior shear and under great tension in the inferior shear. It is usually tender on the side of dysfunction.

The more common iliosacral dysfunctions are the anterior and posterior rotated hip bones. They both have asymmetries of the ASIS and the medial malleolus. The assessment of the ASIS is made to see if one is more anterior or posterior, more superior or inferior, and more medial or lateral than its fellow on the other side. An assessment is made of the length of the medial malleolus in the supine position. The findings are correlated with the positive motion tests of the standing flexion test and the one-legged stork test. The most common are a right anterior hip bone dysfunction and a left posterior hip bone dysfunction. The asymmetry findings are the same and the differentiating finding is the positive motion test, right or left.

The medially or laterally rotated hip bone dysfunctions (in-flare and out-flare) are quite rare and

Table 17.3.
Iliosacral Dysfunctions

Diagnosis		Standing Flexion Test Positive	Anterior Superior Iliac Spine Supine	Medial Malleolus Supine	Posterior Superior Iliac Spine Prone	Sacral Sulcus Prone	Ischial Tuberosity Prone	Sacrotuberous Ligament Prone
Anterior rotated	Right	Right	Inferior right	Long right	Superior right	Shallow right	—	—
	Left	Left	Inferior left	Long left	Superior left	Shallow left	—	—
Rotated posterior	Right	Right	Superior right	Short right	Inferior right	Deep right	—	—
	Left	Left	Superior left	Short left	Inferior left	Deep left	—	—
Rotated lateral (outflare)	Right	Right	Lateral right	—	Medial right	Narrow right	—	—
	Left	Left	Medial left	—	Lateral left	Narrow left	—	—
Rotated medial (inflare)	Right	Right	Medial right	—	Lateral right	Wide right	—	—
	Left	Left	Medial left	—	Lateral left	Wide left	—	—
Superior shear (upslip)	Right	Right	Superior right	Short right	Superior right	—	Superior right	Lax right
	Left	Left	Superior left	Short left	Superior left	—	Superior left	Lax left
Inferior shear (downslip)	Right	Right	Inferior right	Long right	Inferior right	—	Inferior right	Tight right
	Left	Left	Inferior left	Long left	Inferior left	—	Inferior left	Tight left

are only found in those sacroiliac joints that have altered convex-to-concave relationships at S2 with convexity on the sacral side and concavity on the ilial side. They can only be diagnosed after the correction of any hip bone rotational dysfunction that is present. There is a little lateral component to the anterior hip bone and a little medial component to the posterior hip bone dysfunction. If one only looks at the medial and lateral aspects of the ASISs and overlooks the superior-to-inferior and anterior-to-posterior aspects, one can erroneously make a diagnosis of a medial or lateral rotated hip bone.

Symmetry of hip bone rotation, alternately anterior and posterior on each side, is an essential component of the gait cycle. Altered hip bone rotation is frequently associated with altered muscle balance in the trunk and lower extremity. For example, a short tight quadratus femoris muscle is frequently associated with an anterior hip bone on that side, and a short tight hamstring muscle is frequently associated with a posterior hip bone on that side. Treating the joint restriction without also dealing with the muscle imbalance is one reason for chronicity.

MANAGEMENT OF PELVIC GIRDLE DYSFUNCTION

The goal of manual medicine treatment to pelvic girdle dysfunction is to restore the mechanics of the normal walking cycle. In the overall treatment of the patient, one should treat the lumbar spine prior to the treatment of the pelvis because many sacroiliac techniques require the use of the lumbar spine as a lever arm. The pelvis is the bony attachment of many muscles of the trunk above and of the extremities below.

Treatment of the pelvic girdle should always be accompanied by the diagnosis and treatment of muscle imbalance both above and below the pelvis to prevent recurrence of dysfunction and to enhance the therapeutic outcome.

Treatment Sequence

The recommended treatment sequence is symphysis pubis, hip bone shear dysfunction, sacroiliac dysfunction, and iliosacral dysfunction. In the diagnostic sequence, one assesses for pubic dysfunctions early. If dysfunction is found, it should be treated before proceeding with the diagnostic sequence. Recall that the major criterion for sacroiliac dysfunction is identified with the patient in the prone position. If there is residual dysfunction of the symphysis pubis in front, the patient is not symmetric in the prone position on the tripod of the two ASISs and the symphysis pubis.

Following the diagnosis and treatment of the pubic dysfunction, the next major assessment is for the presence of hip bone shear dysfunction. The major index of suspicion occurs with unleveling of the iliac crests in the unloaded position. When a hip bone shear dysfunction is present, it appears to restrict all other motions within that sacroiliac joint. Therefore, it deserves attention early in the diagnostic and treatment process. A second reason for treating the hip bone shear early is the need to have two symmetric hip bones available to assess the sacrum's position in between the bones. Sacroiliac dysfunction is then addressed in order to restore its symmetry to the coronal plane when the patient is supine on the examining table to allow for assessment of each hip bone in relation to the fixed sacrum on the table.

Pelvic Girdle

Symphysis Pubis

Muscle Energy Technique
Supine
  Position: Symphysis either Superior or Inferior ("shotgun technique")

1. Patient supine with hips and knees flexed and feet together.

2. Operator stands at side of table holding patient's knees together.

3. Operator resists two to three patient efforts of knee abduction for 3 to 5 seconds (Fig. 17.52).

4. Operator places forearm between patient's knees (Fig. 17.53).

5. A series of adduction efforts of both knees attempts to distract the symphysis pubis.

6. Retest.

Figure 17.52.

Figure 17.53.

Pelvic Girdle

Symphysis Pubis

Muscle Energy Technique
Supine
    Position: Left Superior Symphysis

1. Patient supine on table with operator standing on left side (Fig. 17.54).
2. Operator slides patient's pelvis to the left side of the table maintaining the left hip bone on the edge. Patient's left arm holds right shoulder for trunk stability (Fig. 17.55).
3. Operator's legs support the patient's freely hanging left leg.
4. Operator's left hand stabilizes right side of patient's pelvis and right hand is placed above the patella over patient's distal left femur.
5. Patient performs a series of three to five repetitions of 3- to 5-second muscle contractions of hip flexion against operator's right hand (Fig. 17.56).
6. After each patient effort, operator engages new barrier by additional left leg extension.
7. Retest.

    Note: With patient's leg in an abducted and extended position, hip flexion activates left adductor muscle group pulling left symphysis inferiorly by concentric isotonic muscle contraction.

Figure 17.55.

Figure 17.54.

Figure 17.56.

Pelvic Girdle

Symphysis Pubis

Muscle Energy Technique
Supine
   Position: Right Symphysis Inferior

1. Patient supine on table with right knee and hip flexed, adducted, and slightly internally rotated.

2. Operator stands on left side and rolls patient's pelvis to the left to place operator's left hand to control patient's right hip bone (Fig. 17.57).

3. Operator places patient's right posterior superior iliac spine between the operator's left middle and ring fingers with heel of hand in contact with the ischial tuberosity (Fig. 17.58).

4. Operator returns patient's pelvis to the table with the right hip bone in contact with the left hand and

a superior and medial compressive force of the heel of the left hand is applied against the ischial tuberosity (Fig. 17.59).

5. Operator resists three to five efforts of a 3- to 5-second muscle contraction by the patient to straighten the right leg in the caudad direction.

6. After each effort, the operator engages new barrier by more hip flexion and compression against the right ischial tuberosity.

7. Alternative operator position with the patient's right knee in the operator's right axilla with right hand holding edge of table (Fig. 17.60).

8. Retest.

Note: Flexion, internal rotation, and adduction of the right hip close packs the right sacroiliac joint so that hip extension effort transmits operator force against the ischial tuberosity in a cephalad and medial direction toward the symphysis pubis.

Figure 17.57.

Figure 17.59.

Figure 17.58.

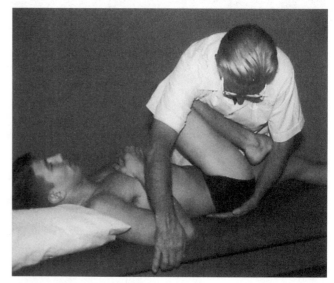

Figure 17.60.

Pelvic Girdle

Iliosacral

Muscle Energy Technique
Supine
Diagnosis
    Position: Left Superior Hip Bone Shear
    Dysfunction

1. Patient supine with feet off end of table.
2. Operator stands at end of table with left thigh against patient's right foot and both hands grasping patient's left leg just proximal to the ankle (Fig. 17.61). An assistant may be used to stabilize the patient's right leg.

3. Operator abducts the extended left leg 10 to 15 degrees to loose pack the left sacroiliac joint (Fig. 17.62).
4. Operator internally rotates the extended, abducted left leg to close pack the left hip joint (Fig. 17.63).
5. Operator puts long-axis extension on the left leg while the patient performs a series of inhalation and exhalation efforts (Fig. 17.64).
6. Three to four respiratory cycles are performed and during the last exhalation effort the patient is instructed to cough while simultaneously the operator tugs left leg in a caudad direction.
7. Retest.

Figure 17.61.

Figure 17.63.

Figure 17.62.

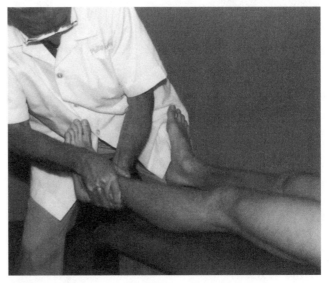

Figure 17.64.

Pelvic Girdle

Iliosacral

Muscle Energy Technique
Lateral Recumbent
    Diagnosis: Right Inferior Hip Bone Shear

1. Patient lies in the left lateral recumbent position.

2. Operator stands in front (or back) of patient with right arm and shoulder supporting the weight of the right lower extremity. An assistant may help by holding the weight of the right leg.

3. Operator's left hand grasps the posterior aspect of the right hip bone from the ischial tuberosity to the posterior superior iliac spine (Fig. 17.65).

4. Operator's right hand grasps the right hip bone from the ischial tuberosity to the inferior pubic ramus (Fig. 17.66).

5. Operator's two hands distract the right hip bone laterally (toward the ceiling) and exert a cephalic directional force on the right hip bone.

6. Patient performs a series of deep inhalation and exhalation efforts while operator maintains distraction of the right hip bone in a cephalic direction.

7. Retest.

Figure 17.65.

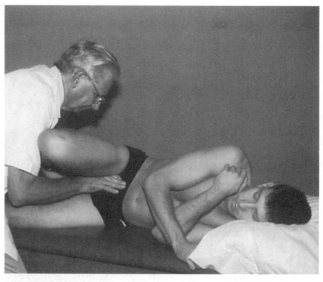

Figure 17.66.

Pelvic Girdle

Iliosacral

Muscle Energy Technique
Prone
Diagnosis
    Position: Right Inferior Hip Bone Shear

1. Patient prone on table with operator standing on the right side.

2. Operator places patient's right foot between the knees and extended right arm and hand controls right knee to loose pack the right sacroiliac joint (Fig. 17.67).

3. Operator's left hand contacts the right ischial tuberosity and maintains a force in a cephalic direction.

4. Patient performs a series of deep inhalation and exhalation efforts.

5. Patient attempts to straighten right arm against a hand contact on the table leg resulting in a caudad force through the trunk.

6. A combination of the operator's force on ischial tuberosity, patient's right arm muscle effort against trunk, and respiratory effort provides superior shearing movement of the right hip bone against the sacrum.

7. Retest.

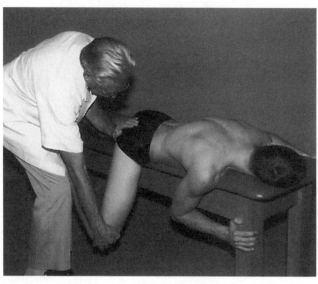

Figure 17.67.

Pelvic Girdle

Sacroiliac

Muscle Energy Technique
  Prone
  Diagnosis
    Position: Left Unilateral Anterior Nutated Sacrum (left sacrum flexed)
    Motion Restriction: Left Unilateral Posterior Nutation

1. Patient prone with operator standing on left side.
2. Operator's fingers of the left hand monitor the left sacral base while operator's right arm introduces abduction of patient's left leg to approximately 15 degrees (Fig. 17.68).
3. Operator internally rotates left leg gapping the posterior aspect of the left sacroiliac joint. Patient holds leg in that position (Fig. 17.69).
4. With right arm straight, operator places heel of hand on left ILA and springs sacrum from above and below and from side to side until point of maximum motion is identified at the left sacral base (Fig. 17.70).
5. Patient takes a maximum inhalation and holds breath as operator maintains a ventral and cephalic compressive force on the left ILA.
6. As patient exhales, operator maintains pressure.
7. Patient performs a series of forced inhalation efforts while operator maintains force on ILA.
8. Retest.

Figure 17.69.

Figure 17.68.

Figure 17.70.

Pelvic Girdle

Sacroiliac

Muscle Energy Technique
    Prone
    Diagnosis
        Position: Right Posterior Nutated Sacrum (right extended sacrum)
        Motion Restriction: Anterior Nutation of Right Sacrum

1. Patient prone on table with operator standing on right side.

2. Operator's right hand monitors the right sacroiliac joint as the left hand abducts right leg to approximately 15 degrees, loose packing right sacroiliac joint (Fig. 17.71).

3. Operator externally rotates right abducted leg gapping the anterior aspect of the right sacroiliac joint. Patient instructed to hold right leg in that position (Fig. 17.72).

4. Patient's trunk is extended by prone prop position while operator's right pisiform is in contact with the right sacral base maintaining a ventral and caudad directional force (Fig. 17.73).

Figure 17.72.

Figure 17.71.

Figure 17.73.

5. Operator's left hand on the right ASIS provides a counterforce against the compression through the right hand (Fig. 17.74).

6. Patient performs a series of forced exhalation efforts while operator maintains ventral and caudad compressive force against the right sacral base.

7. At the end of each exhalation effort, patient is instructed to pull the right ASIS toward the table as a muscle activating force.

8. After three to five repetitions the operator maintains the sacral compression against the counterforce on the ASIS and the patient is instructed to return to the neutral position (Fig. 17.75).

9. Retest.

Figure 17.74.

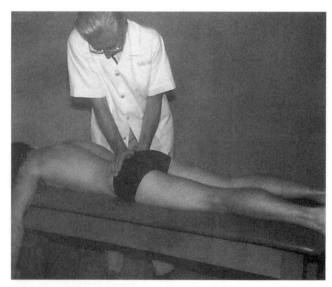

Figure 17.75.

Pelvic Girdle

Sacroiliac

Muscle Energy Technique
  Sims Position
  Diagnosis: Left-on-left Forward (anterior) Sacral
  Torsion
    Position: Sacrum Left Rotated, Right-side Bent
    and Anteriorly Nutated at Right base
    Motion Restriction: Right rotation, left-side bend-
    ing, and posterior nutation of right base

1. Patient prone on table.
2. Operator stands on right side, flexes patient's knees to 90 degrees (Fig. 17.76).
3. Operator rolls patient onto left hip introducing Sims position (Fig. 17.77).
4. Operator controls patient's knees on operator's left thigh, monitors lumbosacral junction with left hand and introduces trunk rotation to the left through the right hand until L-5 begins to rotate left (Fig. 17.78).

Figure 17.77.

Figure 17.76.

Figure 17.78.

5. Operator's right hand now monitors the lumbosacral junction and right sacral base while left hand introduces left-side bending (Fig. 17.79).

6. Operator flexes lower extremities until right sacral base begins to move posteriorly then resists an effort by the patient of lifting both feet toward the ceiling against resistance offered by the left hand (Fig. 17.80).

7. Patient performs three to five muscle contractions of lifting feet to ceiling for 3 to 5 seconds against resistance offered by the operator with engagement of the flexion and side-bending barrier between each effort.

8. Retest.

Figure 17.79.

Figure 17.80.

Pelvic Girdle

Sacroiliac

Muscle Energy Technique
Lateral Recumbent
Diagnosis: Left-on-left Forward (anterior) Sacral Torsion
    Position: Left Rotated, Right-side Bent, Anteriorly Nutated Right Sacral Base
    Motion Restriction: Right Rotation, left-side bending, and posterior nutation of right sacral base

1. Patient lies in right lateral recumbent position with the operator standing in front monitoring the lumbosacral junction (Fig. 17.81).

2. Operator introduces neutral side-bending right, rotation left, through the lumbar spine until L-5 first begins to rotate left (Fig. 17.82).

3. Operator flexes thighs and pelvis until first posterior movement of the right sacral base.

4. Operator introduces left-side bending by lifting the feet toward the ceiling (Fig. 17.83).

5. Patient performs three to five muscle contractions for 3 to 5 seconds by pulling the feet down toward the table.

6. Operator engages new barrier by increasing hip flexion and side bending by lifting knees to the ceiling between each muscle effort.

7. Retest.

Figure 17.82.

Figure 17.81.

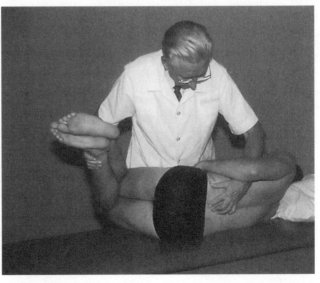

Figure 17.83.

Pelvic Girdle

Sacroiliac

Muscle Energy Technique
Lateral Recumbent
Diagnosis: Right-on-left Backward (posterior) Sacral Torsion
   Position: Right Rotated, Left-side Bent, Posteriorly Nutated Right Sacral Base
   Motion Restriction: Left Rotation, Right-side Bending, and Anterior Nutation of Right Sacral Base

1. Patient lies in left lateral recumbent position with the operator standing in front monitoring the lumbosacral junction with the left hand (Fig. 17.84).

2. Operator pulls patient's left arm anterior and caudad introducing neutral left-side bending and right rotation of the lumbar spine until L-5 first rotates to the right (Fig. 17.85).

3. Operator introduces extension of both legs through the left hand while the right hand monitors the right sacral base until the base first moves anteriorly (Fig. 17.86).

Figure 17.85.

Figure 17.84.

Figure 17.86.

4. Operator drops right leg in front of left knee and places left hand against the patient's distal right femur (Fig. 17.87).

5. Operator's right forearm maintains L5 rotation to the right while left hand resists patient's effort of lifting the right knee toward the ceiling (Fig. 17.88).

6. Patient performs three to five muscle contractions for 3 to 5 seconds with the operator engaging the new barriers between each effort by further extending the bottom leg and dropping the right leg more toward the floor.

7. Retest.

Figure 17.87.

Figure 17.88.

Pelvic Girdle

Sacroiliac

Muscle Energy Technique
Sitting
Diagnosis: Bilateral Anterior Nutated (flexed) Sacrum
    Position: Bilateral Anterior Nutated
      Motion Restriction: Bilateral Posterior Nutation

1. Patient sits on stool with feet apart and legs internally rotated (Fig. 17.89).
2. Patient flexes trunk forward.

3. Operator places heel of right hand over apex of the sacrum and left hand over the patient's thoracic spine (Fig. 17.90).
4. Operator maintains ventral pressure on the sacral apex and resists patient's instruction to lift shoulders toward the ceiling with the patient's breath at full inhalation.
5. Patient performs three to five efforts of 3 to 5 seconds of muscle contraction to restore posterior nutational movement of the sacral base.
6. The full inhalation helps move the sacral base posteriorly.
7. Retest.

Figure 17.89.

Figure 17.90.

Pelvic Girdle

Sacroiliac

Muscle Energy Technique
Sitting
Diagnosis: Bilateral Posterior Nutated (extended) Sacrum
  Position: Bilaterally Posterior Nutated
  Motion Restriction: Bilateral Anterior Nutation

1. Patient sitting on stool with feet together and knees apart externally rotating legs. Arms crossed.
2. Operator stands at side with right hand on sacral base and left hand controlling patient's trunk (Fig. 17.91).
3. Patient is instructed to arch the back by pushing abdomen toward the knees with full exhalation while operator maintains a ventral compressive force with the right hand on the sacral base (Fig. 17.92).
4. Operator's left hand resists three to five repetitions of 3 to 5 second muscle contraction of trunk flexion.
5. The exhalation effort assists in moving the sacral base anteriorly.
6. Retest.

Figure 17.91.

Figure 17.92.

Pelvic Girdle

Iliosacral

Muscle Energy Technique
Supine
    Diagnosis: Left Posterior Hip Bone
        Position: Hip Bone Rotated Posteriorly
        Motion Restriction: Anterior Rotation of Hip
        Bone

1. Patient supine on table with operator standing on left side.
2. Operator slides patient's pelvis until sacrum is at the edge of the table (Fig. 17.93).
3. Operator controls left lower extremity between the knees.
4. Operator stabilizes right side of pelvis at right ASIS (Fig. 17.94).
5. Operator's right hand contacts distal femur above the patella.
6. Operator resists patient's hip flexion effort for 3 to 5 seconds.
7. Operator engages new barrier by dropping the patient's left leg toward the floor and repeats resistance to hip flexion effort three to five times.
8. Retest.

Note: This procedure is similar to that for a superior pubic symphysis dysfunction; the difference is that the sacrum and the posterior aspect of the hip bone are the fixed point on the edge of the table.

Figure 17.93.

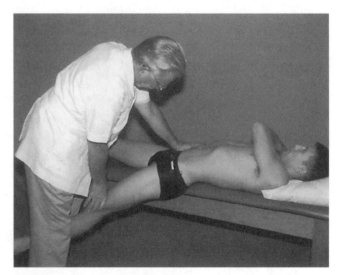

Figure 17.94.

Pelvic Girdle

Iliosacral

Muscle Energy Technique
Prone
Diagnosis: Left Posterior Hip Bone
    Position: Left Hip Bone Rotated Posteriorly
    Motion restriction: Anterior rotation of Left Hip
    Bone

1. Patient prone on table with operator standing on right side.
2. Operator controls patient's left leg by grasping flexed knee in the left hand. Left leg abducted to loose pack left sacroiliac joint.
3. Operator's right hand is on left iliac crest 5 to 6 cm anterior to the posterior superior iliac spine (Fig. 17.95).
4. Operator extends patient's leg to barrier while exerting pressure with right hand in the direction of the iliac crest (Fig. 17.96).
5. Patient's muscle effort is a series of three to five contractions for 3 to 5 seconds of hip flexion (pull leg to table) against operator resistance.
6. After each muscle effort, operator engages new extension barrier.
7. Retest.

Note: This dysfunction frequently accompanies a left sacrum anteriorly nutated (flexed). A combination technique can be performed as the last step of the muscle energy procedure for the left sacrum flexed. While holding the sacrum in the posteriorly nutated position with the right hand, the operator's left extends the left hip, rotating the left hip bone anteriorly and resists the muscle effort of pulling the knee to the table (Fig. 17.97).

Figure 17.96.

Figure 17.95.

Figure 17.97.

Pelvic Girdle

Iliosacral

Muscle Energy Technique
Lateral Recumbent
Diagnosis: Left Posterior Hip Bone
   Position: Left Hip Bone Rotated Posteriorly
   Motion Restriction: Left Hip Bone Anterior Rotation

1. Patient lies in the right lateral recumbent position with operator standing behind.
2. Operator's right hand placed on iliac crest 5 to 6 cm anterior to the posterior superior iliac spine (PSIS) (Fig. 17.98).

3. Operator grasps patient's flexed left knee in the left hand and supporting the left lower extremity loose packs the left sacroiliac joint (Fig. 17.99).
4. Operator extends patient's leg to barrier while exerting anterior pressure along the iliac crest with right hand (Fig. 17.100).
5. Patient provides muscle contraction to pull leg anteriorly against operator's resistance for three to five repetitions of 3 to 5 seconds.
6. Operator engages new extension barrier after each muscle effort.
7. Retest.

Figure 17.99.

Figure 17.98.

Figure 17.100.

Pelvic Girdle

Iliosacral

Muscle Energy Technique
Prone
Diagnosis: Right Anterior Hip Bone
   Position: Right hip Bone Anteriorly Rotated
   Motion Restriction: Posterior Rotation of Right Hip Bone

1. Patient in prone position with operator standing at right side.

2. Operator grasps pelvis and slides patient's lower trunk to the right edge of the table (Fig. 17.101).

3. Operator controls patient's right leg by placing the foot between operator's knees and grasping the right knee with the right hand.

4. Operator's left hand stabilizes the sacrum in the midline with the left index finger monitoring the right sacroiliac joint (Fig. 17.102).

5. Operator controls patient's right leg with abduction, external rotation, and flexion to engage barrier to posterior rotational movement (Fig. 17.103).

6. Patient performs muscle effort for 3 to 5 seconds with three to five repetitions of extending the right leg by pushing the right foot against operator's thigh.

7. Operator engages new barrier of posterior rotation between each patient contraction.

8. Retest.

Figure 17.102.

Figure 17.101.

Figure 17.103.

Pelvic Girdle

Iliosacral

Muscle Energy Technique
Supine
Diagnosis: Right Anterior Hip Bone
    Position: Right Hip Bone Anteriorly Rotated
    Motion Restriction: Posterior Rotation of Right
    Hip Bone

1. Patient in the supine position with the right hip and knee flexed.

2. Operator stands on patient's left side with the heel of the left hand contacting the right ischial tuberosity and with the fingers of the left hand monitoring motion of the sacroiliac joint (Fig. 17.104).

3. Operator flexes, externally rotates, and abducts patient's right leg.

4. Operator exerts a cephalad and lateral force against the right ischial tuberosity.

5. Patient performs three to five muscle contractions for 3 to 5 seconds to extend the right leg against resistance offered by the operator's right hand and trunk (Fig. 17.105).

6. Between each patient effort, operator increases posterior rotation of the right hip bone while monitoring loose-packed position of the right sacroiliac joint with the left hand.

7. Retest.

Note: This procedure is similar to that of an inferior symphysis pubis dysfunction. The differences are loose packing the right sacroiliac joint and the cephalad and lateral force of the left hand on the ischial tuberosity that directs hip bone rotation rather than force toward the symphysis pubis.

Figure 17.104.

Figure 17.105.

Pelvic Girdle

Iliosacral

Muscle Energy Technique
Lateral Recumbent
Diagnosis: Right Anterior Hip Bone
   Position: Right Hip Bone Anteriorly Rotated
   Motion Restriction: Posterior Rotation Right Hip
   Bone

1. Patient in left lateral recumbent position with operator facing patient.
2. Patient's right leg flexed at hip and knee with foot placed against operator's hip.
3. Operator's left hand is placed on the right hip bone with the fingers monitoring motion at the right sacroiliac joint and the heel of the hand against the ischial tuberosity (Fig. 17.106).
4. Operator engages barrier by introducing abduction, external rotation, and flexion of the right leg (Fig. 17.107).
5. Patient performs three to five muscle contractions of 3 to 5 seconds attempting to straighten the right leg against operator resistance.
6. Operator engages new barrier after each patient relaxation.
7. Retest.

   Note: Muscle efforts other than hip extension can be adduction or abduction of the right knee against operator resistance.

Figure 17.106.

Figure 17.107.

Pelvic Girdle

Iliosacral

Muscle Energy Technique
Supine
Diagnosis: Right Hip Bone Internally Rotated (inflare)
    Position: Right Hip Bone Internally Rotated
    Motion restriction: External Rotation of Right Hip Bone

1. Patient supine on table with operator standing on right side.
2. Operator flexes patient's right hip and knee placing the right foot on the left knee (Fig. 17.108).
3. Operator's left hand stabilizes left pelvis at the left ASIS.
4. Operator's right hand on medial side of patient's right knee, externally rotates hip until barrier is engaged (Fig. 17.109).
5. Patient performs three to five muscle contractions for 3 to 5 seconds attempting to internally rotate right leg against resistance by operator.
6. Operator engages new external rotation barrier after each patient contraction.
7. Retest.

Figure 17.108.

Figure 17.109.

Pelvic Girdle

Iliosacral

Muscle Energy Technique
Supine
Diagnosis: Left Hip Bone Externally Rotated
(out-flare)
  Position: Left Hip Bone Externally Rotated
  Motion Restriction: Internal Rotation of Left Hip
  Bone

1. Patient supine on table with operator standing on left side.
2. Operator flexes patient's left hip and knee rolling patient's pelvis to the right. Operator's fingers of the right hand grasp the medial side of the left posterior superior iliac spine (Fig. 17.110).
3. Patient's pelvis returned to neutral with left hip bone resting in operator's hand.

4. Operator's left hand adducts the left femur to the internal rotational barrier of the left hip bone while maintaining lateral traction on the left posterior superior iliac spine by the right hand.
5. Patient performs three to five muscle efforts for 3 to 5 seconds attempting to abduct and externally rotate the left leg against resistance of operator's left hand (Fig. 17.111).
6. Operator engages new internal rotational barrier after each patient relaxation.
7. Retest.

   Note: Operator's left hand also maintains pressure through the left thigh toward the table to prevent the pelvis from rotating to the right during muscle contraction.

Figure 17.110.

Figure 17.111.

Pelvic Girdle

Symphysis Pubis

Mobilization with Impulse Technique
Supine
Diagnosis: Pubic Dysfunction either Superior or
Inferior ("shotgun" technique)

1. Patient supine on table with operator standing at side.

2. Operator's knees and hip flexed with feet on the table.

3. Operator's two hands between patient's knees (Fig. 17.112).

4. Patient is instructed to hold knees together.

5. Operator provides mobilization with impulse thrust by separating both knees with both hands against patient resistance (Fig. 17.113).

6. Retest.

Figure 17.112.

Figure 17.113.

Pelvic Girdle

Sacroiliac

Mobilization with Impulse Technique
Lateral Recumbent
   Diagnosis: Left Unilateral Anterior Nutated Sacrum
(Left Sacrum Flexed)
     Position: Left Sacrum Anteriorly Nutated
     Motion Restriction: Posterior Nutation Left
     Sacral Base

1. Patient in Left Lateral Recumbent Position with Knees and Feet together.

2. Operator stands in front and monitors lumbosacral junction with left hand (Fig. 17.114).

3. Operator's right hand pulls patient's left shoulder anterior and caudad introducing neutral left-side bending right rotation of the lumbar spine until L-5 begins to rotate to the right.

4. Operator's left hand contacts the sacrum with the pisiform on the left ILA and with left forearm parallel to the table.

5. Operator's right hand and forearm stabilize trunk and monitor at lumbosacral junction.

6. Operator performs mobilizing thrust through the left arm in a cephalic direction parallel to the table (Fig. 17.115).

7. An alternate right hand position stabilizes right shoulder for the thrust through the left forearm (Fig. 17.116). This position may offer better leverage for the cephalic thrust through the left arm.

8. Retest.

Figure 17.115.

Figure 17.114.

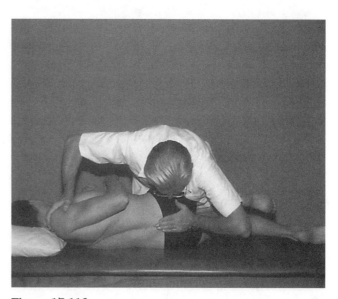

Figure 17.116.

Pelvic Girdle

Sacroiliac

Mobilization with Impulse Technique
Prone
Diagnosis: Left Unilateral Anterior Nutated Sacrum
(Left Sacrum Flexed)
    Position: Left Sacrum Anteriorly Nutated
    Motion Restriction: Posterior Nutation of Left
    Sacral Base

1. Patient prone on table with operator standing on left side.

2. Operator's left hand monitors left sacroiliac joint while right hand abducts left leg to loose pack position (approximately 15 to 20 degrees). Left leg internally rotated and held by patient (Fig. 17.117).

3. Operator's right thenar eminence contacts left ILA .

4. Operator engages posterior nutational barrier by springing the sacrum.

5. Patient deeply inhales and operator delivers a mobilization with impulse thrust in an anterior and superior direction through the right hand (Fig. 17.118).

6. Retest.

Figure 17.117.

Figure 17.118.

Pelvic Girdle

Sacroiliac

Mobilization with Impulse Technique
Left Lateral Recumbent
Diagnosis: Left-on-left anterior (forward) Sacral Torsion
   Position: Sacrum Left Rotated, Right-side bent, and Anteriorly Nutated Right base
   Motion Restriction: Sacral Right Rotation, Left sidebending and Posterior Nutation Right Base

1. Patient in left lateral recumbent position with knees and feet together and shoulders perpendicular to the table.

2. Operator stands in front and flexes and extends lower extremities maintaining neutral mechanics in the lumbar spine and engaging the first posterior nutational barrier of the sacrum (Fig. 17.119).

3. Operator's right hand on right shoulder introduces side-bending right and rotation left of the lumbar spine by pushing the shoulder caudally until L-5 rotates left.

4. Operator's left hand contacts sacrum with left pisiform against the left ILA (Fig. 17.120).

5. The barrier is engaged through the operator's right forearm, and left hand contacting the sacrum with the left pisiform in the direction of the right shoulder.

6. A mobilization with impulse thrust is provided in a scooping fashion of the left hand on the left ILA in the direction of the resistant right hand on the right shoulder.

7. Retest.

Figure 17.119.

Figure 17.120.

Pelvic Girdle

Sacroiliac

Mobilization with Impulse Technique
Supine
Diagnosis: Right-on-left Backward (posterior) Sacral Torsion
   Position: Sacrum Right Rotated, Left-side Bent, and Posteriorly Nutated Right base
   Motion Restriction: Left Rotation, Right side bending, and Anterior Nutation of the Right Sacral Base

1. Patient supine with operator standing on left side of table.
2. Operator translates pelvis from right to left introducing right-side bending of the trunk (Fig. 17.121). Patient clasps hands behind neck.

3. Operator side bends trunk to the right through the lumbar spine, including the sacrum (Fig. 17.122).
4. Operator threads right forearm through patient's right arm. Operator's back of right hand is against sternum (Fig. 17.123).
5. Operator stabilizes right hip bone through left-hand contact on right ASIS.
6. Operator engages barrier by left rotation of the trunk without losing right-side bending (Fig. 17.124).
7. Operator performs mobilization with impulse thrust by enhanced trunk rotation to the left against the stabilized right hip bone resulting in left rotation, right-side bending, and anterior nutation of the right sacral base.
8. Retest.

   Note: This technique is effective for a unilateral right posterior nutated sacrum (extended).

Figure 17.121.

Figure 17.123.

Figure 17.122.

Figure 17.124.

Pelvic Girdle

Sacroiliac

Mobilization with impulse technique
Sitting
Diagnosis: Left-on-left Forward (anterior) Sacral Torsion
  Position: Sacrum left rotated, Right-side bent, Anteriorly Nutated Right Sacral Base
  Muscle Restriction: Right Rotation, Left-side Bending, and Posterior Nutation Right Sacral Base

1. Patient sitting astride table with left hand grasping the right shoulder.

2. Operator stands at right side with right hand grasping patient's left shoulder and right axilla controlling right shoulder.

3. Operator's left pisiform contact is on the left sacral base (Fig. 17.125).

4. Operator's right arm introduces lumbar forward bending, right-side bending, and right rotation (nonneutral mechanics) while left hand prevents left rotation of the left sacral base (Fig. 17.126).

5. Operator's right arm maintains trunk right-side bending as nonneutral mechanics are released into neutral lumbar spine (Fig. 17.127).

6. Left rotation is introduced through the trunk while right-side bent and an anterior thrust is delivered by the left forearm through the contact of the left pisiform on the left sacral base (Fig. 17.128).

7. Retest.

Note: Initially nonneutral lumbar mechanics are used then released into neutral mechanics so that L5 rotates left and the sacrum rotates to the right, bringing the right sacral base posteriorly.

Figure 17.125.

Figure 17.127.

Figure 17.126.

Figure 17.128.

Pelvic Girdle

Sacroiliac

Mobilization with Impulse Technique
Sitting
Diagnosis: Right-on-left Backward (posterior) Sacral Torsion
    Position: Sacrum Right Rotated, Left-side Bent, Posteriorly Nutated Right Sacral Base
    Motion Restriction: Left Rotation, Right-side Bending, and Anterior Nutation Right Sacral Base

1. Patient sitting astride the table with left hand grasping right shoulder.

2. Operator stands at left side with left hand grasping patient's right shoulder and left axilla controlling patient's left shoulder. Operator's right pisiform contacts right sacral base (Fig. 17.129).

3. Operator introduces left-side bending and right rotation of the trunk down to L5 rotating the sacrum to the left. Operator puts anterior compression on right sacral base (Fig. 17.130).

4. Operator reverses trunk mechanics into right-side bending and left rotation down to and including the sacrum (Fig. 17.131).

5. Operator performs mobilizing with impulse thrust through the right forearm to pisiform contact on right sacral base while exaggerating trunk extension while side-bent right and rotated left.

6. Retest

Figure 17.130.

Figure 17.129.

Figure 17.131.

Pelvic Girdle

Iliosacral

Mobilization with Impulse Technique
Supine
Diagnosis: Left Superior Hip Bone Shear

1. Patient supine with operator standing at end of table.
2. Operator grasps distal tibia and fibula above ankle (Fig. 17.132).

3. Patient flexes knee and hip with slight abduction of the left lower extremity but without rotation (Fig. 17.133).
4. When left leg is controlled with left sacroiliac joint plane loose packed, operator provides mobilization with impulse thrust by long-axis extension carrying knee extension, hip extension to left sacroiliac joint (Fig. 17.134).
5. Retest.

   Note: This procedure is not indicated in the presence of knee or hip joint pathology.

Figure 17.133.

Figure 17.132.

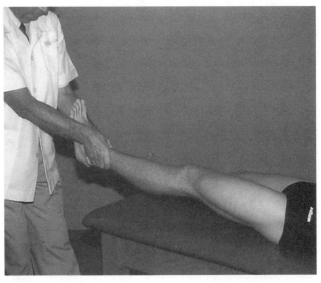

Figure 17.134.

Pelvic Girdle

Iliosacral

Mobilization with Impulse Technique
Lateral Recumbent
Diagnosis: Right Inferior Hip Bone Shear Dysfunction

1. Patient in left lateral recumbent position with operator standing in front monitoring lumbosacral junction (Fig. 17.135).

2. Operator introduces neutral left-side bending right rotation of the lumbar spine down to and including the lumbosacral junction (Fig. 17.136).

3. Operator places patient's right foot in left popliteal space (Fig. 17.137).

4. Operator stabilizes trunk with the right forearm and right hand monitoring at the right sacroiliac joint.

5. Operator's left forearm contacts inferior aspect of the patient's right ischial tuberosity (Fig. 17.138).

6. Operator provides mobilization with impulse thrust in a cephalic direction against the right ischial tuberosity with the plane of the right sacroiliac joint parallel to the table resulting in superior translatory movement of the right hip bone.

7. Retest.

Figure 17.135.

Figure 17.137.

Figure 17.136.

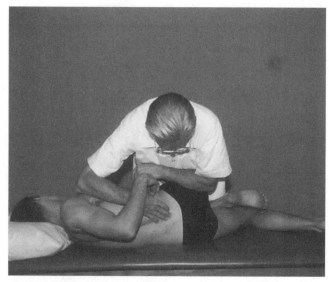

Figure 17.138.

Pelvic Girdle

Iliosacral

Mobilization with Impulse Technique
Diagnosis: Right Anterior Hip Bone
    Position: Right Hip Bone Anteriorly Rotated
    Motion Restriction: Posterior Rotation Right Hip
    Bone

1–4. These steps are identical to the technique for right inferior hip bone shear (Figs. 17.135 to 17.137).

5. Operator's right hand grasps right ASIS and the left hand grasps the right ischial tuberosity (Fig. 17.138).

6. With the plane of the right sacroiliac joint parallel to the table, operator rotates hip bone posteriorly to the barrier and provides a mobilization with impulse thrust with both hands in a counterclockwise direction (Fig. 17.139).

7. An alternate hand position finds the operator's left forearm on the right ischial tuberosity. The right hand stabilizes the trunk with right sacroiliac joint plane parallel to the table. A mobilization thrust is made by the left forearm in an anterior and superior direction rotating the left hip bone posteriorly (Fig. 17.140).

8. Retest.

Figure 17.139.

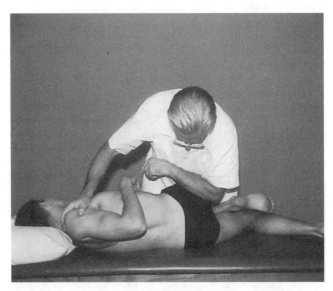

Figure 17.140.

Pelvic Girdle

Iliosacral

Mobilization with Impulse Technique
Lateral Recumbent
Diagnosis: Left Posterior Hip Bone
  Position: Left Hip Bone Posteriorly Rotated
  Motion restriction: Anterior Rotation Left Hip
  Bone

1. Patient in right lateral recumbent position with operator standing in front, monitoring lumbosacral junction (Fig. 17.141).

2. Operator introduces neutral side-bending right, rotation left lumbar curve to include the lumbosacral junction.

3. Operator extends lower extremities until sacral base first starts to move forward (Fig. 17.142). Patient's left knee is placed in right popliteal space.

4. With the left arm stabilizing the trunk and maintaining the plane of the left sacroiliac joint parallel to the table, operator's right pisiform contacts the left posterior superior iliac spine (Fig. 17.143).

5. Operator's body drop provides a mobilization with impulse technique through the right forearm turning the left hip bone anteriorly.

6. An alternate contact is the operator's right forearm along the posterior aspect of the patient's left iliac crest (Fig. 17.144).

7. Operator's body drop provides a mobilization with impulse thrust through the left forearm contact rotating the left hip bone anteriorly.

8. Retest.

Figure 17.141.

Figure 17.143.

Figure 17.142.

Figure 17.144.

MUSCLE DYSFUNCTIONS OF THE PELVIC GIRDLE

Dysfunctions of the pelvic girdle always involve the many muscles to which it is related. Frequently seen is alteration in the pelvic diaphragm. This is particularly common in dysfunctions of the symphysis pubis and the hip bone shear dysfunctions. Widespread symptoms of the lower urinary tract, genitalia, and rectum are frequently present. Restoration of the function of the pelvic diaphragm is described in Chapter 7. Dysfunction of the muscles of the lower extremity and trunk need to be assessed and treated appropriately. These are described in Chapter 20.

CONCLUSION

Dysfunction of the pelvic girdle is complex and not easily understood. It is common to find several dysfunctions within the same pelvic girdle. Each needs to be individually diagnosed and appropriately treated. The diagnostic and therapeutic system described allows the operator to deal with any combination of physical findings that are found within the pelvic girdle. Restoration of pelvic girdle function within the walking cycle is a major therapeutic goal, particularly from the biomechanical postural–structural model.

SUGGESTED READINGS

Alderink GJ. The sacroiliac joint: review of anatomy, mechanics, and function. *J Ortho Sports Phys Ther* 1991;13:71–84.

Beal MC. The sacroiliac problem: review of anatomy, mechanics, and diagnosis. *J Am Osteopath Assoc* 1982;81:667–679.

Bernard TN, Cassidy JD. The sacroiliac syndrome: pathophysiology, diagnosis, and management. In: Frymoyer JW, ed. *The adult spine, principles and practice.* New York: Raven Press, 1991;2107–2133.

Bowen V, Cassidy JD. Macroscopic and microscopic anatomy of the sacroiliac joint until the eighth decade. *Spine* 1981;6:620–628.

Chamberlain WE. The symphysis pubis in the roentgen examination of the sacroiliac joint. *Am J Roentgenol* 1930;24:621–625.

Dihlmann W. *Diagnostic radiology of the sacroiliac joint.* Chicago: Yearbook Medical Publishers, 1980.

DonTigney RL. Function and pathomechanics of the sacroiliac joint. *J Am Phys Ther Assoc* 1985;65:35–44.

Greenman PE. Clinical aspects of sacroiliac function in walking. *J Manual Medicine* 1990;5:125–130..

Greenman PE. Innominate shear dysfunction in the sacroiliac syndrome. *Man Med* 1986;2:114–121.

Lee D. *The pelvic girdle.* Edinburgh: Churchill Livingstone, 1989.

Mitchell FL Sr. *Structural pelvic function.* Carmel, CA: Yearbook of the American Academy of Osteopathy, 1958;71–90.

Mitchell FL Sr. *The balanced pelvis and its relation to reflexes.* Carmel, CA: Yearbook of the Academy Applied Osteopathy, 1948;146–151.

Pitkin HC, Pheasant HC. Sacroarthrogenic telalgia. *J Bone Joint Surg* 1936;18:111–133.

Stevens A: Side-bending and axial rotation of the sacrum inside the pelvic girdle. In: Vleeming A, Mooney V, Snijders CJ, et al., eds. First Interdisciplinary World Congress on Low Back Pain and Its Relation to the Sacroiliac Joint. San Diego CA 5-6 November 1992; 209–230.

Vleeming A, Mooney V, Snijders CJ, et al., eds. *Movement, stability and low back pain: the essential role of the pelvis.* New York: Churchill Livingstone, 1997.

Vleeming A, Pool-Goudzwaard AL, Hammudoghlu D, et al. The function of the long dorsal sacroiliac ligament: its implication for understanding low back pain. *Spine* 1966;21:556–562.

Weisel H. Movement of the sacroiliac joint. *Acta Anat* 1955;23:80–91.

18

UPPER EXTREMITY TECHNIQUE

Highly developed hand dexterity is one of the distinguishing characteristics of humans. Upper extremity function places the hand in positions that allow it to perform its unique intricate movements. The upper extremity is attached to the trunk primarily through muscular attachments. The only articulation of the upper extremity with the trunk is the sternoclavicular joint. The arrangements of the muscular attachments allow the extremity a wide range of movement in relation to the trunk. The upper extremity has a strong interrelationship with the cervical spine, thoracic spine, and thoracic cage through the multiple muscle relationships.

In approaching dysfunctions within the upper extremity, the operator should first examine and treat any dysfunctions within the cervical spine, thoracic spine, and thoracic cage. The cervicothoracic junction is one of the major transitional regions of the body. The relationship of T1 with the first rib and the sternoclavicular joint is of major significance in upper extremity problems. T1 dysfunctions influence the first rib and lead to dysfunctions there. Dysfunctions of the first rib influence the manubrium of the sternum and the sternoclavicular joint. Evaluation of symptoms in the upper extremity should proceed from proximal to distal because of the influence of the cervical spine and thoracic inlet on circulatory and neural functions. Whether the practitioner is using a circulatory or a neurologic model, evaluation of the cervical and thoracic spine is appropriate before moving distally to the upper extremity.

BRACHALGIA

One of the common mistakes the operator makes in evaluating upper extremity complaints is to evaluate only at the joint where the symptom is present and proximal thereto. From the structural diagnostic perspective, a patient with pain in the upper extremity under the general rubric of "brachalgia" has five potential entrapment sites for elements of the brachial plexus.

1. The cervical roots are at risk at the intervertebral foramen as they exit from the vertebral canal.

Productive change of the uncovertebral joint of Luschka and posterolateral protrusion of intervertebral disc material may narrow the intervertebral canal anteriorly, reducing the space available for the roots. Dysfunction or disease of the zygapophysial joints may negatively affect the foraminal size and shape from the posterior direction, reducing space for the nerve roots. In addition to significant osseous change, swelling and congestion from acute or chronic inflammation can also cause entrapment.

2. The roots are transported through the intertransversarii muscles between the transverse processes of the cervical vertebrae. Hypertonicity of these short, fourth-layer spinal muscles, with accompanying chronic passive congestion, may also be a site of potential entrapment. Hypertonicity of these muscles is common with segmental dysfunction at the same level.

3. The roots forming the brachial plexus pass through the scalene muscles. Hypertonicity and passive congestion of these muscles, commonly found in cervical and upper rib cage dysfunction, negatively influence the brachial plexus.

4. As the plexus traverses laterally, it passes through the costoclavicular canal. The lateral portion of the second rib and the posterior aspect of the clavicle bind this triangular-shaped region. Dysfunctions of the second rib, particularly where it is held in an inhalation position in the lateral bucket-handle range, and of the sternoclavicular and acromioclavicular articulations can result in potential entrapment at the costoclavicular canal. A large amount of soft tissue occupies space within this region and if congested, the costoclavicular canal can narrow.

5. More laterally, the neurovascular bundle passes under the insertion of the pectoralis minor tendon to the coracoid process of the scapula. Hypertonicity, shortening, and thickening of the pectoralis muscle and its tendon can compress the nerves as they pass distally.

In addition to the neural structures, the vascular and lymphatic channels are at risk at the scalenes, first rib, costoclavicular canal, and underlying the pectoralis minor tendon. The examiner must thoroughly evaluate the cervical, upper thoracic, and upper rib cage areas before proceeding with the evaluation and management of the distal region of the upper extremity.

The screening examination (see Chapter 2) for the upper extremities involves the patient actively abducting the upper extremities with the elbows extended and attempting to bring the backs of the hands together over the head. Inability to symmetrically accomplish this maneuver demands further diagnostic evaluation. The upper extremities should be evaluated by traditional orthopedic and neurologic testing. A recent addition to testing of the neural structures is the neural dynamic testing of the nervous system for neural and dural restrictions.

There are many systems for the structural diagnosis and manual medicine treatment of the extremities. This author has found many of the procedures found in Mennell's *Joint Pain* to be of considerable therapeutic value. Only a few of these procedures will be repeated here and the reader is encouraged to study Mennell's text.

The shoulder, elbow, and wrist are not single joints; each of the regions contains several articulations. For that reason we will approach the upper extremity on a regional basis and evaluate the specific articulations individually.

SHOULDER REGION

The shoulder region consists of the sternoclavicular, acromioclavicular, and glenohumeral articulations. The scapulocostal junction is not a true articulation. The ability of the concave costal surface of the scapula to smoothly move over the thoracic cage is of major importance in upper extremity function, particularly the shoulder region. The direct restrictors of scapulocostal motion are the muscles and fasciae that hold the scapula to the trunk. These myofascial elements are best approached by soft-tissue and myofascial release techniques. Particular attention must be given to the trapezius, sternocleidomastoid, levator scapulae, rhomboids, serratus anterior, and latissimus dorsi muscles and their fasciae. Evaluation and treatment of these muscles should precede the articulations in the shoulder region.

Sternoclavicular Joint

The medial end of the clavicle articulates with the manubrium of the sternum. Within this joint is a meniscus. The medial end of the clavicle is intimately related to the anterior aspect of the first rib. The joint is polyaxial in its movement with abduction, horizontal flexion, and rotation as the primary motions. As the clavicle is abducted, it externally (posteriorly) rotates, and as it returns to neutral, it internally (anteriorly) rotates. Rotation then becomes a coupled movement with abduction.

Upper Extremity

Sternoclavicular Joint

Diagnosis
Test for Restricted Abduction

1. Patient supine on table with arms resting easily at the side.
2. Operator stands at side or head of table with paired fingers over the superior aspect of the medial end of the clavicle (Fig. 18.1).

3. The patient is asked to actively "shrug the shoulders" by bringing the shoulder tip to the ear bilaterally (Fig. 18.2).
4. The operator's palpating fingers follow the movement at the medial end of the clavicle.
5. The normal finding is equal movement of the medial end of both clavicles in a caudad direction.
6. A positive finding is the failure of one clavicle to move caudad when compared to the opposite. It appears to be held in the original starting position.

   Note: This test can also be done with patient sitting.

Figure 18.1.

Figure 18.2.

Upper Extremity

Sternoclavicular Joint

Mobilization Without Impulse (articulatory treatment)
Diagnosis: Restricted Abduction

1. Patient sits on the examining table or stool.
2. Operator stands behind patient with the thenar eminence of one hand over the superior aspect of the medial end of the dysfunctional clavicle, the other hand grasps the patient's forearm (Fig. 18.3).

3. The operator abducts the extended upper extremity to the resistant barrier (Fig. 18.4) and sweeps it across the patient's torso in the direction of the opposite knee while constant caudad pressure is maintained by the thenar eminence on the medial end of the clavicle (Fig. 18.5).
4. Several repetitions are done, increasing the abduction movement of the patient's extended arm. (A high-velocity thrust by the thenar eminence may be used.)
5. Retest.

Figure 18.4.

Figure 18.3.

Figure 18.5.

Upper Extremity

Sternoclavicular Joint

Muscle Energy Technique
Supine
Diagnosis: Restricted Abduction

1. Patient supine on table with the dysfunctional upper extremity at the edge of the table.

2. Operator stands on the side of dysfunction facing cephalad.

3. Operator places one hand over the medial end of the dysfunctional clavicle while the other grasps the patient's forearm just above the wrist (Fig. 18.6).

4. Operator internally rotates the dysfunctional upper extremity and carries it into extension off the edge of the table to the resistant barrier while monitoring with the opposite hand at the sternoclavicular region (Fig. 18.7).

5. Patient performs a 3- to 5-second muscle contraction to lift the arm toward the ceiling against operator resistance for three to five repetitions.

6. Following each relaxation, the operator increases the extension of the upper extremity to a new resistant barrier and patient again repeats the effort of lifting the arm toward the ceiling.

7. Retest.

   Note: This procedure also increases internal (anterior) rotation at the sternoclavicular joint.

Figure 18.6.

Figure 18.7.

Upper Extremity

Sternoclavicular Joint

Muscle Energy Technique
Sitting
Diagnosis: restricted abduction

1. Patient sitting on table or stool.

2. Operator standing behind patient with the thenar eminence of one hand in contact with the superior aspect of the medial end of the dysfunctional clavicle and the other hand controlling the dysfunctional upper extremity at the elbow (Fig. 18.8).

3. With the elbow at 90 degrees, the upper extremity is externally rotated and abducted to approximately 90 degrees with additional abduction until the resistant barrier is engaged (Fig. 18.9).

4. Patient performs muscle contraction to adduct the upper extremity three to five times for 3 to 5 seconds against resistance offered at the elbow by the operator.

5. After relaxation, operator engages new barrier.

6. Retest.

Note: This procedure also enhances the external (posterior) rotation at the sternoclavicular joint.

Figure 18.8.

Figure 18.9.

Upper Extremity

Sternoclavicular Joint

Diagnosis
Test for Restricted Horizontal Flexion

1. Patient supine on table.
2. Operator stands at side or head of table with fingers symmetrically placed on the anterior aspect of the medial end of each clavicle (Fig.18.10).
3. Patient extends the upper extremities in front of the body by reaching toward the ceiling.

4. Operator evaluates movement of the medial end of each clavicle (Fig. 18.11).
5. The normal finding is for each clavicle to move symmetrically in a posterior direction as the lateral end of the clavicle moves anteriorly.
6. A positive finding is for one clavicle not to move in a posterior direction during the reaching effort.

   Note: This test can also be done with the patient sitting.

Figure 18.10.

Figure 18.11.

Upper Extremity

Sternoclavicular Joint

Mobilization without impulse (articulatory) treatment
Diagnosis: Restricted Horizontal Flexion

1. Patient sitting on table.
2. Operator standing behind with one hand on the anterior aspect of the medial end of the dysfunctional clavicle and the lateral hand grasping the forearm (Fig. 18.12).

3. Operator takes the upper extremity into horizontal extension (Fig. 18.13) and sweeps it forward in horizontal flexion (Fig. 18.14) with increasing arcs of movement, while the thenar eminence of the opposite hand maintains a posterior compressive force on the medial end of the dysfunctional clavicle. (A high-velocity thrust by the thenar eminence may be substituted.)

4. Retest.

Figure 18.13.

Figure 18.12.

Figure 18.14.

Upper Extremity

Sternoclavicular Joint

Muscle Energy Technique
    Supine
    Diagnosis: Restricted Horizontal Flexion

1. Patient supine on table.

2. Operator stands on side of table opposite the dysfunctional sternoclavicular joint.

3. Operator places cephalic hand over the medial end of the dysfunctional clavicle and the caudad hand grasps the patient's shoulder girdle over the posterior aspect of the scapula (Fig. 18.15).

4. Patient's hand grasps back of operator's neck with an extended arm.

5. Patient engages the horizontal flexion barrier by standing more erect and lifting the dysfunctional scapula (Fig. 18.16).

6. Patient pulls down upon the operator's neck with 3 to 5 second muscle effort for three to five repetitions while operator maintains posterior compression on the anterior aspect of the medial end of the dysfunctional clavicle.

7. Operator engages new barrier after each of patient's muscle contraction.

8. Retest.

Figure 18.15.

Figure 18.16.

Upper Extremity

Sternoclavicular Joint

Mobilization without impulse (articulatory)
Technique
Diagnosis: Restricted Horizontal Flexion

1. Patient supine, operator stands on opposite side of dysfunction.
2. Operator places caudad forearm on table between chest and humerus.
3. Patient's opposite hand grasps wrist of dysfunctional extremity. A pull places traction on the clavicle.
4. Operator's cephalic hand applies pressure on medial end of dysfunctional clavicle (Fig. 18.17).
5. Patient pulls on wrist distracting the clavicle while operator springs the medial end of the clavicle posteriorly.
6. Retest.

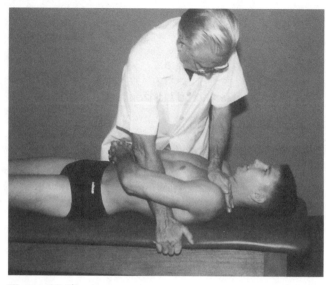

Figure 18.17.

ACROMIOCLAVICULAR JOINT

The acromioclavicular joint contributes only a small amount of motion to the shoulder region, but its contribution to total upper extremity abduction is critical. The primary movements of this articulation are abduction and internal and external rotations. The joint is angled laterally at approximately 30 degrees from before backward. The joint largely depends on ligaments for its integrity and frequently separates during trauma. Productive change at this joint is common. Clinical experience has shown that loss of acromioclavicular joint function is highly significant, particularly the loss of abduction. This is important to remember during motion testing of the shoulder girdle. Dysfunction of this joint is one of the most frequently overlooked in the upper extremity.

Upper Extremity

Acromioclavicular Joint

Diagnosis: Test for Restricted Abduction and Adduction

1. Patient sitting with operator standing behind.
2. Operator's medial hand palpates the superior aspect of the acromioclavicular joint and the lateral hand controls the patient's proximal forearm (Fig. 18.18).

3. Operator introduces adduction and external rotation of the forearm monitoring a gapping movement at the acromioclavicular joint (Fig. 18.19).
4. Absence of the gapping movement is evidence of restriction of adduction movement.
5. Comparison is made with the opposite side.
6. Operator introduces abduction movement while monitoring at the joint for movement (Fig. 18.20).
7. Comparison is made with the opposite side.

Figure 18.19.

Figure 18.18.

Figure 18.20.

Upper Extremity

Acromioclavicular Joint

Muscle Energy Technique
Sitting
   Diagnosis: Restricted Abduction

1. Patient sitting on table or stool with operator standing behind.
2. Operator maintains compressive force on lateral end of the clavicle, medial to the acromioclavicular joint.
3. Operator's lateral hand takes patient's upper extremity to horizontal flexion of 30 degrees and abducts to the barrier (Fig. 18.21).
4. Patient pulls elbow to the side against resistance offered by the operator for 3 to 5 seconds and three to five repetitions.
5. Operator engages new abduction barrier after each muscle effort.
6. Retest.

Figure 18.21.

Upper Extremity

Acromioclavicular Joint

Diagnosis: Test for Restricted Internal and External Rotation

1. Patient sitting on table or stool with operator standing behind.
2. Operator's medial hand palpates the superior aspect of the acromioclavicular joint.

3. Operator's lateral hand moves the upper extremity into horizontal flexion to 30 degrees and abduction to the first barrier (Fig. 18.22).
4. Operator introduces internal rotation (Fig. 18.23) and external rotation (Fig. 18.24) while monitoring mobility of the acromioclavicular joint.
5. Comparison is made with the opposite side.

Figure 18.23.

Figure 18.22.

Figure 18.24.

Upper Extremity

Acromioclavicular Joint

Muscle Energy Technique
Diagnosis: Restricted Internal or External Rotation

1. Patient sitting on table or stool with operator standing behind.
2. Operator's medial hand stabilizes the lateral aspect of the clavicle and monitors the acromioclavicular joint.
3. Operator takes upper extremity to 30 degrees of horizontal flexion and abduction to 90 degrees.

4. External rotational barrier is engaged with the operator's lateral hand grasping the patient's wrist and places forearm to patient's forearm (Fig. 18.25).
5. Operator engages internal rotation barrier by threading lateral forearm under patient's elbow and grasping distal forearm (Fig. 18.26).
6. Patient provides muscle contraction for 3 to 5 seconds and three to five repetitions against resistance of either internal or external rotation.
7. Operator engages new barrier after each muscle contraction.
8. Retest.

Figure 18.25.

Figure 18.26.

GLENOHUMERAL JOINT

The glenohumeral joint has one of the widest ranges of movement of any joint within the body. The depth of the glenoid is increased by the cartilaginous glenoidal labrum. For this joint to perform its normal function it is dependent upon the ability of the scapula to move on the thoracic cage with the glenoid being elevated for upper extremity abduction. For this reason, the muscular attachments to the scapula must perform their normal actions. Tightness and shortening of the levator scapulae and the latissimus dorsi muscles are notoriously found in a dysfunctional upper extremity, particularly the impingement syndrome of the rotator cuff. The articular capsule is normally quite lax and loose, particularly inferiorly, providing for a wide range of movement. Joint integrity is maintained by the intimate attachment of the rotator cuff muscles (supraspinatus, infraspinatus, terres minor, and subscapularis) to the articular capsule.

The extensive movements of this joint are described in relation to the vertical and horizontal planes. In the vertical or neutral plane, the humerus is at the side of the body. Movement then occurs in flexion, extension, internal rotation, and external rotation. In the horizontal plane, with the humerus at 90 degrees to the trunk, it is also possible to have flexion, extension, internal rotation, and external rotation. Adduction moves the humerus toward the body and in front of the chest, and abduction moves the arm away from the body with full range extending so that the elbow can touch the ear. All of these motions should be tested and compared with the opposite side. The primary movement loss in the glenohumeral joint involves the functions of external rotation and abduction. The humeral head must move from cephalad to caudad on the glenoid during abduction. Loss of this ability to track from superior to inferior during abduction results in major restriction at the glenohumeral joint.

Because the vast majority of dysfunctions within the glenohumeral joint are muscular in origin, muscle energy diagnostic and therapeutic techniques are most effective. The principles of diagnosis and treatment are (a) to evaluate range of motion in all of the motion directions described above, (b) to evaluate the strength of each of the muscle groups, (c) to treat restricted range of movement by postisometric relaxation technique at the restrictive barrier, and (d) if weakness is identified, to treat by means of a series of concentric isotonic contractions. Each motion should be compared with that available on the opposite side.

Glenohumeral Joint

Muscle Energy Procedure

1. Patient sits on table or stool with operator standing behind.

2. Range of motion is tested in all directions by engaging the restrictive barrier. Comparison is made with the opposite side.

3. If motion is restricted, operator engages resistant barrier. Patient performs three to five repetitions of a 3 to 5 second isometric contraction against operator resistance.

4. The operator performs strength testing by having the patient contract the muscle in the direction of operator resistance. Comparison is made with the opposite side. If one muscle group is weak, the patient performs a series of three to five concentric isotonic contractions through the total range of movement against progressively increasing resistance by the operator.

5. Operator's medial hand stabilizes the shoulder girdle with the fingers on the coracoid process, the web of the hand over the acromioclavicular joint, and the thumb posterior and inferior over the spine of the scapula.

6. Operator's lateral hand controls patient's elbow and forearm.

7. Operator introduces the following motions and treats accordingly:

   - Neutral flexion (Fig. 18.27)
   - Neutral extension (Fig. 18.28)
   - Neutral external rotation (Fig. 18.29)
   - Neutral internal rotation, stage 1 (Fig. 18.30)
   - Neutral internal rotation, stage 2 (Fig. 18.31)
   - Adduction (Fig. 18.32)
   - Abduction (Fig. 18.33)
   - Horizontal flexion (Fig. 18.34)
   - Horizontal extension (Fig. 18.35)
   - Horizontal internal rotation (Fig. 18.36)
   - Horizontal external rotation (Fig. 18.37)

8. Retest.

Figure 18.27.

Figure 18.28.

Figure 18.29.

Figure 18.30.

Figure 18.31.

Figure 18.32.

Figure 18.33.

Figure 18.34.

Figure 18.36.

Figure 18.35.

Figure 18.37.

Glenohumeral Joint

Glenoidal Labrum (Green's) Technique

This technique enhances movement of the humeral head within the glenoid and glenoid labrum and is useful as the initial treatment in a patient with adhesive capsulitis (frozen shoulder).

1. Patient prone with the involved arm off the edge of the table and operator sitting at side facing dysfunctional shoulder (Fig. 18.38).

2. Operator grasps distal humerus in both hands and applies caudad and anterior traction with internal and external rotation two to three times (Fig. 18.39).

3. Operator next grasps patient's humeral neck with thumbs on the greater tuberosity, the index and middle fingers on the attachment of the rotator cuff, and the ring and little fingers surrounding the proximal shaft, controlling the humeral shaft against the thenar eminences (Fig. 18.40).

4. Operator applies movement through the humeral head in an anterior–posterior, cephalic–caudal, and medial and lateral traction—distraction directions.

5. Operator induces circular and figure-eight motions, enhancing range in all directions.

6. Operator emphasizes increase in caudal translatory movement of the humeral head on the glenoid.

7. Retest.

Figure 18.39.

Figure 18.38.

Figure 18.40.

Glenohumeral Joint

Spencer Seven-Step Technique

The principle is a sequential, direct action, mobilization without impulse (articulatory) technique against motion resistance.

1. Patient in lateral recumbent position with affected shoulder uppermost, head supported, and knees flexed.
2. Operator stands facing patient.
3. Operator's proximal hand stabilizes the shoulder girdle including the clavicle and scapula.

4. Step 1: Operator gently flexes (Fig. 18.41) and extends arm (Fig. 18.42) in the sagittal plane with the elbow flexed. Repetitions are made within limits of pain provocation.
5. Step 2: Operator flexes patient's arm in the sagittal plane with elbow extended in a rhythmic swinging movement, increasing range so that patient's arm covers the ear (Fig. 18.43).
6. Step 3: Operator circumducts patient's abducted humerus with the elbow flexed. Clockwise and counterclockwise concentric circles with gradual increase in range are made within limits of pain (Fig. 18.44).

Figure 18.41.

Figure 18.43.

Figure 18.42.

Figure 18.44.

7. Step 4: Operator circumducts patient's humerus with elbow extended in clockwise and counterclockwise circles, increasing range as permitted by pain (Fig. 18.45).

8. Step 5: Operator abducts patient's arm with elbow flexed with gradual increases of range of abduction against the stabilized shoulder girdle (Fig. 18.46).

9. Step 6: Operator places patient's hand behind the rib cage and gently springs elbow forward and inferior, increasing internal rotation of the humerus (Fig. 18.47).

10. Step 7: Operator grasps patient's proximal humerus with both hands and applies lateral and caudad traction in a pumping fashion (Fig. 18.48).

11. Retest.

Figure 18.45.

Figure 18.47.

Figure 18.46.

Figure 18.48.

ELBOW REGION

There are three joints at the elbow region: the humeroulnar joint, the humeroradial joint, and the proximal radioulnar joint. The primary movements are flexion and extension, pronation and supination, and a small amount of abduction–adduction. All joints participate in elbow function. Flexion–extension is the primary movement at the humeroulnar joint, and pronation–supination is a combined humeroradial and proximal radioulnar joint movement. Abduction–adduction movement is primarily a joint play movement at the humeroulnar joint, and, when dysfunctional, reduces the flexion–extension range. The elbow region has a number of related pain syndromes that are frequently described as "tennis elbow." Many of these patients present with pain on the lateral aspect of the elbow, radiating into the forearm, which is aggravated by activity. Dysfunction of the radial head involving the proximal radioulnar and humeroradial joints is a frequent finding. Radial head dysfunction is the most common somatic dysfunction within the elbow region.

Elbow Region

Diagnosis: Restricted Abduction–Adduction (humeroulnar joint)

1. Patient sitting on table with operator standing in front.
2. Operator's two hands circumferentially grasp proximal radioulnar region.
3. Operator supports patient's hand and wrist between medial side of elbow and trunk.
4. Operator's hands introduce translatory movement medially (Fig. 18.49) and laterally (Fig. 18.50) through the arc from flexion to extension testing for resistance.
5. Comparison made with the opposite side.
6. A direct action mobilization without impulse, progressively carried through to mobilization with impulse, has operator engage either the adduction or abduction barrier while extended (Fig. 18.51). Mobilization without impulse repetitions are made against resistant barrier with final mobilization with impulse performed.
7. Retest.

   Note: Adduction restriction is more common than abduction.

Figure 18.50.

Figure 18.49.

Figure 18.51.

Elbow Region

Muscle Energy Technique
Restricted Elbow Extension

1. Patient sitting on table with operator standing in front.
2. Operator's medial hand grasps patient's distal supinated forearm with lateral hand stabilizing the elbow.
3. Patient's elbow extension barrier is engaged (Fig. 18.52).
4. Patient performs a series of three to five muscle contractions for 3 to 5 seconds against operator's resistance.
5. Operator progressively engages elbow extension barrier after each muscle contraction (Fig. 18.53).
6. Retest.
7. An alternate technique has patient perform a series of isotonic contractions of the triceps muscle through full flexion-to-extension arc.
8. Operator fully flexes the elbow, stabilizing elbow with lateral hand, grasping distal forearm to provide resistance to isotonic contraction (Fig. 18.54).
9. Patient performs three to five repetitions with progressively increasing resistance by the operator's medial hand until full elbow extension is achieved (Fig. 18.55).
10. Retest.

Figure 18.52.

Figure 18.54.

Figure 18.53.

Figure 18.55.

Elbow Region

Muscle Energy Technique
Restricted Pronation and Supination

1. Patient sitting on table with operator standing in front.
2. Operator's medial hand stabilizes patient elbow flexed to 90 degrees. Lateral hand grasps distal forearm, wrist, and hand with patient's thumb pointing vertically (Fig. 18.56).

3. Operator introduces supination (Fig. 18.57) and pronation (Fig. 18.58) testing for restriction.
4. Comparison is made with the opposite side.
5. Treatment of restricted supination has operator's lateral hand stabilizing the flexed elbow and monitoring the radial head while medial hand supinates forearm to resistant barrier (Fig. 18.59).
6. Patient performs three to five muscle contractions for 3 to 5 seconds against resistance offered by operator's medial hand.

Figure 18.56.

Figure 18.58.

Figure 18.57.

Figure 18.59.

7. Operator engages new supination barrier after each patient effort.

8. Treatment of restricted pronation has operator's two hands in same location but engaging pronation barrier (Fig. 18.60).

9. Patient performs three to five muscle contractions for 3 to 5 seconds against operator resistance.

10. Operator engages new pronation barrier after each muscle contraction.

11. Retest.

   Note: Restricted pronation and supination of the forearm combines motion of the humeroradial, proximal radioulnar, and distal radioulnar articulations. Supination is the most common restriction.

Elbow Region

Diagnosis of Radial Head Dysfunction
Test 1: Palpation for Asymmetry

1. Patient sitting on table, elbows flexed to 90 degrees, forearm supinated and supported in lap.

2. Operator stands in front and palpates the radial head posteriorly with the index fingers and the soft tissues anteriorly with the thumbs (Fig. 18.61).

3. Operator assesses the symmetric relationship of the radial head to the capitulum of the humerus.

4. In addition to asymmetry, the dysfunctional side is usually tender with tension of the periarticular tissues.

Figure 18.60.

Figure 18.61.

Elbow Region

Diagnosis of Radial Head Dysfunction
Test 2: Motion of the Radial Head

1. Patient sitting on table with elbow flexed to 90 degrees.

2. Operator stands in front with lateral hand palpating the radial head at the humeroradial articulation with the index finger posteriorly and the thumb anteriorly.

3. Operator's medial hand grasping distal radius and ulna introduces supination (Fig. 18.62) and pronation (Fig. 18.63).

4. Comparison is made with the opposite side. In dysfunction, asymmetry is identified in the motion between the radial head and the capitulum.

Figure 18.62.

Figure 18.63.

Elbow Region

Diagnosis of Radial Head Dysfunction
Test 3: Motion Test

1. Patient sits on table with forearms supinated.
2. Patient flexes and brings elbows to front of chest with medial margins of forearm and hand approximated (Fig. 18.64).
3. Patient attempts to extend elbows while maintaining forearms together (Fig. 18.65).
4. Pronation of the forearm during elbow extension identifies radial head dysfunction.

Elbow Region

Muscle Energy Technique
    Diagnosis
        Position: Radial Head Posterior
        Motion Restriction: Supination

1. Patient sitting on table with elbow flexed to 90 degrees.
2. Operator stands in front with lateral hand supporting the proximal forearm and index finger over the posterior aspect of the radial head.

3. Operator's medial hand grasps distal forearm and introduces supination to the barrier (Fig. 18.66).
4. Patient pronates the hand against operator resistance for 3 to 5 seconds for three to five repetitions.
5. Operator engages new supination barrier after each patient effort.
6. With last patient muscle effort, an attempt is made to flex the elbow against resistance in addition to pronation.
7. Retest.

Figure 18.65.

Figure 18.64.

Figure 18.66.

Elbow Region

Mobilization with Impulse Technique
   Diagnosis
      Position: Radial Head Posterior
      Motion Restriction: Supination

1. Patient sitting on the table.
2. Operator stands in front grasping proximal forearm with index finger of lateral hand overlying posterior aspect of radial head (Fig. 18.67).

3. Operator controls patient's distal forearm, hand, and wrist between elbow and chest wall.
4. Operator engages barrier of extension, supination, and slight adduction (Fig. 18.68).
5. Operator performs mobilization with impulse thrust in a lateral and anterior direction.
6. Retest.

Figure 18.67.

Figure 18.68.

Elbow Region

Mobilization with Impulse Technique
   Diagnosis
      Position: Radial Head Anterior
      Motion Restriction: Pronation

1. Patient standing or sitting on table.

2. Operator stands in front with medial hand grasping proximal forearm and thumb of lateral hand over the anterior aspect of the radial head (Fig. 18.69).

3. Operator pronates and flexes patient's forearm while thumb holds radial head posteriorly (Fig. 18.70).

4. When barrier is engaged, an increasing elbow flexion mobilization with impulse thrust is performed.

5. Retest.

Figure 18.69.

Figure 18.70.

WRIST AND HAND REGION

Like the elbow, the wrist is not a single articulation but a combination of many. They include the radiocarpal joint with the distal radius articulating with the carpal scaphoid and lunate, the distal radioulnar joint, the ulnar-meniscal-triquetral, the intercarpal joint, the carpometacarpal joints, and the proximal and distal interphalangeal joints. Movements at the wrist region include dorsiflexion, palmar flexion, adduction (ulnar deviation), abduction (radial deviation), and pronation and supination. Pronation and supination occur primarily at the distal radioulnar joint and are related to similar pronation–supination movement at the elbow region.

Wrist and Hand Region

Diagnosis

1. Patient sitting on table with operator standing in front.

2. Patient's arms at the side with elbows flexed to 90 degrees.

3. Operator introduces palmar flexion (Fig. 18.71), dorsiflexion (Fig. 18.72), ulnar deviation pronated (Fig. 18.73), radial deviation pronated (Fig. 18.74), radial deviation supinated (Fig. 18.75), and ulnar deviation supinated (Fig. 18.76) testing for restricted range of movement.

4. Muscle strength testing can be performed in the same directions.

Figure 18.71.

Figure 18.72.

Figure 18.73.

Figure 18.75.

Figure 18.74.

Figure 18.76.

Wrist and Hand Region

Muscle Energy Technique

1. Patient sitting on table with operator standing in front.

2. Operator's proximal hand stabilizes patient's distal forearm while distal hand engages resistant barrier of wrist and hand motion.

3. Operator engages resistant barriers in palmar flexion (Fig. 18.77), dorsiflexion (Fig. 18.78), pronated radial deviation (Fig. 18.79), pronated ulnar deviation (Fig. 18.80), supinated radial deviation (Fig. 18.81), and supinated ulnar deviation (Fig. 18.82).

4. Patient performs 3 to 5 second muscle contractions against operator resistance for three to five repetitions.

5. Operator engages new barrier after each patient effort.

6. Retest.

Figure 18.78.

Figure 18.77.

Figure 18.79.

Figure 18.80.

Figure 18.81.

Figure 18.82.

Wrist and Hand Region

Mobilization with Impulse Technique

1. Patient sitting on table with operator standing in front.

2. Operator's two hands grasps patient's hand and wrist with operator's thumbs contacting dorsal aspect of the scaphoid and lunate (Fig. 18.83) and index fingers grasping volar aspect of the scaphoid and lunate (Fig. 18.84).

3. Operator engages dorsiflexion barrier and applies mobilization with impulse thrust by taking patient's wrist toward the floor (Fig. 18.85).

Figure 18.84.

Figure 18.83.

Figure 18.85.

4. Operator engages palmar flexion barrier and provides a mobilization with impulse thrust by carrying wrist toward the ceiling (Fig. 18.86).

5. Operator engages radial deviation barrier and performs mobilization with impulse thrust while taking the wrist laterally (Fig. 18.87).

6. Operator engages ulnar deviation barrier and provides mobilization with impulse thrust by taking the wrist medially (Fig. 18.88).

7. Retest.

Wrist and Hand Region

Joint Play: Long-Axis Extension
Radiocarpal Joint

1. Patient sitting or standing on table with operator in front.

2. Operator's proximal hand stabilizes patient's elbow flexed to 90 degrees.

3. Operator's distal hand grasps radiocarpal joint just distal to the radial and ulnar styloid processes (Fig. 18.89).

4. Operator takes up long-axis extension to barrier.

5. Operator performs a long-axis extension thrust by the distal hand.

6. Retest.

Note: This technique also performs joint play movement at the proximal radioulnar and humeroradial joints.

Figure 18.86.

Figure 18.88.

Figure 18.87.

Figure 18.89.

Wrist and Hand Region

Joint Play
Distal Radioulnar and Ulna-meniscal-triquetral
Articulations

1. Patient standing or sitting on table with operator in front.
2. Operator stabilizes patient's hand and radiocarpal region by placing index finger in the web of the patient's thumb (Fig. 18.90) and the thenar eminences and middle, ring, and little fingers grasping the distal radius and proximal carpals (Fig. 18.91).
3. Operator grasps distal ulna between thumb and pads of the fingers (Fig. 18.92).
4. Operator provides anteroposterior glide and medial and lateral rotary joint play movements of the distal ulna (Fig. 18.93).

Figure 18.90.

Figure 18.92.

Figure 18.91.

Figure 18.93.

5. Using the same handhold to stabilize the distal radius and carpals, operator places the right thumb over the dorsal surface of the distal ulna and the proximal interphalangeal joint of the right index finger over the pisiform bone (Fig. 18.94).

6. Operator squeezes thumb and index finger providing an anteroposterior glide joint play movement at the ulnar-meniscal-triquetral joint (Fig. 18.95).

7. The maneuver is a squeeze-and-release process through operator's right hand.

8. Retest.

Wrist and Hand Region

Joint Play
Midcarpal Joint

1. Patient standing or sitting on table with operator at side.

2. Operator's proximal hand grasps distal radius and ulna and the fingers contact the proximal row of the carpal bones.

3. Operator's distal hand controls patient's hand and distal row of carpal bones.

4. Operator's knuckles of the index fingers and thumbs of both hands are together.

5. Operator introduces approximately 15 degrees of palmar flexion to loose pack the midcarpal joint (Fig. 18.96).

6. While maintaining stability with the proximal hand, the distal hand moves toward the ceiling and to the floor providing an anteroposterior glide of the midcarpal joints.

7. Retest.

Figure 18.95.

Figure 18.94.

Figure 18.96.

Wrist and Hand Region

Joint Play
Midcarpal Joint Dorsal Tilt

1. Patient standing or sitting on table with operator standing in front.

2. Operator's right thenar eminence is placed transversely across the proximal crease of the patient's right wrist stabilizing the distal radius, ulna, and proximal row of carpals (Fig. 18.97).

3. Operator identifies dorsal aspect of head of capitate by coursing left index finger proximally between the shafts of the patient's second and third metacarpal bones (Fig. 18.98).

4. Operator places left pisiform over the head of patient's capitate with the rest of the hand stabilizing patient's hand (Fig. 18.99).

5. Operator's two arms are parallel with each other, and by moving both elbows medially, a joint play dorsal tilt of the head of the capitate is performed.

6. Retest.

Figure 18.98.

Figure 18.97.

Figure 18.99.

Wrist and Hand Region

Joint Play
First Carpometacarpal Joint

1. Operator's left hand stabilizes patient's wrist and hand (Fig. 18.100).

2. Operator grasps patient's thumb and first metacarpal bone, placing operator's to patient's first metacarpals (Fig. 18.101).

3. Operator performs joint play mobilizing thrust by tilting with the right hand toward the patient, resulting in an anteroposterior tilt of the first carpometacarpal joint.

4. Retest.

Figure 18.100.

Figure 18.101.

Wrist and Hand Region

Myofascial Release

1. Patient sitting on table with operator standing in front.

2. Operator's two hands grasp patient's hand with one hand holding the thumb (Fig. 18.102) and the other holding the ulnar side of the patient's hand (Fig. 18.103).

3. Operator's hand applies abduction and extension load to the thumb while the other hand introduces radioulnar deviation and palmar–dorsiflexion loads in a circular fashion, seeking direct and indirect barriers.

4. Operator localizes to individual carpal bones by contacting dorsal surface with the tip of the thumb and the volar surfaces with the finger pads (Fig. 18.104).

5. Retest.

Figure 18.103.

Figure 18.102.

Figure 18.104.

Wrist and Hand Region

Myofascial Release
Wrist Retinaculi

1. Patient sitting on table with operator standing in front.
2. Operator's two hands grasp the patient's hand with the thumbs over the lateral attachments of the wrist retinaculum (Fig. 18.105). Fingers overlie the dorsal aspect of the wrist.
3. Operator's hands introduce dorsiflexion of the patient's wrist (Fig. 18.106).
4. Operator applies lateral distraction load until release is achieved (Fig. 18.107).

Figure 18.106.

Figure 18.105.

Figure 18.107.

Wrist and Hand Region

Flexor Retinaculi and Flexor Tendons

1. Patient sitting on table with operator standing in front.

2. Operator interlaces the fingers of both hands applying a thenar eminence contact across distal radius and ulnar on the dorsal side and the wrist retinaculum on the volar side (Fig. 18.108).

3. Operator maintains anteroposterior compression over wrist while patient actively flexes and extends fingers (Fig. 18.109).

4. Patient repeats flexion and extension efforts several times, mobilizing flexor tendons under the flexor retinaculum while operator's two hands maintain compression resulting in distraction.

5. Retest.

Figure 18.108.

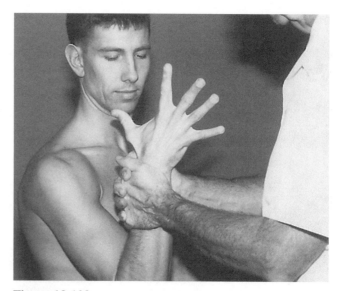

Figure 18.109.

UPPER LIMB NEURAL TENSION TESTS AND DURAL MOBILIZATION

The work of Selvy and Butler has generated an interest in the upper and lower extremities neural tension tests and the use of these diagnostic maneuvers for dural mobilization. The peripheral nervous system has an extensive connective-tissue interface that can be subjected to restriction, altered tension, and mobility. The diagnostic tests add another dimension to the neurologic tests of reflex testing, sensory examination, and muscular weakness (strength) testing. Restriction of the peripheral nervous system and its dura is frequently seen in association with somatic dysfunction of the vertebral complex from which the nerve roots emerge and from their course through the extremities. These maneuvers can be used as an additional activating force in mobilizing areas of somatic dysfunction. Although Butler does not describe the relationship of the peripheral tests and mobilizing procedures with the cranial dura, others knowledgeable about the craniosacral system have found that there is clearly an association, and the use of peripheral dural mobilizing procedures can profoundly influence the dural component of the craniosacral system.

In the upper extremity, there are three upper limb tension tests that are biased toward the median, radial, and ulnar distributions. When using the ma-neuvers therapeutically in the presence of restricted neural and dural mobility, a gentle on and off of the tension is applied. One does not attempt to "stretch" the nerve, but enhance its mobility within its connective tissue.

Upper Limb Tension Test 1: Median Nerve Bias

1. Patient supine on the table with operator standing at the side.
2. Operator's left hand depresses patient's left shoulder to prevent elevation during abduction of the upper extremity by the operator's left thigh (Fig. 18.110).
3. Operator's right hand introduces external rotation of the humerus (Fig. 18.111) and supination of the forearm and wrist with extension of the fingers (Fig. 18.112).

Figure 18.111.

Figure 18.110.

Figure 18.112.

4. Operator extends the elbow (Fig. 18.113) sensing for restriction in tension and the initiation of painful discomfort in the arm.

5. Patient side bends the head to the left and assessment is again made to see if there is change in the arm symptom (Fig. 18.114). Usually, the tension and discomfort are lessened.

6. Patient side bends the head to the right (Fig. 18.115) and assessment is again made. This maneuver usually enhances the sensation of tension and patient symptoms.

7. If used as a therapeutic maneuver, the on and off of elbow extension is done within the limits of the tension.

Figure 18.114.

Figure 18.113.

Figure 18.115.

Upper Limb Tension Test 2: Radial Nerve Bias

1. Patient supine with operator standing at head of table.

2. Patient's left arm off side of table with operator's right thigh stabilizing patient's left shoulder to prevent elevation.

3. Operator's right hand holds the patient's arm and the left hand controls the left wrist (Fig. 18.116).

4. Operator's left hand flexes patient's wrist and thumb and applies ulnar deviation (Fig. 18.117).

5. Operator abducts arm with elbow straight sensitizing radial nerve.

Figure 18.116.

Figure 18.117.

Upper Limb Tension Test 3: Ulnar Nerve Bias

1. Patient supine on table with operator standing at side.
2. Operator stabilizes shoulder and arm at ninety degrees as in upper limb tension test 1 (Fig. 18.110).
3. Patient's wrist is extended, the forearm pronated, and the elbow flexed (Fig. 18.118).
4. Patient's shoulder is abducted directing the patient's left hand toward the left ear (Fig. 18.119).

SUMMARY

Frequent complaints in the upper extremity include bursitis, tendonitis, epicondylitis, tennis elbow, golfer's elbow, carpal tunnel syndrome, and many others. Dysfunction in the symptomatic joint regions is commonly found as are proximal and distal dysfunc-tions. The examiner should always assess, and appropriately treat, any dysfunction in the trunk proximal to the extremity before addressing the extremity. The identification and appropriate treatment of dysfunctions within the entire upper extremity is helpful in the management of these patients.

SUGGESTED READINGS

Butler DS. *Mobilization of the nervous system.* Melbourne: Churchill Livingstone, 1991.

Kaltenborn FM. *Manuelle Therapie der Extremitatengelenke.* Oslo: Norlis Bokhandel, 1976.

Mennell J McM. *Joint pain.* Boston: Little, Brown and Company, 1964.

Mennell J McM. *The musculoskeletal system: differential diagnosis from symptoms and physical signs.* Gaithersburg, MD: Aspen Publishers, 1992.

Figure 18.118.

Figure 18.119.

19

LOWER EXTREMITY TECHNIQUE

The primary function of the lower extremity is ambulation. The complex interactions of the foot, ankle, knee, and hip regions provide a stable base for the trunk in standing and a mobile base for walking and running. Dysfunction in the lower extremities alters the functional capacity of the rest of the body, particularly the pelvic girdle. The screening examination (see Chapter 2) evaluated the lower extremities while standing, during walking, performing the squat test, the straight leg-raising test (for hamstring length), the standing flexion test, and the one-legged stork test. A positive finding of any of these screening tests requires that the examiner proceed to further evaluation of the hip, knee, foot, and ankle. This chapter deals with the lower extremity from the hip to the distal regions. From the functional perspective, the lower extremity begins at the sacroiliac joint rather than the hip joint. The hip bone functions as a lower extremity bone during the walking cycle. Assessment of lower extremity function must include the pelvic girdle.

As with the upper extremities, evaluation should proceed from proximal to distal for several reasons. First, when considering the respiratory–circulatory model, it is appropriate to proceed from proximal to distal to enhance venous and lymphatic return. If edema and inflammation are part of the restrictive process, this sequence assists fluid movement. Second, proceeding from proximal to distal provides the examiner a point of reference for evaluating one bone in relation to another at an articulation. Structural examination of the lower extremities should be combined with standard orthopedic and neurologic tests and, particularly, some of the newer neural and dural tension signs found within the system of mobilization

of the nervous system. The ultimate goal of evaluation and treatment of the lower extremities is to return the most symmetric walking cycle that is possible. Anatomic variation in the bones of the lower extremity can result in the "short leg" and pelvic tilt syndromes that have clinical significance in somatic dysfunction of the vertebral column and pelvic girdle. Alteration in the mechanics of the foot with flattening of the medial, transverse, and lateral arches; of the knee region, including the tibiofemoral and proximal tibiofibular articulations; and the hip may alter function within the vertebral axis and pelvic girdle.

As with the upper extremity, several of Mennell's diagnostic and therapeutic joint play techniques are presented. A thorough study of that system is highly recommended and can be found in publications by Mennell, including *Joint Pain, Foot Pain,* and *The Musculoskeletal System: Differential Diagnosis from Symptoms and Physical Signs.*

HIP JOINT

The hip joint is a ball-and-socket articulation that has polyaxial movement. There is a cartilaginous lip surrounding the acetabulum, and the hip capsule is intimately related to the extensive musculature surrounding the hip joint. Hip joint movement includes flexion–extension, abduction–adduction, and internal rotation–external rotation. The musculature surrounding the hip joint can be divided into six groups, each responsible for one of the movement directions. In addition to dysfunction of muscle, there are joint play dysfunctions and capsular restrictions that need to be assessed and treated in order to achieve muscle balance surrounding the hip joint.

Hip Joint

Supine

Assessment of Hip Capsular Pattern

1. Patient supine with operator standing at side of table.

2. Operator's distal hand grasps the ankle region while the proximal hand controls the flexed hip and flexed knee.

3. Operator introduces circumduction in clockwise (Fig. 19.1) and counterclockwise directions (Fig. 19.2).

4. Operator increases the circumduction arc seeking to see if the capsular pattern is smooth in all directions.

5. A positive finding is to have a hitch or delay in movement during the circumduction arc that frequently is reported by the patient as being pinching and painful.

Figure 19.1.

Figure 19.2.

Hip Joint

Supine

Joint Play

1. Patient supine with operator standing at side of table.
2. Operator flexes patient's hip and knee to 90 degrees.
3. Operator drapes flexed knee over shoulder and grasps the anterior aspect of the proximal femur with interlaced hands.
4. When all slack is taken up, a mobilizing joint play distraction thrust is applied in a caudad direction by the two hands (Fig. 19.3).
5. Operator drapes knee over the neck and with interlaced fingers grasps medial side of proximal femur.
6. When slack is taken out in a medial-to-lateral direction, a joint play thrust is applied in lateral distraction by the two hands (Fig. 19.4).
7. Reassess.

Hip Joint

Supine

Acetabular Labrum Technique (example, left hip)

1. Patient supine with operator standing at side of table.
2. Operator flexes knee and hip and controls left lower extremity with the left arm, axilla, and trunk.

3. Operator places heel of right hand against the lateral aspect of the patient's left greater trochanter (Fig. 19.5).
4. Operator applies a series of impaction compressive forces through the right arm in the direction of the femoral head and hip joint, while alternately providing an anteroposterior compressive force through the left arm contact, with some cephalic-to-caudad distraction as well.
5. Various degrees of adduction–abduction and internal–external rotation are used to fine-tune against the resistant barrier.
6. The activating force is mobilization without impulse.
7. Retest.

Figure 19.4.

Figure 19.3.

Figure 19.5.

Hip Joint

Prone

Mobilization of Anterior Capsule (Example: right hip)

1. Patient prone with operator standing at side of table.

2. Operator flexes right knee and grasps anterior aspect of distal right femur with the right hand and arm.

3. Operator's left hand contacts the posterior aspect of the proximal right femur with the left arm fully extended (Fig. 19.6).

4. Operator gently lifts the right knee off the table and applies a series of mobilizing without impulse forces in an anterior direction against the proximal femur.

5. Operator fine-tunes against resistant barrier by internally and externally rotating the right femur and by applying medial and lateral directional forces through the left hand.

6. Retest.

Figure 19.6.

Hip Joint

Supine

Mobilization of Posterior Hip Capsule (Example: right hip)

1. Patient supine with operator standing on right side.
2. Operator's right hand is placed over the ischial tuberosity with the left hand controlling the flexed hip and knee (Fig. 19.7).
3. Operator abducts and adducts and internally and externally rotates the right hip against the restrictive barrier.
4. Operator's activating force is repetitive mobilization without impulse in a posterior direction through the shaft of the femur.
5. An alternate position has the operator on the left side of the patient and the patient's left hip bone on the edge of the table.
6. Operator's two hands are on the patient's flexed left knee and fine-tunes adduction–abduction, and internal–external rotation against the barrier, and then provides repetitive posterior mobilization without impulse through the shaft of the left femur (Fig. 19.8).
7. Reassess.

The primary dysfunctions of the hip joint are imbalances of length and strength of the six muscle groups. Structural diagnosis and muscle energy techniques for these muscle imbalances are as follows:

1. Operator passively takes the hip joint through a range of motion, evaluating quantity of range, quality of movement during the range, and quality of the end feel.
2. Comparison is made on the opposite side.
3. Asymmetry may be due to shortening of the muscle group on the restricted side or weakness of the contralateral muscle group with increased range.
4. Strength testing is performed by asking the patient to maximally contract the muscle against equal and opposite resistance, comparing one side to the other.
5. Treatment of short and tight muscle groups is achieved by a series of 3 to 5 second isometric contractions against operator's equal and opposite resistance. After each patient effort, the operator engages the next resistant barrier with gradual lengthening of the shortened muscle by the principle of postisometric relaxation.
6. Treatment of functional weakness of a muscle group is accomplished by asking the patient to perform a series of three to five concentric isotonic contractions made through the total range of movement against an operator counterforce that is yielding in nature, but with progressive increase in resistance with each effort.
7. Retest for length and strength of comparable muscle groups.

Figure 19.7.

Figure 19.8.

Hip Joint

Muscle Energy Technique

Motion Tested: Abduction
Muscles Tested: Adductors (adductor magnus, adductor brevis, adductor longus)

1. Patient supine on table with operator standing at end grasping lower extremity at the ankle.

2. Operator abducts extended lower extremity to the end point, evaluating total range and quality of movement during the range (Fig. 19.9). During motion testing, the operator prevents the extended leg from moving into external rotation.

3. Operator tests for adductor strength by offering resistance against the patient's extended leg with the knee fully extended. Operator's resistance is above the knee joint to protect the medial collateral ligament (Fig. 19.10).

4. Treat shortness or weakness as appropriate.

5. Retest.

Figure 19.9.

Figure 19.10.

Hip Joint

Muscle Energy Technique

Motion Tested: Adduction
Muscles Tested: Abductors (gluteus medius, gluteus minimis)

1. Patient supine on table with operator standing at end.
2. Operator adducts the extended leg across the front of the opposite leg, testing for range and quality of movement (Fig. 19.11).

3. Operator tests for strength by asking the patient to maximally abduct the leg against resistance offered by the operator holding the leg in the adducted position (Fig. 19.12).
4. Comparison is made with the opposite leg.
5. Treatment for shortness or tightness is accomplished as appropriate.
6. Retest.

Note: An alternate method is to lift the leg not being tested (Fig. 19.13) and adduct the extended leg being tested beneath it (Fig. 19.14). Testing in this position also evaluates the tensor fascia lata muscle.

Figure 19.11.

Figure 19.13.

Figure 19.12.

Figure 19.14.

Hip Joint

Muscle Energy Technique

Motion Tested: External rotation with hip flexed to 90 degrees

Muscles Tested: Internal Rotators (gluteus medius, gluteus minimis)

1. Patient supine on table with operator standing at side next to extremity being tested.

2. Operator holds lower extremity with 90-degree flexion at both the hip and the knee (Fig. 19.15).

3. Operator externally rotates the femur by carrying the foot and ankle medially, evaluating range and quality of movement (Fig. 19.16).

4. Operator performs strength testing by having the patient internally rotate the femur against equal and opposite resistance (Fig. 19.17).

5. Comparison is made with the opposite side.

6. Shortness or weakness is treated as appropriate.

7. Retest.

Figure 19.16.

Figure 19.15.

Figure 19.17.

Hip Joint

Muscle Energy Technique

Motion Tested: Internal Rotation with Hip Flexed to 90 degrees
Muscles Tested: External Rotators (primarily piriformis)

1. Patient supine on table with operator standing at side next to extremity being tested.

2. Operator holds the lower extremity with 90-degree flexion at both the hip and knee (Fig. 19.15).

3. Operator introduces internal rotation testing for range and quality of movement (Fig. 19.18).

4. Operator performs strength testing by asking the patient to externally rotate against resistance offered by the operator (Fig. 19.19).

5. Comparison is made with the opposite side.

6. Shortness or tightness is treated as appropriate.

7. Retest.

Figure 19.18.

Figure 19.19.

Hip Joint

Muscle Energy Technique

Motion Tested: Partial Hip Flexion (straight leg raising)

Muscles Tested: Hip extensors, primarily hamstring muscles (semitendinosus, semimembranosus, biceps femoris)

Note: Gluteus maximus and adductor magnus become hip extensors when thigh is flexed.

1. Patient supine on table with operator standing at side of table.
2. Operator monitors anterior superior iliac spine on side opposite leg being tested.
3. Operator lifts extended leg introducing hip flexion, testing for range and quality of movement with the end point being the first movement of the opposite anterior superior iliac spine (Fig. 19.20).
4. Shortness and tightness are treated by a series of isometric contractions against resistance with the patient effort being to pull the heel toward the buttock (Fig. 19.21).

   Note: An alternative position has the patient holding the posterior aspect of the distal thigh while the operator extends the knee and resists a knee flexion effort by the patient against the operator's resistance (Fig. 19.22).

5. Strength testing is performed by having the patient prone on the table with the operator resisting patient attempts at knee flexion in a bilateral fashion.
6. Weakness is treated by a series of concentric isotonic contractions through the full range of knee flexion against progressively increasing operator resistance.
7. Retest.

Figure 19.21.

Figure 19.20.

Figure 19.22.

Hip Joint

Muscle Energy Technique

Motion Tested: Hip Extension
Muscle Tested: Iliopsoas

1. Patient supine with pelvis close to the end of the table so that lower extremity below the knee is free of the table.
2. Operator stands at end of table facing patient.
3. Patient's hips and knees are flexed.
4. Patient holds leg opposite that being tested in a flexed position while operator passively extends the leg being tested (Fig. 19.23).
5. The normal range is for the back of the thigh to strike the table with the knee fully flexed (Fig. 19.24).
6. Patient performs strength testing by attempting to lift the knee to the ceiling against operator resistance.
7. Comparison is made with the opposite side.
8. Shortness is treated by isometric contraction against operator resistance. Patient is instructed to perform hip flexion. Operator also resists attempts at external rotation of the hip by offering a resist-ance with leg against the medial side of the patient's foot and ankle (Fig. 19.25).
9. Weakness is treated by a series of concentric isotonic contractions of hip flexion and external rotation.
10. Retest.

Note: Before testing for length and strength of the iliopsoas, the lumbar spine should be evaluated and treated appropriately. This iliopsoas test puts stress on the lumbar spine, particularly the lumbosacral junction.

Figure 19.24.

Figure 19.23.

Figure 19.25.

Hip Joint

Muscle Energy Technique

Motion Tested: Knee Flexion
Muscles Tested: Quadriceps group (rectus femoris, vastus lateralis, vastus intermedius, vastus medialis)

1. Patient prone on table with operator standing at foot facing patient.
2. Operator flexes both knees while holding patient's ankles (Fig. 19.26).

3. Test is made for range and quality of movement.
4. Operator performs strength testing by asking the patient to extend the knees against resistance with both sides contracting simultaneously.
5. Shortness is treated by a series of isometric contractions against resistance (Fig. 19.27).
6. Weakness is treated by a series of concentric isotonic contraction against progressively increasing operator resistance.
7. Retest.

Figure 19.26.

Figure 19.27.

Hip Joint

Muscle Energy Technique

Motion Tested: Internal Rotation with Hips in Neutral
Muscles Tested: External Rotators (obturator internus, obturator externus, gemellus superior, gemellus inferior, quadratus femoris, and piriformis)

1. Patient prone on table with operator standing at foot of table facing patient.
2. Operator flexes patient's knees to 90 degrees (Fig. 19.28).
3. Operator tests for range and quality of internal rotation by allowing the feet to drop laterally (Fig. 19.29).
4. Operator performs strength testing by asking the patient to bilaterally pull the feet together against resistance.

5. Shortness is treated by operator holding the opposite leg with the knee flexed and hip internally rotated while the patient performs external rotation of the leg in the 90-degree flexed position against operator resistance (Fig. 19.30).
6. Weakness is treated by a series of concentric isotonic contractions through a range of external rotation with the knee at 90 degrees.
7. Retest.

Note: This muscle group is intimately attached to the posterior hip capsule and frequently needs attention with an altered hip capsular pattern.

Figure 19.29.

Figure 19.28.

Figure 19.30.

Hip Joint

Muscle Energy Technique

Motion Tested: External rotation with the hips at neutral

Muscles Tested: Internal rotators (gluteus medius, gluteus minimis, tensor fascia lata)

1. Patient prone on table with operator standing at foot facing patient.

2. Operator stabilizes leg opposite one being tested with slight knee flexion and hip external rotation.

3. Leg being tested is flexed to 90 degrees and externally rotated looking for range and quality of movement (Fig. 19.31).

4. The opposite side is tested in a similar manner (Fig. 19.32).

5. Operator performs strength testing by asking the patient to internally rotate against resistance.

6. Shortness and tightness are treated by a series of isometric contractions of internal rotation against resistance (Fig. 19.33).

7. Weakness is treated by a series of concentric isotonic contractions against increasing operator resistance.

8. Retest.

The balancing of the hip musculature is an important part of the treatment of the patient's musculoskeletal system, particularly those patients with lower back and lower extremity pain syndromes. Many experts debate the exact treatment sequence but this author has found it most effective to treat shortness and tightness before treating weakness. Clinical observation finds that the short, tight group of muscles reflexly inhibits the antagonist, resulting in apparent weakness of the antagonist muscle. Once the shortness and tightness of the agonist are removed, the apparent weakness of the antagonist is frequently no longer present. If a muscle still appears to be functionally weak after treating the shortness and tightness of its antagonist, it should be treated for weakness using the techniques described. Muscle imbalance patterns are frequently seen in the six muscle groups. It is common to find the right adductors tight with apparent weakness of the left adductors and weakness of the right abductors. The psoas and rectus femoris muscles are frequently tight and need to be stretched so that appropriate hip extension can occur during the walking cycle. The imbalance of tightness and weakness between agonist and antagonist is consistent with the tight–loose concept found when using the myofascial release system of diagnosis and treatment.

Figure 19.32.

Figure 19.31.

Figure 19.33.

KNEE JOINT

The primary movement at the knee joint is flexion and extension of the tibia under the femur. The lengths of the medial and lateral femoral condyles are different resulting in an internal–external rotational component to the flexion–extension arc. During extension, the tibia rotates externally, and during flexion, the tibia rotates internally. Dysfunction of the internal–external rotation interferes with normal flexion–extension. The flexion–extension and the internal–external rotation movements depend on a small anteroposterior glide and medial-to-lateral gapping of the opposing joint surfaces. These minor joint play movements are present within the constraints of normal ligamentous stability. The movements are increased when there is ligamentous or cartilage damage within the knee. The primary somatic dysfunctions of the knee joint are at the medial meniscus and the internal–external rotation of the tibia on the femur.

Knee Joint

Supine

Medial Meniscus Technique
Mobilization without Impulse

1. Patient supine on table with operator standing at side near dysfunctional knee.

2. Operator holds patient's distal leg between upper arm and chest with both hands surrounding the proximal tibia.

3. Operator's thumbs are placed over the medial joint space with the knee in flexion (Fig. 19.34).

4. Operator's lateral hand exerts a medial compression on the distal femur while operator's thumbs maintain posterolateral compressive force on the medial meniscus and the leg is carried into extension (Fig. 19.35).

5. Several repetitions of this procedure may be necessary to release restriction of the medial meniscus.

6. Retest.

Figure 19.34.

Figure 19.35.

Knee Joint

Supine

Medial and Lateral Meniscus Technique
Mobilization without Impulse Technique

1. Patient supine on table with operator standing at caudal end facing patient.
2. Operator supports the patient's dysfunctional leg between the thighs over the edge of table.
3. Operator's two hands grasp proximal tibia with the thumbs over the anteromedial or anterolateral joint space depending on whether the restriction is of the lateral or medial malleolus (Fig. 19.36).
4. For medial meniscus dysfunction, operator performs a circumduction movement beginning in flexion, in-cluding medial translation with thumb compression over the medial meniscus, while carrying the knee into full extension (Fig. 19.37).
5. For restriction of the lateral meniscus, operator places the thumbs overly the anterolateral aspect of the knee. The circumduction movement begins in flexion and includes lateral translation while carrying the distal leg into extension.
6. Several repetitions may be necessary.
7. Retest.

Note: Restriction of the medial meniscus is much more common than restriction of the lateral meniscus.

Figure 19.36.

Figure 19.37.

Knee Joint

Supine

Medial and Lateral Meniscal Tracking
Joint Play

1. Patient supine on table with operator standing at side closest to dysfunctional knee.

2. Operator controls dysfunctional leg at 90-degree hip and 90-degree knee flexion positions with the distal hand controlling dorsiflexion of the ankle for close packing while the proximal hand controls the distal femur with the thumb over the lateral meniscus and the index and middle fingers over the medial meniscus (Fig. 19.38).

3. Operator medially and laterally rotates the tibia through the close-packed ankle joint with progressive extension of the hip and knee (Fig. 19.39).

4. Several repetitions are necessary. The amount of medial and lateral rotation gradually decreases as the knee extends.

5. Retest.

Knee Joint

Supine

Extension Compression Test

1. Patient supine on table with operator standing at side of dysfunctional leg.

2. Operator's proximal hand stabilizes the distal femur.

3. Operator's distal hand grasps patient's heel (Fig. 19.40).

4. Operator carries the distal leg into increased extension at the knee against the stabilizing proximal hand.

5. Comparison is made with the opposite side.

6. Restriction of extension with pain provocation is a positive test and indicates restriction of external rotation and extension of the knee joint or meniscal injury.

Figure 19.39.

Figure 19.38.

Figure 19.40.

Knee Joint

Sitting

Diagnosis
Restriction of Internal–External Rotation

1. Patient sits on edge of table with lower legs dangling with operator sitting in front of patient.

2. Operator grasps feet and dorsiflexes ankle to close-pack position.

3. Operator introduces external rotation (Fig. 19.41) and internal rotation (Fig. 19.42), testing for range, quality of range, and end feel.

4. Operator performs strength testing by asking the patient to internally and externally rotate tibia against resistance.

Knee Joint

Sitting

Muscle Energy Technique
Diagnosis
    Position: Tibia Internally Rotated
    Motion Restriction: External Rotation of Tibia

1. Patient sitting on edge of table with lower legs dangling and operator sitting in front of patient.

2. Operator grasps heel of foot in one hand and forefoot in the other.

3. Operator dorsiflexes foot at ankle and introduces external rotation to barrier (Fig. 19.43).

4. Patient internally rotates forefoot against operator resistance for 3 to 5 seconds and three to five repetitions.

5. After each patient effort, operator externally rotates tibia to the new barrier.

6. Retest.

Figure 19.42.

Figure 19.41.

Figure 19.43.

Knee Joint

Sitting

Muscle Energy Technique
Diagnosis
   Position: Tibia Externally Rotated
   Motion Restriction: Internal Rotation of the Tibia

1. Patient sits on edge of table with lower legs dangling with operator sitting in front of patient.

2. Operator grasps heel of foot in one hand and forefoot in the other.

3. Operator dorsiflexes foot at ankle and introduces internal rotation to barrier (Fig. 19.44)

4. Operator externally rotates forefoot against operator resistance for 3 to 5 seconds and three to five repetitions.

5. Following each patient effort, operator internally rotates tibia to the new barrier.

6. Retest.

Knee Joint

Prone

Muscle Energy Technique

   Diagnosis of Internal–External Rotation

1. Patient prone on table with knees flexed to 90 degrees and operator standing at end of table grasping each foot in each hand.

2. Operator introduces dorsiflexion of the ankle and externally rotates (Fig. 19.45) and internally rotates tibia (Fig. 19.46) testing for range, quality of range, and end feel.

3. Operator performs strength testing by asking the patient to internally or externally rotate the foot against resistance offered by the operator.

Figure 19.45.

Figure 19.44.

Figure 19.46.

Knee Joint

Prone

Muscle Energy Technique
Diagnosis: Tibia Internally Rotated
    Motion Restriction: External Rotation of the Tibia

1. Patient prone on table with operator standing on side of dysfunctional extremity.
2. Operator flexes knee to 90 degrees and grasps heel and forefoot in each hand.
3. Operator dorsiflexes ankle and externally rotates foot to barrier (Fig. 19.47).
4. Patient internally rotates forefoot against operator resistance for 3 to 5 seconds and three to five repetitions.
5. Following each patient effort, operator externally rotates foot to new barrier.
6. Retest.

Knee Joint

Prone

Muscle Energy Technique
Diagnosis
    Position: Tibia Externally Rotated
    Motion Restriction: Internal Rotation of Tibia

1. Patient prone on table with operator standing at side of dysfunctional extremity.
2. Operator flexes knee to 90 degrees and grasps heel and forefoot of patient.
3. Operator dorsiflexes ankle and internally rotates the tibia to the barrier (Fig. 19.48).
4. Patient externally rotates forefoot against operator resistance for 3 to 5 seconds and three to five repetitions.
5. Following each patient effort, operator internally rotates foot to new barrier.
6. Retest.

Figure 19.47.

Figure 19.48.

PROXIMAL TIBIOFIBULAR JOINT

This articulation is intimately related to the knee joint and is equally important in its relation to the ankle. The proximal tibiofibular joint has an anteroposterior glide and is influenced by the action of the biceps femoris muscle inserting at the fibular head. The proximal tibiofibular joint can be restricted either anteriorly or posteriorly. Restoration of the normal anteroposterior glide and its normal relationship to the tibia are the goals of treatment.

Restoration of normal internal–external rotational movement of the tibia on the femur is accomplished before addressing the proximal tibiofibular joint.

The plane of the joint is approximately 30 degrees from lateral to medial and from before backward. Testing for the anteroposterior movement of the proximal tibiofibular joint must be within the plane of the joint and can be accomplished with the patient in the supine or sitting position.

Proximal Tibiofibular Joint

Testing for Anteroposterior Glide

1. Patient sits on table with both feet flat for fixation (Fig. 19.49) or patient sits on edge of table with the operator sitting in front holding the medial sides of both feet together (Fig. 19.50).

2. Operator grasps the proximal fibula between the thumb or thenar eminence and the fingers of each hand being careful not to compress the peroneal nerve against the fibular head.

3. Operator translates the fibular head anteriorly and posteriorly within the plane of the joint, testing for comparable range on each side, the quality of movement, and end feel.

4. A fibular head that resists anterior translatory movement is positionally a posterior fibular head, and a fibular head that resists posterior translatory is positionally an anterior fibular head.

Figure 19.49.

Figure 19.50.

Proximal Tibiofibular Joint

Sitting

Muscle Energy Technique
Diagnosis
    Position: Fibular Head Posterior
    Motion Restriction: Anterior Glide of the Fibular
    Head

1. Patient sits on edge of table with dysfunctional leg dangling and operator sitting in front with the medial hand grasping the patient's forefoot.

2. Operator inverts and internally rotates the patient's foot while the lateral hand exerts an anterolateral force on the posterior aspect of the fibular head (Fig. 19.51).

3. Patient is instructed to evert and dorsiflex the foot against resistance offered by the operator's medial hand for 3 to 5 seconds and three to five repetitions.

4. Operator engages new barrier after each patient effort.

5. Retest.

Proximal Tibiofibular Joint

Sitting

Muscle Energy Technique
Diagnosis
    Position: Fibular Head Anterior
    Motion Restriction: Posterior Glide of the Fibular
    Head

1. Patient sitting on edge of table with dysfunctional leg dangling and operator sitting in front with the medial hand grasping the patient's forefoot.

2. Operator inverts and externally rotates the patient's foot while the lateral thumb exerts a posteromedial force against the anterior aspect of the fibular head (Fig. 19.52).

3. Patient everts and plantar flexes the foot against operator resistance for 3 to 5 seconds and three to five repetitions.

4. Operator engages a new barrier after each patient effort.

5. Retest.

Figure 19.51.

Figure 19.52.

Proximal Tibiofibular Joint

Supine

Mobilization with Impulse Technique
Diagnosis
    Position: Posterior Fibular Head
    Motion Restriction: Anterior Glide of Fibular Head

1. Patient supine on table with operator standing at side of dysfunction with caudal hand controlling patient's foot and ankle.

2. Operator's cephalic hand supports the flexed knee with the metacarpophalangeal joint of the index finger posterior to the fibular head (Fig. 19.53).

3. Operator engages barrier by externally rotating the flexed knee and pinching the metacarpophalangeal joint between the distal femur and the fibular head.

4. Operator performs a mobilization with impulse thrust by exaggerating the knee flexion bringing the fibular head anterior (Fig. 19.54).

5. Retest.

Figure 19.53.

Figure 19.54.

Proximal Tibiofibular Joint

Prone

Mobilization with Impulse Technique
Diagnosis
  Position: Posterior Fibular Head
  Motion Restriction: Anterior Glide of the Fibular
  Head

1. Patient prone on table with operator standing at side of dysfunction with distal hand controlling the foot and ankle.
2. Operator's proximal hand is laid over the popliteal space with the metacarpophalangeal joint of the index finger posterior to the fibular head (Fig. 19.55).
3. Operator's knee is flexed pinching the metacarpophalangeal joint between the fibular head and the femur.
4. The barrier is engaged by slight external rotation to the leg and flexion of the knee and the operator performs a mobilization with impulse thrust by exaggerating knee flexion (Fig. 19.56).
5. Retest.

Proximal Tibiofibular Joint

Supine

Mobilization with Impulse Technique
Diagnosis
  Position: Fibular Head Anterior
  Motion Restriction: Posterior Glide of the Fibular
  Head

1. Patient supine on table with operator standing on side of dysfunction.

2. Operator's distal hand controls the lower leg in knee extension and internally rotates to approximately 30 degrees.
3. The thenar eminence of the operator's proximal hand is placed over the anterior aspect of the proximal fibula (Fig. 19.57).
4. Operator engages barrier of the anteroposterior motion of the fibular head by downward compression through the extended arm.
5. When barrier is engaged, the operator performs a mobilization with impulse thrust by dropping the body weight of the operator through the extended arm onto the anterior aspect of the fibular head.
6. Retest.

Figure 19.56.

Figure 19.55.

Figure 19.57.

ANKLE REGION

The ankle region consists of the distal tibiofibular articulation, the articulation of the superior aspect of the talus with the tibiofibular joint mortise, and the talocalcaneal (subtalar) articulation. Although the talocalcaneal joint is frequently classified as being in the foot, it is the key to functional movement of the talus. Talar restriction, from either above or below, significantly restricts ankle motion. The talus is of interest because it has no direct muscular attachments. Its movement is determined by muscle action on bones above and below. Dysfunction of the talus at the tibiofibular joint mortise is one of the more common dysfunctions in the lower extremity. Another important anatomic feature of the talus is that its superior surface is wedge-shaped, with the posterior aspect being narrower than the anterior, as it articulates with the tibiofibular joint mortise. The ankle is more stable when dorsiflexed than when plantar flexed. The most common dysfunction at this joint is restricted dorsiflexion.

The distal tibiofibular joint is quite stable and does not have a synovial capsule. It is infrequently dysfunctional. The distal tibiofibular joint is associated with the function of the proximal tibiofibular articula-

tion. Appropriate treatment at the proximal tibiofibular articulation frequently restores function at the distal tibiofibular articulation. Appropriate evaluation and treatment of the proximal and distal tibiofibular articulations should be performed before addressing the talotibiofibular mortise articulation.

Ankle Region: Distal Tibiofibular Joint

Supine

Diagnosis: Distal Tibiofibular Dysfunction

1. Patient supine on table with operator standing at foot with the medial hand grasping the posterior and medial aspects of the patient's ankle and heel.

2. Operator's lateral hand grasps the lateral malleolus between the thumb and index finger (19.58).

3. Operator's right hand glides the lateral malleolus anteriorly and posteriorly against the fixed foot and ankle.

4. Restriction of anterior movement is a posterior distal tibiofibular joint, and restriction of posterior movement is an anterior distal tibiofibular joint.

5. Comparison is made with the opposite side.

Figure 19.58.

Ankle Region: Distal Tibiofibular Joint

Supine

Mobilization with Impulse Technique
Diagnosis
    Position: Anterior Distal Tibiofibular Joint
    Motion restriction: Posterior Movement of the Lateral Malleolus

1. Patient supine on table with operator standing at foot.

2. Operator's medial hand grasps the patient's heel and maintains the ankle at 90-degree flexion. Thumb is placed over the anterior aspect of the lateral malleolus (Fig. 19.59).

3. The thenar eminence of the operator's lateral hand is superimposed on the thumb with the fingers curled around the posterior aspect of the ankle (Fig. 19.60).

4. When the barrier is engaged, a mobilization with impulse thrust is performed in a posterior direction against the anterior aspect of the lateral malleolus by a combined effort of the thenar eminence of the lateral hand and the thumb of the medial hand.

5. Retest.

Figure 19.59.

Figure 19.60.

Ankle Region: Distal Tibiofibular Joint

Prone

Mobilization with Impulse Technique
Diagnosis
   Position: Posterior Distal Tibiofibular Joint
   Motion Restriction: Anterior Movement of the
   Lateral Malleolus

1. Patient prone with feet over edge of table with operator standing at foot facing cephalad.
2. Operator's medial hand grasps the foot and ankle maintaining dorsiflexion at the ankle. The thumb is placed over the posterior aspect of the lateral malleolus (Fig. 19.61).
3. Operator's lateral hand places the thenar eminence against the opposing thumb (Fig. 19.62).
4. The barrier is engaged in an anterior direction and a mobilization with impulse thrust is performed by combined activity of the lateral hand's thenar eminence and the medial hand's thumb carrying the lateral malleolus toward the floor.
5. Retest.

Ankle Region: Talotibial Joint

Diagnosis

1. Patient sitting on table with legs dangling and operator sitting in front of patient.
2. Operator grasps forefoot and plantar flexes to the barrier evaluating each side for restriction.

3. Each thumb is placed on the anterior aspect of the neck of the talus with the fingers under the forefoot and the operator passively swings the foot toward the table resulting in dorsiflexion of the talotibial joint (Fig. 19.63). Restriction of dorsiflexion is compared from side to side. Frequently the neck of the talus on the dysfunctional side will be tender.
4. A frequent cause of restricted dorsiflexion of the talotibial joint is shortness and tightness of the gastrocnemius and soleus muscles in the calf.

Figure 19.62.

Figure 19.61.

Figure 19.63.

Ankle Region: Talotibial Joint

Sitting

Muscle Energy Technique
Diagnosis
Position: Talus Plantar Flexed
Motion Restriction: Dorsiflexion of the Talus

1. Patient sitting on edge of table with feet dangling and operator sitting in front of the dysfunctional talus.
2. Operator places medial hand under the plantar surface of the forefoot with the web of the lateral hand overlying the neck of the talus (Fig. 19.64).
3. The dorsiflexion barrier is engaged through a combined dorsiflexion movement of the foot and a posterior force on the talar neck.
4. Patient performs plantar flexion muscle effort against equal and opposite resistance for 3 to 5 seconds and three to five repetitions (Fig. 19.65).
5. After each patient effort, additional dorsiflexion is introduced against the resistant barrier.
6. Retest.

Note: It is helpful to have the operator cross the lower legs under the patient's forefoot to assist in resistance of plantar flexion.

Ankle Region: Talotibial Joint

Supine

Mobilization with Impulse Technique
Diagnosis
Position: Talus Plantar Flexed
Motion Restriction: Dorsiflexion of the Talus

1. Patient supine with operator standing at foot of table.
2. Operator's hands encircle patient's foot with middle fingers overlapping the superior aspect of the talar neck and the thumbs on the sole of the foot (Fig. 19.66).
3. Operator engages barrier by dorsiflexing and long-axis traction.
4. A mobilization with impulse thrust is made by long-axis extension through both hands.
5. Retest.

Figure 19.65.

Figure 19.64.

Figure 19.66.

Ankle Region: Talotibial Joint

Mobilization with Impulse Technique

Diagnosis
Position: Dorsiflexed or Plantar Flexed Talus
Motion Restriction: Dorsiflexion or Plantar Flexion of Talus

1. Patient supine on table with operator sitting on edge on dysfunctional side facing caudad.

2. Patient's hip is flexed to 90 degrees and externally rotated. The knee is flexed to 90 degrees with the thigh against the operator's posterior trunk.

3. The webs of operator's thumb and index fingers are placed on the neck of the talus anteriorly and the tubercle of the talus posteriorly through the Achilles tendon (Fig. 19.67).

4. The talus is dorsiflexed or plantar flexed against the resistant barrier.

5. When the barrier is engaged, a direct action mobilization with impulse thrust is made in a long-axis distraction direction.

6. Retest.

Ankle Region: Talocalcaneal (Subtalar) Joint

Testing for anteromedial-to-posterolateral glide

1. Patient supine on table with operator standing at end facing dysfunctional ankle.

2. Operator's proximal hand grasps the ankle region with the web of the thumb and index finger over the neck of the talus, the fingers grasping the medial malleolus and the thumb over the lateral malleolus stabilizing the talus.

3. Operator's distal hand grasps the calcaneus, maintains the foot and ankle at 90 degrees and translates the calcaneus anteromedially and posterolaterally under the talus sensing for restricted movement (Fig. 19.68).

4. Comparison is made with the opposite side.

Figure 19.67.

Figure 19.68.

Ankle Region: Talocalcaneal (Subtalar) Joint

Supine

Mobilization with Impulse Technique
Diagnosis
Position: Anteromedial or Posterolateral Talus
Motion Restriction: Posterolateral or Anteromedial
Glide of the Talus

1. Patient supine on table with operator sitting on table facing caudally.

2. Patient's hip is flexed to 90 degrees and externally rotated with the knee flexed to 90 degrees and the posterior aspect of the thigh being against the operator's trunk.

3. The web between the thumb and index finger of the operator's medial hand contacts the superior aspect of the calcaneus.

4. The web of the thumb and index finger of the operator's lateral hand grasps the anterior and lateral aspect of the calcaneus and incorporates the cuboid. The thumb is on the tarsal navicular.

5. In the presence of an anteromedial talus (calcaneus posterolateral), the calcaneus is medially rotated (inverted to the barrier) (Fig. 19.69).

6. In the presence of a posterolateral talus (calcaneus anteromedial), the calcaneus is laterally rotated (everted) (Fig. 19.70).

7. When the barrier is engaged, a mobilization with impulse thrust is performed through both hands by a long-axis distraction maneuver.

8. Retest.

Figure 19.69.

Figure 19.70.

FOOT

The foot is a complex structure incorporating the tarsals, metatarsals, and phalanges. There are four arches within the foot. The lateral, weight-bearing arch runs from the calcaneus, through the cuboid, to the fourth and fifth metatarsal bones, and to the fourth and fifth toes. The key to the lateral weight-bearing arch is the cuboid that rotates medially and laterally around the anterior articulation of the calcaneus. The medial spring arch includes the talus, the navicular, the medial cuneiform, the first metatarsal, and the great toe. The medial and lateral rotations of the navicular around the head of the talus determine the function of the medial spring arch. The transverse arch includes the cuboid laterally and the navicular medially and the accompanying cuneiforms.

The major restrictors of the transverse arch are dysfunction of the cuboid laterally and the navicular medially. The most common dysfunction of the transverse arch is at the cuboid being rotated internally and pronated.

The metatarsal arch is not a true arch but refers to the relation of the heads of the five metatarsals. Restrictions of the metatarsal heads at the metatarsal arch are usually secondary to dysfunction of the other arches of the foot and are accompanied by restriction of the soft tissues of the foot, primarily the plantar fascia.

Dysfunction at the navicular is either internal or external rotational restriction. Dysfunction usually accompanies that of the cuboid and the most common dysfunction is for the navicular to rotate externally with elevation of its medial tubercle. A less common dysfunction is with the navicular rotating internally with depression of the medial tubercle.

The cuneiforms respond to normal motion or dysfunction of the navicular and the cuboid. The first cuneiform rotates internally and externally on the navicular. The remaining cuneiforms glide on each other and when dysfunctional, there is usually depression with flattening of the transverse arch.

The first tarsometatarsal joint has movement similar to those of the navicular on the talus and the first cuneiform on the navicular. The remaining tarsometatarsal joints have a dorsal-to-plantar joint play glide motion in response to the transverse tarsal arch. A second joint play movement is medial and lateral rotation.

The metatarsal heads form the pseudometatarsal arch. The second metatarsal appears to be the axis of the forefoot and the first metatarsal is moved on the second, the third on the second, the fourth on the third, and the fifth on the fourth. The joint play movements are dorsal and plantar glide as well as rotation. The most common area of restriction is between the second and third metatarsal heads. When the metatarsal heads are restricted, there is frequent tension and tenderness of the interosseous muscles.

The metatarsophalangeal and interphalangeal joints have primary motions of dorsiflexion and plantar flexion. There are also minor play movements of these joints with medial and lateral tilt and rotation. Restoration of the joint play movements frequently restores pain-free flexion and extension of the metatarsophalangeal and interphalangeal joints.

The primary goals of manual medicine treatment of the foot are to restore functional capacity of the entire mechanism particularly of the cuboid laterally, the navicular medially, the tarsometatarsal joints, the metatarsal heads, and the joints of the phalanges. Appropriate diagnosis and treatment of dysfunctions of the foot frequently restore pain-free movement. Treatment of these dysfunctions strongly influences the remaining lower extremity joints and trunk during the walking cycle.

Calcaneocuboid Joint

Supine

Diagnosis: Cuboid Dysfunction

1. Patient supine on table with operator standing at end.
2. Operator palpates plantar surface of each cuboid looking for prominence of the tuberosity on the dysfunctional side.
3. Operator palpates plantar surface of each cuboid for tenderness and tension.
4. Operator motion tests cuboid on each side by having the medial hand grasp the calcaneus and holding the foot in 90 degrees at the ankle. The lateral hand grasps the lateral side of the forefoot encircling the cuboid. Internal and external rotations of the forefoot are performed while monitoring for movement at the calcaneocuboid joint (Fig. 19.71).

Calcaneocuboid Joint

Prone

Mobilization with impulse technique (J-stroke technique)
Diagnosis
   Position: Cuboid Pronated (internally rotated)
   Motion Restriction: Cuboid Supination (external rotation)

1. Patient prone with dysfunctional leg off side of table with operator standing at side on dysfunctional side facing cephalad.
2. Operator's two hands grasp the forefoot.

3. The thumb of the lateral hand is placed over the plantar surface of the cuboid and is reinforced with the thumb of the medial hand (Fig. 19.72).
4. Operator swings the foot in a series of oscillating movements, plantar flexing the forefoot.
5. With engagement of the barrier, the foot is "thrown" toward the floor with acute plantar flexion of the forefoot with the reinforced thumbs carrying the cuboid dorsally and into external rotation (Fig. 19.73).
6. Retest.

Figure 19.72.

Figure 19.71.

Figure 19.73.

Calcaneocuboid Joint

Supine

Muscle Energy Technique and Mobilization with Impulse Technique
Diagnosis
    Position: Cuboid Pronated (internally rotated)
    Motion Restriction: Supination (external rotation) of the Cuboid

1. Patient supine on table with operator standing at foot facing dysfunctional foot.

2. Medial hand grasps the calcaneus and maintains the foot in 90 degrees of ankle flexion.

3. Operator's lateral hand grasps the lateral aspect of the foot with the middle and ring fingers overlying the plantar aspect of the cuboid and the hypothenar eminence over the dorsal aspect of the fourth and fifth metatarsal shafts (Fig. 19.74).

4. Operator engages the resistant barrier by lifting with the middle and ring fingers and depressing the metatarsals with the hypothenar eminence.

5. Patient is instructed to perform dorsiflexion of the little toe against resistance for 3 to 5 seconds with three to five repetitions.

6. Operator engages a new barrier after each effort.

7. With the same localization, the operator performs a mobilization with impulse thrust by an acute lifting maneuver with the reinforced middle and ring fingers and depression of the fourth and fifth metatarsals (Fig. 19.75).

8. Retest.

Figure 19.74.

Figure 19.75.

Talonavicular Joint

Diagnosis: Internal or External Rotation
of the Navicular

1. Patient supine on table with operator standing at end facing cephalad.

2. Operator palpates the medial tubercle of each navicular for symmetry, tension, and tenderness of the medial and plantar surface.

3. Operator's proximal hand grasps the neck of the talus between the web of the thumb and index finger. The web and index finger of the distal hand surround the navicular. Operator stabilizes the proximal hand and internally and externally rotates with the distal hand in a "ringing" motion testing for the capacity for internal rotation (Fig. 19.76) and external rotation (Fig. 19.77).

4. Comparison is made with the opposite side.

Talonavicular Joint

Muscle Energy Technique and Mobilization with Impulse Technique
Diagnosis
    Position: Navicular Internally Rotated or Externally Rotated
    Motion Restriction: Internal or External Rotation of the Navicular

1. Patient and operator positions the same as for the diagnostic procedure.

2. With the navicular externally rotated, the operator's distal hand internally rotates the navicular against the resistant barrier (Fig. 19.76). Patient is instructed to invert the foot against resistance for 3 to 5 seconds and repeat three to five times.

3. After each muscle effort, the new barrier is engaged.

4. With the navicular internally rotated, the distal hand externally rotates the navicular to the resistant barrier. The patient is instructed to exert the foot against resistance for 3 to 5 seconds and three to five repetitions (Fig. 19.77).

5. Operator engages new barrier after each patient effort.

6. A mobilization with impulse thrust activating force can be substituted for the muscle energy activity by mobilizing the distal hand against the proximal.

7. Retest.

Figure 19.76.

Figure 19.77.

Cuneiform Bones (Intertarsal Joints)

Diagnosis: Cuneiform Dysfunction

1. Patient supine on table with operator standing at foot facing cephalad.

2. Each cuneiform is grasped between the thumb and index finger. While stabilizing one cuneiform, the other is tested for dorsi-to-plantar joint play movement (Fig. 19.78).

3. With the thumbs on the dorsum of the cuneiforms and the fingers of both hands on the plantar surface of the foot, a plantar force is exerted through the thumbs ascertaining the presence or absence of springing movement.

4. Both sides are tested for comparison.

5. Operator can perform a joint play treatment procedure by grasping cuneiform and moving the adjacent one in a dorsal-to-plantar joint play direction.

Cuneiform Bones (Intertarsal Joints)

Muscle Energy Technique

Diagnosis
Position: Depression of Cuneiforms
Motion Restriction: Dorsal Arching of the Cuneiforms

1. Patient supine on table with operator standing at foot facing cephalad.

2. Operator's proximal hand stabilizes the hind foot with the thumb against the plantar surface of the dysfunctional cuneiform exerting a dorsal force.

3. Operator's distal hand stabilizes the forefoot with the hypothenar eminence over the dorsal aspect of the metatarsal shafts.

4. The barrier is engaged by plantar flexing the forefoot (Fig. 19.79).

5. Patient is instructed to perform a muscle effort of lifting the toes cephalad against equal and opposite resistance for 3 to 5 seconds and three to five repetitions (Fig. 19.80).

6. A new barrier is engaged after each patient effort.

7. Retest.

Note: In the presence of dysfunction of the first cuneiform to the navicular, the muscle energy and mobilization with impulse technique of the navicular on the talus can be modified by the proximal hand grasping the navicular and the distal hand the first cuneiform.

Figure 19.79.

Figure 19.78.

Figure 19.80.

Tarsometatarsal Joints

Joint Play

Diagnosis: Restoration of Dorsal-to-Plantar Glide

1. Patient supine with operator standing at foot of table.
2. Operator's two thumbs are on the plantar surface of adjacent metatarsal bases with the fingers on the dorsal side of the proximal metatarsal shafts.
3. Operator holds one metatarsal while the other is moved in a dorsal-to-plantar glide fashion (Fig. 19.81).
4. If restriction is noted, a mobilizing without impulse joint play maneuver is performed enhancing gliding movement between the bases of the metatarsal bones and the tarsometatarsal articulations.
5. Each metatarsal base and shaft are evaluated and treated sequentially.
6. Comparison is made with the opposite side for symmetry.

Tarsometatarsal Joints

Joint Play

Diagnosis: Evaluation and restoration of medial and lateral rotations

1. Patient supine with operator standing at foot of table.
2. Operator's proximal hand stabilizes the cuneiform bones through the web of the thumb and index finger.
3. Operator's distal hand dorsiflexes forefoot and introduces eversion of the forefoot (Fig. 19.82) and inversion of the forefoot (Fig. 19.83).
4. Comparison of eversion and inversion of each foot is made.
5. In the presence of restriction in either direction, a mobilizing with impulse joint play maneuver is performed against the resistant barrier.
6. Retest.

Figure 19.82.

Figure 19.81.

Figure 19.83.

Metatarsal Heads

Joint Play

Diagnosis: Restriction of Joint Play at Metatarsal Heads

1. Patient supine with operator standing at end of table.

2. Operator's medial hand grasps the shaft of the second metatarsal while the lateral hand grasps the shaft of the third metatarsal (Fig. 19.84).

3. While stabilizing the second metatarsal, operator's lateral hand dorsi and plantar moves the metatarsal head seeking resistance to motion and provides joint play mobilization if restricted. Comparison is made with the opposite side.

4. Operator's medial hand holds the shaft of the second metatarsal and the lateral hand holds the shaft of the third metatarsal. The lateral hand is rotated medially and laterally testing for rotary capacity of the metatarsal heads. Comparison is made with the opposite side. Joint play rotary mobilization is performed in the presence of restricted motion.

5. Sequentially the fourth metatarsal is moved on the third, the fifth metatarsal is moved on the fourth, and the first metatarsal is moved on the second in similar fashion.

Metatarsophalangeal Joints and the Interphalangeal Joints

Motion Testing and Joint Play
Example: First Metatarsophalangeal Joint

1. Patient supine with operator standing at foot of table.

2. Operator stabilizes proximal bone (first metatarsal) with thumb and fingers.

3. Operator grasps distal bone (proximal phalanx of the first toe).

4. Flexion–extension, anterior–posterior glide, medial and lateral rotation, medial and lateral tilt are performed, testing for resistance to movement (Fig. 19.85).

5. Comparison is made with the opposite side.

6. Sequential joint play motions are performed to restore all joint play movements.

7. All other interphalangeal joints can be treated in similar fashion by stabilizing the proximal bone and moving the distal upon it.

Figure 19.84.

Figure 19.85.

LOWER LIMB TENSION TESTS

As with the upper extremity, the lower extremity has peripheral nerves encased in connective tissue, and the nerves need mobility within the covering connective tissue. The reader is encouraged to study the system of neural tension testing and neural and dural mobilization through the work of Butler.

The primary lower extremity tests are really variations of the interpretation of straight leg raising. There are tests using a bias for the femoral nerves as well, but those shown here have been most helpful diagnostically and therapeutically for this author. They are helpful in differentiating pain in the lower extremity coming from neural, muscular, or joint problems. As in many problems of the musculoskeletal system, they are multifactorial. The lower limb tension test maneuvers can be used therapeutically as they are

in the upper extremities. It has been observed that the lower limb dural mobilizing maneuvers can profoundly influence the cranial dura when used with traditional cranial technique.

Lower Limb Tension Test (Sciatic Bias)

1. Patient supine on the table with operator standing on side to be tested.

2. Operator grasps lower leg at the ankle and stabilizes the thigh into knee extension (Fig. 19.86).

3. Operator raises leg sensing for tension and the provocation of pain (Fig. 19.87). The most common area of pain is in the posterior thigh about two thirds down from the hip joint and relates to tightness of the hamstring muscles. The pain from the

Figure 19.86.

Figure 19.87.

neural system is more to the lateral aspect of the knee.

4. Operator increases the tension by adducting and internally rotating the extended leg (Fig. 19.88).

5. Operator can use dorsiflexion of the foot on the ankle for additional neural and dural tension (Fig. 19.89).

6. When using these maneuvers for dural and neural mobilizations, it is imperative to use an on and off of the tension at the restrictive barrier. Do not use a sustained application of force.

CONCLUSION

The foot of the lower extremity is the bottom block of the postural structural model. Intrinsic dysfunction within the foot or dysfunction secondary to other dysfunctions within the lower extremity can influence the biomechanical function of the total musculoskeletal system. Lower extremity joint function is essential for symmetric gait. The sole of the foot is a sense organ for sensory motor balance. Evaluation and restoration of function to the foot and lower extremity are essential components of the treatment of patients with musculoskeletal problems.

SUGGESTED READINGS

Butler DS. *Mobilization of the nervous system.* Melbourne: Churchill Livingstone, 1991.

Kaltenborn FM. *Manuelle Therapie der Extremitatengelenke.* Oslo: Norlis Bokhandel, 1976.

Mennell J McM. *Foot pain.* Boston: Little, Brown and Company, 1964.

Mennell J McM. *Joint pain.* Boston: Little, Brown and Company, 1964.

Mennell J McM. *The musculoskeletal system: differential diagnosis from symptoms and physical signs.* Gaithersburg, MD: Aspen Publishers, 1992.

Figure 19.88.

Figure 19.89.

Section III

CLINICAL INTEGRATION
AND CORRELATION

20 EXERCISE PRINCIPLES AND PRESCRIPTIONS

Exercise has a long history in the healing arts. Exercise has been used for the maintenance of general health and for the prevention of disease by both Eastern and Western cultures. The ancient Greeks originated the Olympic movement to honor those with exceptional athletic skills. Modern Olympians continue that tradition, spending enormous time and energy enhancing their level of expertise and maximizing their performance potential.

Today there is an ever-increasing interest in exercise and sporting activities. There continues to be an increase in the numbers of health spas, athletic centers, and clubs dedicated to the principle that exercise is a fundamental good that is not only essential for one's health but is also an enjoyable leisure past time.

Health professionals of many disciplines, particularly physical therapists, have increasingly used exercise. William's flexion exercises and Mackenzie's extension program have been widely used for lower back pain. There is more to William's program than flexion and more to Mackenzie's program than extension, but these systems, and many similar programs, are designed to enhance the strength and flexibility in the patient who suffers from lower back pain from a variety of causes. In the management of lower back pain, a great emphasis has been placed on the principle of core stability. Recent work from Australia has demonstrated the significant role of the transversus abdominus muscle contraction in core stability.

There are many texts on procedures for manual muscle testing, stretching, and strengthening. More recently, video series on the topic have been developed, for health professionals and laypersons, to assist in the maintenance of health and as part of therapeutic treatment plan.

Numerous diagnostic and therapeutic exercise equipment systems have been developed and are currently on the market. This equipment objectively measures range of motion and muscle strength in various physical activities. Some machines have been developed to exercise specific areas of the body and related muscle groups, whereas other equipment is designed for the maintenance of aerobic capacity and restoration of fitness after bouts of injury or disease.

Despite all of the activities described, it has been this author's observation that many health professionals, in a variety of disciplines, have limited knowledge and understanding of how to prescribe exercises that are appropriate for their patients. While there are a number of programs that have generic value, each patient is an individual and requires an exercise program specific for his or her problem. The practitioner needs the skill to identify problems of the patient's neuromusculoskeletal system and to prescribe appropriate exercises just as they prescribe appropriate medication, manual medicine, or surgical intervention. The following principles and procedures are those that this author has found effective and are the results of the contributions of numerous authors and colleagues.

PRINCIPLES OF MUSCLE IMBALANCE

As stated in Chapter 1, the goal of manipulation is to restore maximal, pain-free movement of the musculoskeletal system in postural balance. When the manipulative intervention has achieved maximum mobility, the question remains, how is it maintained? The obvious answer is an appropriate exercise program the patient can perform that maintains the functional capacity of the musculoskeletal system within the constraints of the available anatomy. The manual medicine practitioner is limited by the available anatomy, which may be altered by genetic development, single or repetitive trauma, and surgical intervention. Despite the altered anatomy and pathology present, it is surprising and satisfying to both the practitioner and the patient to see the amount of functional capacity that can be restored and maintained by an appropriate exercise program.

An appropriate exercise prescription provides the patient with the ability, and responsibility, to maintain a high level of neuromusculoskeletal health. It is important that the patient understands and commits to perform the necessary exercise program. While being as comprehensive as necessary, it should be simple and be performed without depending on specialized equipment or facilities. Obviously, if appropriate equipment is available, its use can be beneficial. Of utmost importance is that patients understand that following a disabling musculoskeletal condition, it is imperative to continue an active exercise program for the rest of their lives.

PRINCIPLES OF MOTOR CONTROL

Muscle Pathology

Functional pathology of muscle results from a perturbation of a highly complex neurologic control system. A disturbance of musculoskeletal function initiates a series of events beginning with stimulation to mechanoreceptors and nociceptors resulting in afferent neural activity initiating a variety of reflexes at the cord, brainstem, and cortical levels. The final common pathway is the alpha motor neuron that stimulates the muscle fiber to contract, and through the gamma system, the muscle spindle to adapt, resulting in alteration in muscle tone. Chronic articular or a muscle dysfunction feeds the afferent loop with more nociception and abnormal mechanoreceptor information, perpetuating ongoing aberrant muscle tone. Interruption and reprogramming of this vicious cycle contribute to improvement of overall muscle tone and maintenance of balance.

Morphology

The work of Wyke and colleagues has led to an increased appreciation of the morphology and functional characteristics of articular receptor systems.

Receptors

There are four different types of receptors (Table. 20.1). These receptors are found in joint capsules, ligaments, and articular fat pads. They have different sizes, shapes, clusters, and nerve fibers that range from small unmyelinated fibers to very small, small, medium, and large myelinated fibers. Their different behaviors include responses to static and dynamic change, with low or high thresholds, and range from rapidly adapting to slow adapting to nonadapting. In simplistic terms, this system provides the central nervous system information on the three-dimensional position of joints and the rate of change in relationship. This articular information, combining impulses from muscle spindles and Golgi tendon organs, reporting on muscle length and tension, is transmitted to the spinal cord for central processing. Afferent fibers from nociceptors and mechanoreceptors enter the dorsal horn where numerous neuronal reflexes are initiated and mediated.

Neurons

There are numerous combinations of neuronal connections acting on the motor neuron of the final common pathway. Divergence describes the process of a single neuron synapsing with several target end organs, either directly or through interneurons. Convergence describes the process where a motor neuron receives and summates inputs from a variety of fibers, including afferents, interneurons, and descending fibers from other spinal and supraspinal regions. Gating is the process of altering the output from the motor neuron via inhibitory interneurons or inhibiting neurons from descending control signals. Occasionally, the gate can be initiated by presynaptic inhibition, an example is the descending inhibitory control signals acting on the presynaptic terminals of afferent fibers.

Four Components of the Motor System

There are four hierarchically organized components of the motor system. From above downward they include the premotor cortical regions, the motor cortex, the brainstem, and the spinal cord. It is through the spinal cord that many activities of the motor system are initiated and maintained. The cord is programmed to respond to peripheral and central stimulations. The spinal cord has the capacity to learn. Preprogrammed normal behavior can be replaced by abnormal response if the cord has repetitive aberrant stimulation. This process can be viewed as both good and bad, because the cord that learns to perpetuate abnormal mechanical behavior through persistence of structural and functional pathology can be reprogrammed to activity that is more normal through appropriate manual medicine and exercise procedures.

All four components of the motor system are functionally interrelated. A stimulus from the periphery initiates afferent input to segmental spinal reflexes and carries information centrally to the brainstem and cortical areas. The cord level information proceeds through efferent spinal pathways to muscle groups resulting in force generation to displace a load. Response to this activity returns by afferent loops, joining with the original afferent stimulation, to continue information processing at the cord level. The initial afferent input stimulates cortical and brainstem levels

Table 20.1.
Four Types of Articular Receptors

Shape	Nerve	Characteristic
1. Globular	Small myelinated	Static and dynamic mechanoreceptors
2. Conical	Large myelinated	Dynamic mechanoreceptor
3. Fusiform	Medium myelinated	Mechanoreceptor
4. Plexus	Unmyelinated	Nociceptor

thus initiating descending pathways from the brainstem and the motor cortex. These complex descending pathways are modulated through the basal ganglion and cerebellar systems thereby changing brainstem activity, which descends through the cord, modulates cord reflexes, and ultimately influences muscle activity.

Spinal Cord. The spinal cord has intricate neuronal interconnections through long and short propriospinal pathways that influence motor neuron pools to the muscles of the axial skeleton and the extremities. The neuronal pools for the axial muscles are oriented medially, those for the extremities more laterally, with the proximal limb being central and the distal limb more lateral. These neuronal pathways are both ipsilateral and contralateral and course up and down through several levels of the spinal cord.

Brainstem Pathways. There are two groups of descending brainstem pathways. The first is the ventral medial group, which includes the reticulospinal, the vestibulospinal, and the tectospinal tracts. The dorsolateral pathways are primarily those related to the red nucleus. The rubrospinal tract crosses centrally and descends in the contralateral dorsolateral funiculus of the cord. These descending pathways provide much of the information for central control of cord and spinal column activity.

Cortical Pathways. The descending cortical pathways include the crossed and uncrossed systems. The lateral cortical spinal tract crosses in the pyramidal desiccation and terminates in the lateral aspect of the cord. This system has considerable input to the rubrospinal tracts of the brainstem. The ventral cortical spinal tract is uncrossed and terminates more centrally in the ventral portion of the cord. Influence from this tract occurs through the ventral medial brainstem pathways. Most cortical influence on cord activity occurs through the brainstem pathways rather than directly at cord level. The information descending from the cortex and brainstem is designed to initiate muscle action and modulate the action on the basis of response. Much of the descending information is inhibitory to the programmed cord response so that the resultant action is controlled, smooth, and appropriate for the desired result.

Alpha Motor Neuron. Stimulation to the alpha motor neuron, the final common pathway, results in muscle activity. The resultant action is reported through a complex feedback system to determine both muscle length and muscle tension. Control of muscle length is primarily determined by the response of the muscle spindle. When the muscle is stretched, increasing discharge from the spindle reports to the cord that the muscle is lengthening. When the muscle contracts with shortening of the extrafusal fibers, there is initial momentary electrical silence from the spindle, followed by

rapid stimulation to the spindle to shorten in response to the shortening of the extrafusal fibers. The spindle has both nuclear bag and nuclear chain fibers, each having their own afferent control. The spindle responds to change in static length as well as dynamically in the rate of change of length. Control of muscle tension is primarily mediated through the Golgi tendon apparatus. While the muscle spindles are parallel to the extrafusal fibers, the Golgi tendon organs are in series. The Golgi tendon organ responds to muscle stretch and contraction. It discharges most actively during muscle contraction and initiates an inhibitory reflex arc preventing overload of the muscle and the musculotendinous junction.

The alpha motor neuron is controlled by central demand and through feedback loops. The central control of the gamma motor neuron establishes the length of the muscle spindle and sets the anticipated activity of the positive stimulation to the alpha motor neuron. After the alpha motor neuron is stimulated, changes in muscle length and tension occur. The spindle compares the response to the anticipated activity. Feedback loops to the spinal cord modulate the continued central control of the alpha motor neuron. Differences between anticipated and actual change result in appropriate muscle length and tension through the activity. Feedback loops from the spindle report difference in length, while the Golgi tendon organ reports difference in force. Feedback loops can be either excitatory or inhibitory to the alpha motor neuron so that the final action of muscle is appropriate.

Another Reflex Pathway

Another basic reflex pathway governs reciprocal innervation and inhibition. Stimulation to both limb flexor and extensor muscles is called cocontraction and stabilizes a joint and restricts its movement. During joint flexion, the flexor contracts, and by reciprocal inhibition, the extensor muscle group relaxes, allowing controlled flexion activity. The reverse is true for extension: The extensor contracts and the flexor is inhibited and relaxes. This reciprocal inhibition occurs contralaterally and ipsilaterally. When the ipsilateral flexor contracts, there is reflex inhibition of the contralateral flexor. The harder a muscle contracts, the more it inhibits its antagonist. This phenomenon occurs ipsilaterally and contralaterally. Through this reflex pathway, facilitated muscle contracts and is maintained in a shortened position, resulting in inhibition of its antagonist, which becomes weakened.

Muscle Fiber Type

Fiber type, either slow or fast twitch, characterizes muscles. Slow-twitch muscle uses oxidative metabolism and has a high capillary density giving it its characteristic red color. The twitch speed is slow and the function of these muscles is described as tonic or postural. Muscles that have high-density slow-twitch fibers react to functional disturbance by shortening and tightening. Fast-twitch fibers use a glycolytic metabolic pathway, fatigue rapidly, have low capillary density, and a white color. Muscles of this type are phasic in function and react to disturbance by weakening. All muscles have a mixture of slow- and fast-twitch fibers, but some muscles have more of the slow-twitch fibers whereas others have more of the fast-twitch variety. Muscles with primary postural or tonic function in the pelvic and hip regions include the hamstrings, iliopsoas, rectus femoris, tensor fascia lata, thigh adductors, and piriformis. Phasic muscles in the pelvic and hip region include the vastus medialis and lateralis of the anterior thigh and the gluteus medius, maximus, and minimus. In the trunk, the postural, tonic muscles are the erector spinae group, primarily in the lumbar and cervical regions, the quadratus lumborum, and the scalenes. The phasic muscles of the trunk are the erector spinae muscles in the mid-thoracic region. In the lower extremity, the gastrocnemius and soleus muscles are tonic and the tibialis anterior and peroneal muscles are phasic. In the shoulder girdle, the postural, tonic muscles are the pectoralis major, levator scapulae, upper trapezius, and biceps brachii. The phasic muscles are the rhomboids, lower trapezius, and triceps brachii. An understanding of muscle function, either phasic or tonic, is important for the prescription of an appropriate exercise program.

THEORETIC CAUSES OF MUSCLE IMBALANCE

Malregulation of the Central Nervous System

Muscle imbalance consists of shortening and tightening of muscle groups (usually the tonic muscles), weakness of certain muscle groups (usually the phasic muscles), and loss of control of integrated muscle function. Alteration in length, strength, and motor control can occur from a variety of causes. Muscle balance is continually adapting the body's posture to gravity. Faulty posture results in alteration of the center of gravity, which initiates mechanical responses requiring muscle adaptation. Change in a joint's mechanical behavior causes neuroreflexive alteration in muscle function through aberrant afferent mechanoreceptor stimulation of articular reflexes. Long-term activation of abnormal articular reflexes causes change in cord memory from a normal to an abnormal adaptive program, resulting in muscle imbalance. Muscle imbalance results from malregulation by the central nervous system, either at the cord level or higher centers, from altered agonist and antagonist reactions and responses to dysfunction of the limbic system. Muscle balance is altered in response to noxious stimuli through central-mediated pathways and

segmental reflexes. Central mediation through the lateral reticular system alters activity of gamma motor neurons resulting in hyperreflexia and altered time-activation sequences of muscle action. At a segmental level, nociception facilitates alpha motor neurons to the flexors in the limbs and to the extensors in the neck and trunk. Muscle balance responds to the physical demands placed on the muscle. Depending on its metabolic pathway, muscle responds to fatigue in different ways. Tonic muscles fatigue more slowly than phasic muscles. In the presence of altered movement patterns through chronic overuse, some muscles will become tight and abnormal muscle pattern habits result. It is for this reason that motor programming through appropriate exercise is so important. Psychological factors can influence muscle balance and tone. Who is not aware of the tightness and fatigue that result when we are "uptight"? Muscle imbalance is clearly a multifactorial problem and can be highly complex. In simplistic terms, the result of muscle imbalance is that tight muscles become tighter, weak muscles become weaker, and motor control becomes more asymmetric. Each of these factors needs to be addressed in an exercise program.

Scientific-Clinical Theory of Janda

Much of the following material is based on the work of the late Professor Vladimir Janda, a rehabilitation specialist and previous chairperson of Rehabilitation Medicine at the University of Charles, Prague, Czech Republic, who researched normal and abnormal muscle function at the basic science and clinical levels. He determined that muscle dysfunction is not a random occurrence, but that muscles respond in characteristic patterns.

Pseudoparesis. Postural/tonic muscles respond to dysfunction by facilitation, hypertonicity, and shortening. Dynamic/phasic muscles respond to dysfunction by inhibition, hypotonicity, and weakness. Janda describes this weakness as "pseudoparesis." The weakness of the muscle is due to inhibition rather than intrinsic weakness. There are multiple patterns of muscle response to dysfunction in which certain muscles become inhibited and weak, whereas others become facilitated and tight. In the hip region, the weak muscles are the gluteus medius and maximus and the facilitated tight muscles are the iliopsoas, rectus femoris, piriformis, adductors, and tensor fascia lata. In shoulder dysfunction, the weak muscles are the supraspinatus, deltoid, infraspinatus, rhomboids, lower trapezius, and serratus anterior and the facilitated, tight muscles are the levator scapula, upper trapezius, and pectorals.

Muscle Firing Patterns. Muscle dysfunction is characterized by facilitation and inhibition as well as by the manner in which muscles sequentially fire. Altered muscle firing pattern shows delay in activation

Figure 20.1.
a: Hip extension firing pattern beginning position. **b:** Hip extension firing pattern during patient muscle contraction.

and in the amplitude of the electromyographic activity of the dynamic/phasic muscles. Continued exercise in the presence of abnormal muscle firing sequence perpetuates hypertonicity, tightness, and shortening of the tonic muscles with continued and progressive inhibition of the phasic muscles. Janda's research work has identified the normal and abnormal muscle firing patterns in the movement patterns of hip extension, hip abduction, and shoulder abduction. He reported the normal firing pattern of prone hip extension as hamstrings, gluteus maximus, contralateral lower lumbar erector spinae, and ipsilateral lower lumbar erector spinae. Other studies have failed to replicate his firing sequence but have shown that the pathology increases as asymmetry in the pattern and firing delays of the gluteus maximus increase. The most common alteration of this normal pattern is failure of activation and weakness of the gluteus maximus with substitution by the hamstrings and erector spinae musculature, particularly in the upper lumbar and lower thoracic regions (Fig. 20.1).

The muscle firing sequence for hip abduction in the side-lying posture is gluteus medius, tensor fascia lata, ipsilateral quadratus lumborum, and erector spinae. The most common substitution pattern is weakness of the gluteus medius with early firing of the tensor fascia lata or the quadratus lumborum. Early firing of the tensor fascia lata results in internal rotation and flexion of the hip during hip abduction. The worst scenario is that the motion is initiated by the firing of the quadratus lumborum (Fig. 20.2).

Figure 20.2.
a: Hip abduction firing pattern beginning position. **b:** Hip abduction firing pattern during patient muscle contraction.

The firing sequence for shoulder abduction while seated is supraspinatus, deltoid, infraspinatus, mid and lower trapezius, and contralateral quadratus lumborum muscles. The most common substitution pattern is for shoulder elevation by the levator scapulae and upper trapezius and early firing of the quadratus lumborum, even on the ipsilateral side (Fig. 20.3).

Muscle Imbalance Syndromes. Janda also described three different syndromes resulting from muscle imbalance. They are the lower crossed syndrome in the pelvic girdle, the upper crossed syndrome in the shoulder girdle, and the layer syndrome from caudad to cranial. The upper and lower cross syndromes will be described subsequently. The layer syndrome is characterized by alternate bands of muscle tightness and weakness on the dorsal surface of the body beginning from below upward (Fig. 20.4). The layer syndrome is usually characterized by tightness of the gastrocnemius and soleus muscles, tightness of the hamstrings, weakness of the glutei and the lower lumbar erector spinae, tightness of the lower thoracic and upper lumbar erector spinae, weakness of the rhomboids and lower trapezius, and tightness of the upper trapezius and levator scapulae. Another feature of the layer syndrome is "banding" in erector spinae musculature. With close observation, the examiner can identify sequential areas of hypertonicity and inhibition in various groups of the erector spinae muscle mass, particularly the longissimus. These reflect themselves as layers of fullness and small divots when observing tangentially along the erector spinae mass (Fig. 20.5).

PRINCIPLES IN TREATMENT OF MUSCLE IMBALANCES

In treating muscle imbalances, the fundamental principles are to restore length, strength, and control of muscle function. Many exercise systems address length and strength, but few address the issues of motor control. A successful exercise program restores nervous system control of muscle function as much as possible. Of fundamental concern is the sequence of muscle firing. To achieve the result, the most useful sequence is as follows:

1. Sensory motor balance training;
2. Stretching of short, tight, hypertonic muscle to symmetry;
3. Strengthening (retraining) of inhibited weak muscles to balance; and
4. Aerobic conditioning.

GOALS OF TREATMENT OF MUSCLE IMBALANCES

In manual medicine practice, the goal for an exercise program is to maintain the enhanced functional capacity of the musculoskeletal system that has been achieved by appropriate manual medicine intervention. Appropriate exercise assists the patient in assuming control of his or her musculoskeletal system and its associated painful conditions. Improved muscle balance helps to protect the osteoarticular system and reduce the strain on joints and their capsules and ligaments. Appropriate muscle balance of agonist and

Figure 20.3.
a: Shoulder abduction firing pattern beginning position. **b:** Shoulder abduction firing pattern during patient muscle contraction.

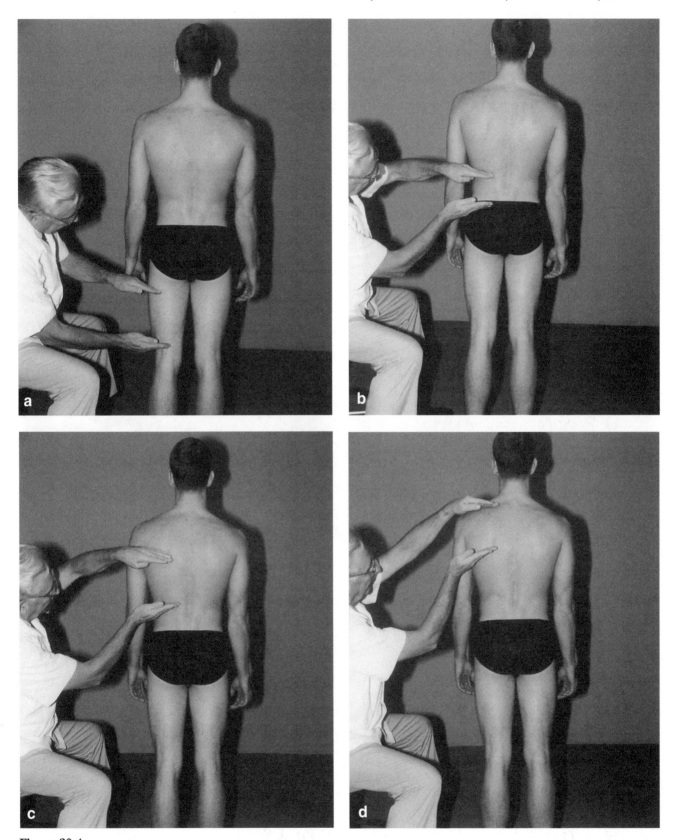

Figure 20.4.
a: Layer syndrome, hamstrings. **b:** Layer syndrome, lumbar spine. **c:** Layer syndrome, thoracolumbar spine. **d:** Layer syndrome, upper thoracic spine.

Figure 20.5.
Muscle banding.

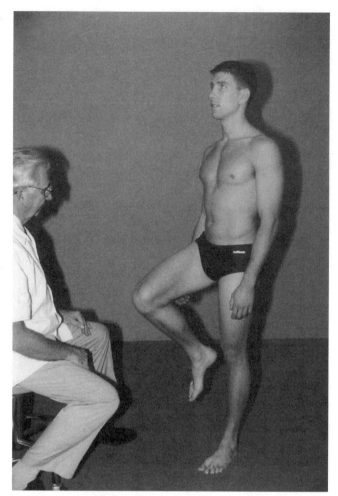

Figure 20.6.
Balance testing, level one.

antagonist provides shock absorption and prevents impact loading of joint surfaces. Lewit has noted that dysfunction of the musculoskeletal system appeared earlier than degenerative morphologic change. It is hypothesized that the establishment and maintenance of length and strength of the hip flexors and extensors might prevent degenerative hip joint disease.

SENSORY MOTOR BALANCE TRAINING

Sensory motor balance training helps restore symmetric muscle firing patterns for control of motor function. Restoration of normal muscle firing sequences provides an opportunity to successfully stretch hypertonic shortened muscle and to strengthen inhibited muscle.

Body balance is a complex function and is the result of three primary afferent systems. Our orientation in three-dimensional space results from the visual system, the vestibular system, and the proprioceptive input from the soles of the feet. The body adapts to loss of vision by enhanced proprioception from the extremities and greater dependence on the vestibular mechanism. The visual system compensates for reduced efficiency of proprioceptive input from contact with the ground by the soles of the feet.

Indications for Training

The first indication that a patient may need sensory motor balance training occurs during the screening and scanning examinations, particularly the function of the pelvic girdle. During the one-legged stork test, the patient stands on a single foot. If the patient is so unsteady that it is impossible to perform the test smoothly, an index of suspicion is high that the pa-

tient has deficit of proprioceptive sensitivity of the sole of the foot. Initial diagnostic testing includes asking the patient to stand in bare feet, first on one foot and then on the other to see if there is equal balance from right to left (Fig. 20.6). A second level of difficulty of this test is to ask the patient to stand on one leg with arms crossed (Fig. 20.7). This removes the balancing assistance of the upper trunk and extremities. A third level of difficulty is to ask the patient to stand on one leg with arms crossed and then close the eyes (Fig. 20.8). The removal of visual perception greatly increases the difficulty. Ideally, the patient should be able to symmetrically stand on one leg with arms crossed and eyes closed for 30 seconds.

Retraining

Sensory motor retraining should be done with bare feet on a carpeted surface. One of the primary goals is to stimulate the proprioceptors of the sole of the foot. One begins by practicing to shorten the foot. The "short foot" is obtained by attempting to grasp the

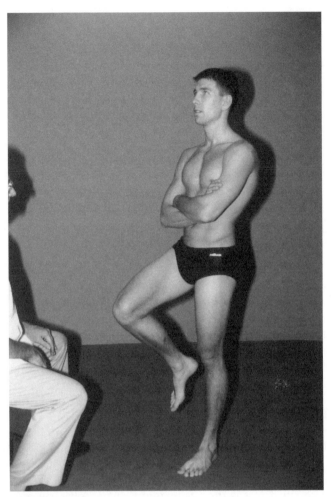

Figure 20.7.
Balance testing, level two.

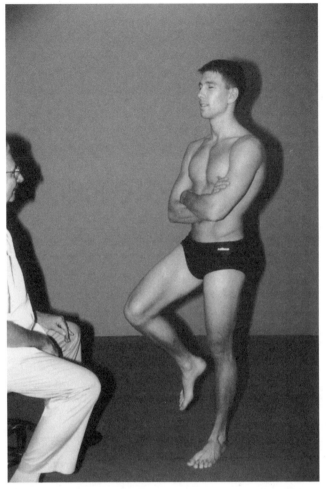

Figure 20.8.
Balance testing, level three.

floor with the sole of the foot without excessive curling of the toes. The shortened foot elevates the medial longitudinal arch and enhances the sensitivity of the sole of the foot. All exercises should be done with a shortened foot. A simple home program for sensory motor retraining is shown in Table. 20.2.

The goal of sensory motor balance training is the capacity to symmetrically stand on one leg with arms crossed and eyes closed for 30 seconds. The more severe the deficit, the more difficult it will be to achieve the goal. Right-to-left symmetry is the primary objective and the ultimate goal is to achieve the highest level of difficulty with arms crossed, eyes closed, and length of time. The presence of a neurologic deficit of a lower extremity, which frequently follows a lumbar radiculopathy, can make this exercise difficult. Even in the presence of a neurologic deficit, it is advisable to achieve the maximum possible functional capacity to assist in the restoration of more normal muscle firing pattern sequences.

EVALUATION AND TREATMENT OF THE LOWER QUARTER

The muscle imbalances of the lower extremity include facilitation, hypertonicity, and shortening of the iliopsoas, rectus femoris, tensor fascia lata, quadratus lumborum, short thigh adductors, piriformis, hamstrings, and lumbar erector spinae muscles. The dynamic muscles involved with inhibition, hypotonicity, and weakness are the gluteus maximus, medius, and minimus; rectus abdominus; external and internal obliques; peroneals; vastus medialis and lateralis; and tibialis anterior. Janda's lower crossed syndrome includes weakness of the gluteus maximus, tightness of the hip flexors, weak abdominals, short erector spinae, weak gluteus medius and minimus with short tensor fascia lata and quadratus lumborum, increased lumbar lordosis and anterior pelvic tilt with hypermobility of the lower lumbar levels, and altered functional activities, which include curling up and sitting up from supine and forward-bent postures.

Table 20.2.
Sensory Motor Examination and Retraining Program

DO ALL ACTIVITIES WITH BARE FEET

1. Sitting—practice shortening both feet
2. Standing—feet aligned with the hips, neutral pelvis, trunk erect, both knees slightly flexed, practice shortening both feet

DO THE FOLLOWING ACTIVITIES WITH A NEUTRAL PELVIS, ERECT TRUNK, AND SHORTENED FEET

1. Standing on one leg
   A. Eyes open, arms down
   B. Eyes open, arms crossed
   C. Eyes closed, arms down
   D. Eyes closed, arms crossed
2. Standing—feet aligned with the hips, practice slight squatting, keep heels on surface, gradually increase to semisquat (up to 90 degrees)
3. Standing—on one leg—practice squatting
   A. Eyes open, arms down
   B. Eyes open, arms crossed
   C. Eyes closed, arms down
   D. Eyes closed, arms crossed
4. Standing on a rocker board or rebounder
   A. Feet parallel about one foot apart, shift weight from side to side, bringing trunk over each foot
   B. One foot places a short step in front of the other, shift weight from back to front alternate feet
   C. Do both with arms crossed
   D. Do both with eyes closed and arms crossed
5. Standing on one foot on a rocker board or rebounder, repeat with arms crossed and then eyes closed
6. Walk on the floor/balance beam—place one foot directly in front of the other (heel to toe), done first with eyes open and then with eyes closed
7. Walk on the floor/balance beam—place one foot directly behind the other (toe to heel), done first with eyes open and then with eyes closed

SIX DIAGNOSTIC TESTS

Diagnosis of muscle imbalance and faulty postural control of the lower quarter uses six tests.

Test 1

The evaluation begins with three-dimensional assessment of pelvic control by the use of a pelvic clock maneuver in the supine position (Fig. 20.9). The examiner monitors the patient's anterosuperior iliac spine with thumb contact while the patient moves the pelvis from the 12-o'clock to 6-o'clock positions through a range of anterior and posterior pelvic tilts. In the presence of good pelvic control, the anterosuperior iliac spines stay symmetric from neutral to 12 o'clock and to 6 o'clock. In the presence of poor pelvic control, the anterosuperior iliac spine becomes more asymmetric at the 12-o'clock or 6-o'clock position. A common dysfunctional pattern is to find that the right anterosuperior iliac spine does not proceed as far

cephalically as the left at 12 o'clock and that the left anterosuperior iliac spine does not travel as far caudally as the right at 6 o'clock. This is followed by assessment of the anterosuperior iliac spine as the pelvis is moved from 3 o'clock to 9 o'clock. This maneuver frequently reproduces lower back pain. Good pelvic control finds that the pelvis rolls symmetrically across the horizontal plane from 3 to 9 o'clock and from 9 to 3 o'clock. Poor trunk control is identified when there is elevation of one anterosuperior iliac spine by hip hiking and substitution by lumbar spine extension.

Test 2

The second test is to evaluate passive hip abduction and external rotation in the supine position (Fig. 20.10). The examiner places the thumbs under the anterosuperior iliac spines and asks the patient to do a posterior pelvic tilt in the 12-o'clock-position maneuver. While holding the posterior pelvic tilt, the patient is asked to drop the knees apart. Loss of control in maintaining the posterior pelvic tilt is indicative of muscle imbalance, particularly tightness of the short hip abductors. One of the most common patterns that is seen is that the right anterosuperior iliac spine cannot be maintained in a cephalic direction during hip abduction and external rotation and travels in a caudad direction during the maneuver. This muscle imbalance is commonly seen in pubis dysfunction.

Test 3

The third test is the performance of a pelvic tilt and heel slide in the supine position (Fig. 20.11). The patient is asked to lie supine with the knees flexed, maintain a posterior pelvic tilt at the 12-o'clock position, slowly extend first one leg and then the other, ascertaining if it is possible to maintain a posterior pelvic tilt during eccentric lengthening of the iliopsoas. In the presence of a tight iliopsoas muscle, the patient is unable to maintain the lumbar spine flat on the examining table. This test also assesses the strength of the abdominal musculature in a lengthened position. A second variation of this test has the patient maintain a neutral lumbar lordosis by voluntary contraction of the transversus abduminus muscle and then eccentrically lengthen the iliopsoas on each side.

Test 4

The fourth test is active trunk rotation in the supine position (Fig. 20.12). With the knees and hips flexed, the patient is asked to maintain the knees and feet together and drop the knees first to one side then the other. With the trunk fully rotated, the patient is asked to return the knees to the midline by the use of abdominal control and not hip rotation. The patient is asked to bring each of the spinal segments to the table from above downward without any arching of the lower thoracic and lum-

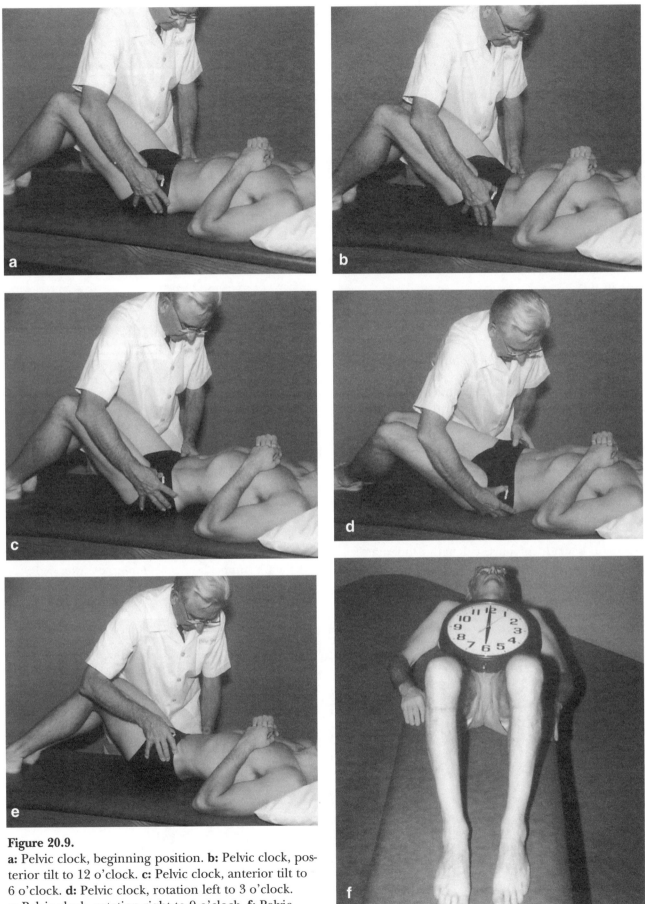

Figure 20.9.
a: Pelvic clock, beginning position. **b:** Pelvic clock, posterior tilt to 12 o'clock. **c:** Pelvic clock, anterior tilt to 6 o'clock. **d:** Pelvic clock, rotation left to 3 o'clock. **e:** Pelvic clock, rotation right to 9 o'clock. **f:** Pelvic clock, body orientation.

Figure 20.10.
Hip abduction, external rotation holding 12-o'clock position.

bar spines. This test assesses the control of the abdominal obliques and short deep lumbar musculature. Loss of this lumbar spine segmental control is frequently associated with nonneutral lumbar spine dysfunctions and may cause exacerbation of lower back pain.

Tests 5 and 6

The fifth and sixth tests are the muscle firing pattern sequences of hip extension and hip abduction previously described.

MUSCLE ASSESSMENT

Assessment is made of muscle length, and manual stretching followed by self-stretches at home treats shortness and tightness. The commonly tight muscles

Figure 20.11.
a: Pelvic tilt and heel slide, beginning position. **b:** Patient slides heel while holding 12-o'clock position.

Figure 20.12.
a: Active trunk rotation right. **b:** Active trunk rotation left.

can be treated by a sustained stretch in the test position for 20 to 30 seconds with two or three repetitions. A second process can be postisometric relaxation. A 5 to 7 second muscle contraction against resistance is followed by a slow sustained stretch to engage a new motion barrier. Manual stretches are followed by self-stretches using a 20 to 30 second sustained hold with two or three repetitions or a series of 5 to 7 second isometric contractions repeated three to five times. Test position, manual stretching, and self-stretches for the lower quarter are shown in Figs. 20.13 through 20.28. After short and tight muscles are stretched, muscles that are inhibited can undergo retraining. Lower quadrant retraining exercises are found in Figs. 20.29 through 20.40. As in all manual medicine procedures, following assessment, stretching, and strengthening, reevaluation of faulty movement patterns of the lower quadrant is done.

Figure 20.13a.
Psoas Muscle
Length test and manual stretch position supine
Modified Thomas position
1. Patient supine with buttocks at the end of the table and with operator standing at side.
2. Patient holds leg not being tested in a flexed position.
3. Operator extends hip of leg being tested. The back of the thigh should contact the table. If not, psoas shortening is present.
4. To stretch shortness and tightness, operator resists a 5 to 7 second contraction of hip flexion for five to seven repetitions, with the operator increasing hip extension after each effort.

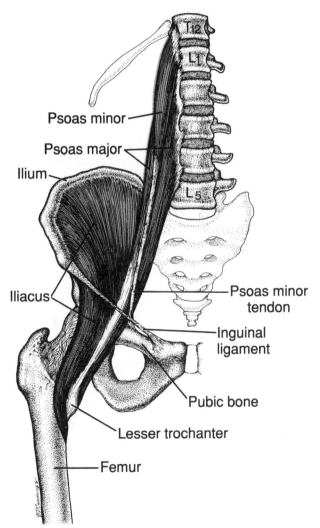

Figure 20.13b.
Attachments of the right psoas major, psoas minor, and iliacus muscles. The psoas major crosses many articulations including T12, the lumbar spine and the lumbosacral, sacroiliac, and hip joints. It does not attach to L5. The psoas minor does the same, except that it does *not* cross the hip joint. The iliacus, on the other hand, crosses only the hip joint.

Figure 20.13c.

Psoas Muscle

Self-stretch position kneeling

1. Patient kneels and internally rotates femur on the side to be stretched with the opposite hip and knee flexed to 90 degrees.
2. Patient places hand on the buttock, voluntarily contracts the gluteus maximus, flattens the stomach, and maintains a 12-o'clock posterior pelvic tilt.
3. Patient maintains trunk in an upright position, uses the opposite leg to pull the body forward, leading with the involved hip and maintaining contraction of the gluteal muscles throughout the stretch that is felt in the front of the hip and thigh.
4. Patient performs a series of contract–relax stretches for 1 to 2 minutes or a sustained 30-second stretch repeated two or three times. The opposite side should be stretched in the same manner to achieve symmetric balance.

Figure 20.14a.

Rectus Femoris Muscle

Supine length test and manual stretch position.

Modified Thomas position

1. Patient supine with buttocks on end of table and operator standing at end of table.
2. Patient holds leg not being tested in a flexed position with the thigh of the tested leg on the table.
3. Operator assesses flexion at the knee. If less than 90 degrees, rectus femoris shortness is present.
4. Operator treats shortness and tightness by resisting a 5 to 7 second contraction of knee extension, for five to seven repetitions, with the operator increasing knee flexion after each patient effort.

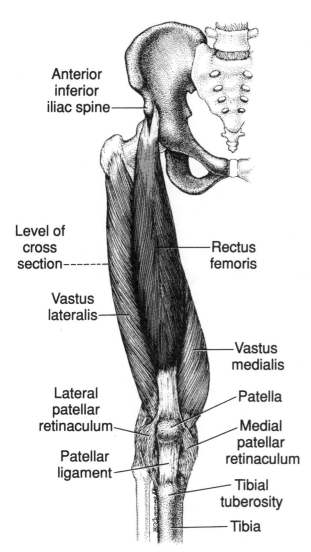

Figure 20.14b.
Rectus femoris muscle
Attachments (front view) of the right rectus femoris muscle in relation to the vastus lateralis and vastus medialis muscles.

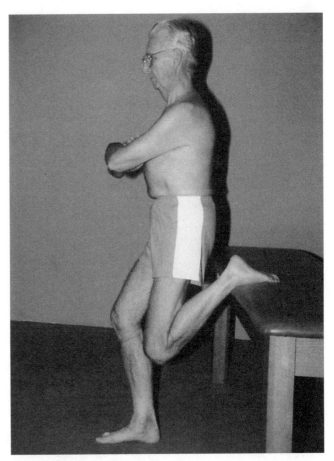

Figure 20.14c.
Rectus Femoris Muscle
Self-stretch standing
1. Patient stands with foot of leg to be stretched on a table or chair with the knee flexed.
2. Patient contracts abdominal and gluteal muscles in the 12-o'clock position. If stretch is felt in the anterior thigh, maintain for 10 to 15 seconds and repeat three times.
3. As length increases, additional stretch is obtained by flexing the opposite knee. Stretch is felt in the anterior thigh.
4. This is repeated on the opposite side for symmetric muscle balance.
5. A dual outcome results with stretching of one side, while strengthening on the side of active knee flexion.

Psoas and Rectus Femoris Muscles Prone Position

The prone position has the advantage of maintaining better control of the lumbar spine in the neutral position and avoiding the potential stress on the lumbar spine by the Thomas position.

Figure 20.16.

Psoas Muscle

Length test and manual stretch position prone

1. Patient and operator in the same position as that for testing rectus femoris muscle.
2. Operator lifts patient's leg with knee flexed while blocking pelvic motion at the ischial tuberosity until engaging barrier. Normally the knee can be lifted 6 in. (15.24 cm) off the table. If less, tightness and shortness of the psoas are present.
3. In the presence of shortness and tightness, operator resists a 5 to 7 second patient effort of hip flexion (knee to table) for five to seven repetitions, with reengagement of the barrier after each effort.

   Note: It is frequently useful to stretch the anterior hip capsule before stretching the rectus femoris and psoas muscles. Stretching of tightness of the anterior hip capsule (see Chapter 19, Fig. 19.6) frequently results in increased length of the rectus femoris and psoas muscles.

Figure 20.15.

Rectus Femoris Muscle

Testing and manual stretch position prone

1. Patient prone and the leg not tested flexed at the hip and the foot on the floor (Fig. 20.15a).
2. Operator stands at side of table and flexes the knee until resistance is felt. Normally, the heel of the tested leg touches the buttock. If not, tightness of the rectus femoris is present (Fig. 20.15b).
3. Operator treats shortness and tightness by resisting a 5 to 7 second patient effort of knee extension at the flexion barrier with five to seven repetitions. Operator engages a new flexion barrier after each patient effort.
4. Operator may substitute an on-and-off pumping maneuver against the barrier instead of the patient's contract–relax effort.
5. Operator must be cautious in knee flexion to avoid abnormal stretch of the femoral nerve. If knee flexion causes severe pain to the patient with an empty end feel, be suspicious of a femoral nerve problem and not rectus femoris tightness.

Figure 20.17a.
Tensor Fascia Lata Muscle
Length test and manuals stretch position supine
Modified Thomas position
1. Patient supine with buttocks on end of table and operator standing at the end of the table.
2. Patient holds leg not being tested in the flexed position with the thigh of the tested leg on the table.
3. Operator introduces external rotation of the femur and internal rotation of the tibia, sensing for resistance, and monitors the contour of the lateral thigh. If resistance is encountered and the lateral thigh shows a groove, tightness of the tensor fascia lata is present.
4. Operator treats shortness and tightness by maintaining external rotation of the femur, internal rotation of the tibia, adduction of the thigh, and resisting five to seven repetitions of a 5 to 7 second patient effort of hip flexion. The operator engages a new barrier after each patient effort.

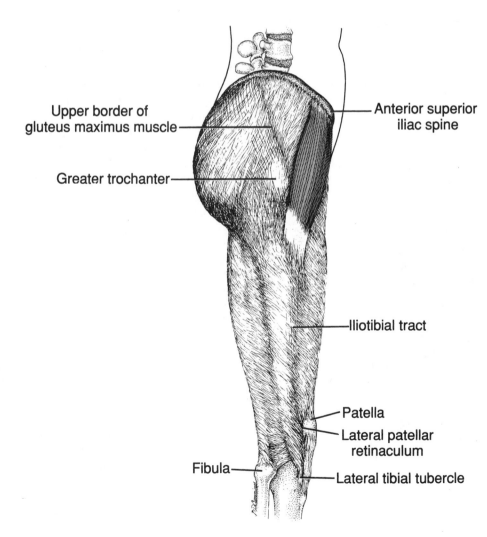

Upper border of
gluteus maximus muscle

Greater trochanter

Anterior superior
iliac spine

Iliotibial tract

Patella

Lateral patellar
retinaculum

Fibula

Lateral tibial tubercle

Figure 20.17b.
Tensor Fascia Lata Muscle
Side view of attachments of the right tensor fascia lata muscle. The muscle attaches along and below the crest of the ilium just posterior to the anterosuperior iliac spine. The anteromedial tendinous fibers attach to the fascia of the knee, and the posterolateral tendinous fibers anchor to the iliotibial tract, which continues down to the lateral tubercle of the tibia.

Figure 20.17c.
Tensor Fascia Lata Muscle
Self-stretch position kneeling
1. Patient position starts the same as for the self-stretch of the psoas muscle with the knee of the leg to be stretched on the floor and the opposite hip and knee flexed to 90 degrees.
2. Patient externally rotates the leg to be stretched.
3. Patient places hand on the buttocks, contracts the stomach, and maintains a 12-o'clock posterior pelvic tilt.
4. While maintaining the trunk in an upright position, patient pulls the trunk forward leading with the involved hip, maintaining gluteal contraction, and then adds a translatory motion of the pelvis toward the involved side resulting in trunk side bending away from the involved hip.
5. A sustained 30-second hold is repeated two to three times.

Figure 20.18a.
Piriformis Muscle and External Rotators of the Hip
Piriformis Muscle
Length test and manual stretch position below 90 degrees, supine position
1. Patient supine on table with operator standing on the opposite side of the leg being tested.
2. Operator flexes tested leg at the hip and knee and places the foot outside of the opposite knee. Operator stabilizes anterosuperior iliac spine on side being tested. (Fig. 20.18b)
3. Operator introduces internal rotation and adduction of the tested leg to the barrier and compares with the opposite side. Reduced range and a tight end feel indicate shortness and tightness of the piriformis being tested.
4. Operator treats shortness and tightness by resisting a 5 to 7 second patient effort of knee abduction and external rotation repeated five to seven times with the operator engaging a new barrier after each effort.
5. Operator maintains a compressive force toward the hip joint while stabilizing the anterosuperior iliac spine.

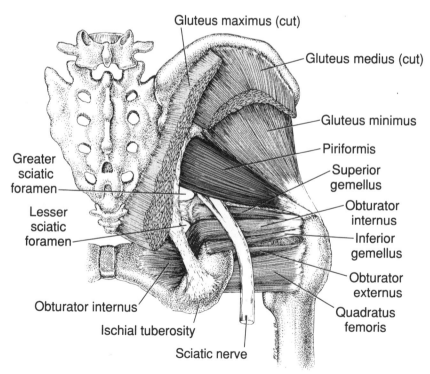

Gluteus maximus (cut)

Gluteus medius (cut)

Gluteus minimus

Piriformis

Superior gemellus

Obturator internus

Inferior gemellus

Obturator externus

Quadratus femoris

Sciatic nerve

Ischial tuberosity

Obturator internus

Lesser sciatic foramen

Greater sciatic foramen

Figure 20.18b.
Piriformis Muscle
Length Test and Manual Stretch above 90 degrees
Supine
1. Patient supine and the operator standing on same side as leg being tested.
2. Operator grasps patient's knee and ankle of leg being tested and introduces hip flexion and external rotation. (Fig. 20.18c)
3. Resistance to further hip flexion and external rotation, compared with the opposite side, indicates shortness and tightness of the piriformis muscle. Normally the knee should touch the chest.
4. In the presence of shortness and tightness, the operator resists a 5 to 7 second patient effort of extending the leg against two hands for five to seven repetitions. Operator engages a new barrier after each effort.

Figure 20.18c.

Figure 20.18d.
Piriformis Muscle Below 90 Degrees
Self-stretch Position Supine
1. Patient supine with leg on involved side flexed at the hip and knee and with the foot lateral to the opposite knee. (Fig. 20.18d)
2. Patient grasps the distal thigh and maintains adduction and internal rotation of the leg while stabilizing the pelvis with the other hand on the anterosuperior iliac spine. If the arm is too short, a belt or towel can be placed around the distal thigh to offer resistance.
3. Patient pushes knee laterally against resistance and without rotating pelvis.
4. Patient performs a series of contract–relax muscle efforts of 5 to 7 seconds with five to seven repetitions.

Figure 20.18e.
Piriformis Muscle Above 90 Degrees
Self-stretch position supine
1. Patient lies on back and grasps with both hands the ankle and knee of involved side.
2. The knee is pulled toward the opposite shoulder until a stretch is felt in the buttock.
3. Patient performs a sustained 30-second stretch repeated twice or a series of 5 to 7 second contract–relax muscle efforts repeated five to seven times.
4. The opposite side is stretched to balance.

Figure 20.18f.
Piriformis Muscle
Self-stretch position prone
1. Patient begins on hands and knees and places foot of involved side in front of the opposite knee, with the foot pointing toward the ceiling and the knee lateral to the trunk. The involved leg is flexed, externally rotated, and abducted.
2. The opposite leg is stretched distally while keeping the pelvis level until stretch is felt in the buttock.
3. A sustained 30-second stretch is repeated twice.
4. The position is reversed to stretch the opposite side to balance.

Figure 20.18g.
External Rotators of the Hip
Self-stretch position supine
The external rotators of the hip beside the piriformis are assessed and treated in relation to the posterior hip capsule (see Chapter 19, Figs. 19.7 and 19.8). The manual stretch for this group of external hip rotator muscles is found in Chapter 19 (Figs. 19.29 and 19.30).
1. Patient supine on table with uninvolved leg crossed over the involved leg and serving as a stabilizer.
2. Patient rotates pelvis away from the involved hip sufficient to get the buttocks off the table.
3. With the uninvolved leg preventing movement of the involved leg, the patient attempts to pull the buttock of the involved side back to the table by a 5 to 7 second contraction repeated five to seven times.
4. The pelvis is rotated away from the involved hip by the other leg between each contraction.

Figure 20.19.

Quadratus Lumborum Muscle

Length test and manual stretch position lateral recumbent

1. Patient in the lateral recumbent position with the leg not being tested in the flexed position and the leg being tested straight and slightly behind the trunk (Fig. 20.19a).
2. Operator stands behind the patient and stabilizes the twelfth rib with the proximal hand while relaxing the quadratus muscle be abducting the lower extremity (Fig. 20.19b).
3. Operator allows leg to drop toward the floor and assesses length of the quadratus lumborum muscle (Fig. 20.19c). Comparison is made with the opposite side.

4. Operator treats shortness and tightness by again stabilizing the twelfth rib with tension off the quadratus lumborum muscle (Fig. 20.19d).
5. Operator stabilizes leg against barrier with distal hand and resists patient's attempt to lift the leg for 5 to 7 seconds repeated five to seven times (Fig. 20.19e) engaging a new barrier after each effort.

Figure 20.20

Quadratus Lumborum Muscle

Self-stretch position lateral recumbent

1. Patient lies in the lateral recumbent position with the involved side uppermost.
2. Patient's bottom leg is flexed to 90 degrees, with the involved leg extended and adducted off the side of the table or bed.
3. Patient's arm on the involved side reaches overhead, adding to the stretch by the weight of the involved leg.
4. The stretch is held for 10 to 15 seconds and repeated three times or a sustained stretch for 30 seconds.
5. The opposite side is stretched to balance.

Figure 20.21.

Quadratus Lumborum Muscle

Self-stretch position standing

1. Patient stands with the arm of the involved side stretched overhead (Fig. 20.21a).
2. Patient laterally translates the pelvis toward the involved side as the trunk is side bent away from the involved side (Fig. 20.23b).
3. The position is sustained for 15 to 30 seconds and repeated two to three times.
4. The opposite side is stretched to symmetry.

Figure 20.22.
Quadratus Lumborum and Latissimus Dorsi Muscles
Self-stretch position kneeling
1. Patient on hands and knees reaches forward with the hand of the involved side and grasps a chair or stool with the hand internally rotated.
2. Patient shifts the pelvis laterally toward the involved side and then sits back, elongating the involved side with each repetition and increasing the diagonal drop of the pelvis.
3. The stretch is held for 10 to 15 seconds and repeated three to four times.
4. Externally rotating the hand adds an increase in the stretch of the latissimus dorsi.
5. The opposite side is stretched to balance.

Figure 20.23.
Hamstring Muscles
Length test and manual stretch position supine
1. Patient supine on table with operator standing on same side as leg being tested.
2. Operator monitors the opposite anterosuperior iliac spine while lifting the tested leg to the barrier of hip flexion. Comparison is made with the opposite side. If asymmetric, shortness and tightness are present in the involved hamstring muscles.
3. Operator performs the test with the leg adducted and abducted to test the difference in tightness of the medial and lateral hamstrings.
4. If short and tight, operator resists a 5 to 7 second patient effort of hip extension for five to seven repetitions with the operator engaging a new barrier after each effort.
Note: This test also affects the neural and dural mobility of the sciatic nerve. Frequently, the barrier to hip flexion is dural tension rather than hamstring tightness (see Chapter 19).

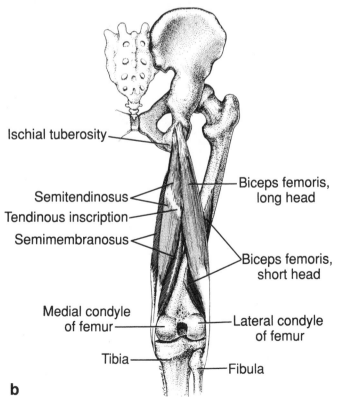

Ischial tuberosity

Semitendinosus
Tendinous inscription
Semimembranosus

Biceps femoris, long head

Biceps femoris, short head

Medial condyle of femur

Lateral condyle of femur

Tibia

Fibula

b

Figure 20.24.
Hamstring Muscles
Self-stretch position supine
1. Patient lies on back with the lumbar spine in neutral. A towel or pillow may be necessary.
2. Patient grasps the back of the thigh with both hands with the hip at 90 degrees.
3. Patient actively extends the knee, reaching with the foot toward the ceiling.
4. Dorsiflexion of the ankle increases the stretch.
5. Patient performs a series of contract–relax muscle efforts for 5 to 7 seconds repeated five to seven times.
6. This procedure can be used to mobilize the sciatic nerve complex.

Figure 20.25.
Hamstring Muscles
Self-stretch position sitting
1. Patient sits with the buttocks on a pillow or rolled towel to assist in maintaining the pelvis in an anteriorly rotated (6 o'clock) position.
2. A belt or towel is placed around the forefoot.
3. Beginning with the knees flexed, patient actively extends knees, feeling stretch in the posterior leg. It is important to maintain neutral lumbar mechanics during the stretch.
4. Patient performs a series of contract–relax knee extension muscle efforts or 5 to 7 seconds repeated five to seven times.
5. The patient may need to begin by sitting on a step to maintain neutral lumbar spinal mechanics.

Figure 20.26.
Hamstring Muscles
Self-stretch position standing
1. Patient stands with the feet 6 in. (15.24 cm) apart with the hands on the wall (Fig. 20.26a).
2. Patient bends hips to 90 degrees and flexes knees so that the trunk can become straight and arms fully extended. It is important to obtain a straight spine by dropping the chest and assuming a 6-o'clock position for the lumbar spine and pelvis.
3. Patient extends knees in an attempt to lift the buttocks toward the ceiling and elongate the spine.
4. Patient performs a series of contract–relax knee extension muscle efforts repeated five to seven times.
5. Patient may have to begin with the hands farther up the wall to keep the spine straight without dropping the head.
6. As progress is made, the hands are lowered on the wall until the trunk is horizontal to the floor. The hands may now be placed on a table or stand (Fig. 20.26b).
7. Patient pushes against the wall of the table during knee extension efforts.
Note: This exercise is also valuable as a self-mobilization of the dural tightness of the sciatic nerve.

Pectineus
(cut ends)

Adductor magnus
(posterior attachment)

Adductor brevis
(posterior attachment)

Adductor longus
(posterior attachment)

Adductor magnus
(posterior attachment)

Femur

Adductor magnus
(adductor minimus part)

Obturator foramen

Pubis

Adductor brevis

Adductor longus

Adductor magnus
(middle part)

Adductor magnus
(ischiocondylar part)

Tendinous (adductor)
hiatus

Patella

Figure 20.27.
Hip Adductor Muscles
Manual stretch position supine
1. The test for tightness of these muscles was performed in Test 2 of the lower quarter (Fig. 20.10).
2. To manually stretch tight adductor muscles, the operator stabilizes the patient's pelvis on the affected side by hooking thumb under the anterosuperior iliac spine.
3. The patient's involved leg is flexed at the hip and knee and externally rotated to the barrier.
4. Operator resists adduction and internal rotation of the involved leg with the distal hand on the medial knee (Fig. 20.27a).
5. Patient performs a series of five to seven muscle contractions for five to seven repetitions with the operator engaging a new barrier of abduction after each effort.

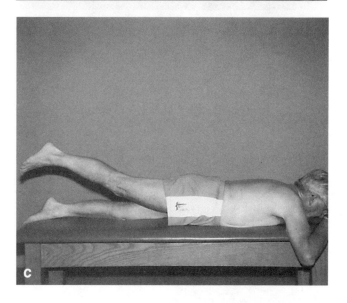

Figure 20.28.

Hip Adductor Muscles

Self-stretch position sitting

1. Patient sits with the buttocks as close to the wall as possible with the lumbar spine in neutral. A pillow or towel may be placed under the ischial tuberosities to provide an anterior pelvic tilt. The patient may begin by sitting on a low step.
2. Patient puts soles of feet together, pulling the feet toward the body, and actively externally rotates and abducts both legs.
3. Patient places both hands behind hips to assist in lifting and anteriorly rotating the pelvis and assuming the 6-o'clock position.
4. The stretch is held for 10 to 15 seconds and repeated three to four times with increasing external rotation and abduction with each effort.

Figure 20.29.

Gluteus Maximus Muscle

Retraining: Step 1

1. Patient prone and places toe on table (Fig. 20.29a).
2. Patient voluntarily contracts gluteus maximus.
3. When able to contract muscle, patient attempts to straighten knee (Fig. 20.29b).
4. When the patient is able to voluntarily contract the gluteus maximus muscle (Fig. 20.29c), proceed to Step 2.

Gluteus medius

Gluteus maximus

d

Figure 20.30.
Gluteus Maximus Muscle
Retraining: Step 2

1. Patient prone on table with the involved leg over the edge of the table with the operator supporting the leg at the flexed knee.
2. Operator monitors gluteus maximus for voluntary contraction (Fig. 20.30a).
3. When patient can sustain a gluteal muscle contraction, the operator removes the knee support and the patient holds leg steady by gluteal contraction (Fig. 20.30b).
4. When sufficient strength has returned, patient lifts flexed leg toward the ceiling (Fig. 20.30c) and slowly allows leg to descend toward the floor. Several repetitions are performed.
5. The gluteus maximus is exercised concentrically and eccentrically by this maneuver.
6. It is important that the patient maintains the pelvis level and the lumbar spine stable in neutral during this exercise. (Fig. 20.30d)

Figure 20.31.

Gluteus Maximus Muscle

Retraining: Step 3

1. Patient lies on back with knees flexed and feet flat.
2. Patient stabilizes the trunk by voluntary contraction of the transversus abdominus muscle, squeezes the buttocks together, and lifts the buttocks from the table (Fig. 20.31a). The pelvis should remain level and the lumbar spine in neutral.
3. Patient holds position for 5 to 7 seconds, slowly returns to the table, and repeats five to seven times.
4. When able to perform easily, patient progresses to straighten one leg while in the bridged position (Fig. 20.31b) and repeats the 5 to 7 second hold for five to seven repetitions on each side. It is important that the pelvis remain level during the one-legged bridge.

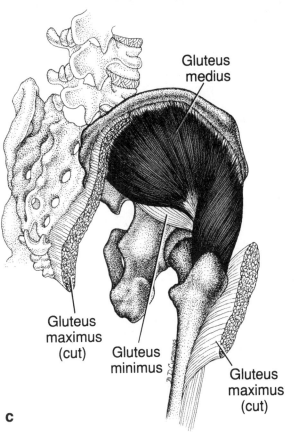

Gluteus medius

Gluteus maximus (cut)

Gluteus minimus

Gluteus maximus (cut)

Figure 20.32.

Gluteus Medius Muscle
Retraining

1. Patient lies in the lateral recumbent position with the knees flexed to 45 to 60 degrees and the upper hand overlying the gluteus medius muscle (Fig. 20.32a).
2. Maintaining the feet together, patient lifts top knee toward the ceiling, holds for 5 to 7 seconds, slowly lowers leg, and repeats five to seven times (Fig. 20.32b).
3. This muscle (Fig. 20.32c) may fatigue rapidly with this exercise, and the patient must be cautious about the number of repetitions.
4. The knee should not be elevated too far because this will increase the contraction of the piriformis muscle as the external rotator.
5. Repeat on the opposite side for balance.

Figure 20.33.
Gluteus Medius Muscle
Retraining
1. Patient in the lateral recumbent position against the wall with the shoulders and pelvis perpendicular to the table or floor and the upper leg extended.
2. Patient's upper arm is placed on and pushes into the table or floor while dorsiflexing the upper foot.
3. Patient slowly raises the upper leg to hip level keeping the heel in contact with the wall, holds for 5 to 7 seconds, and lowers leg slowly. This is repeated five to seven times.
4. Externally rotating the leg reduces the influence of the tensor fascia lata muscle, and elongating the leg reduces the influence of the quadratus lumborum muscle and isolates action more to the gluteus medius.
5. Repeat on the opposite side for symmetric balance.
6. As progress is made, the exercise may be done with the knees at 90 degrees. Added difficulty is to raise both legs toward the ceiling.

Figure 20.34.
Gluteus Medius Muscle
Retraining
1. Patient begins in the hands and knees position and diagonally sits back. The pelvis should translate laterally and the spine on the side to be stretched should elongate.
2. Patient holds the position for 5 to 7 seconds, returns to the starting position, and repeats five to seven times on both sides.
3. As strength returns, patient can sink further back. The direction and distance should be symmetric on each side.
4. The arms should be passive and the control should come from the buttocks.
Note: This exercise also stretches the quadratus lumborum muscle on the side of the hip sink.

ABDOMINAL MUSCLES

The abdominal muscles as a group are notoriously weak and inhibited. They are essential for the maintenance of core stability, particularly the transversus abdominus. Recent research has found that the transversus abdominus muscle is the first to contract when movement occurs in the upper or lower extremity. In patients with lower back pain, the activation of the transversus abdominus is delayed. There are a large number of exercises for strengthening the abdominal muscles, but few exercise all components of the abdominals.

There are several ways to learn to control and strengthen the transversus abdominus. One is to lay supine, place your hand under your lumbar lordosis, and contract the transversus abdominus by pulling the navel posteriorly without losing the lumbar lordosis. Another is to be on the hands and knees with a neutral lumbar lordosis and lift the navel without changing the lumbar curve. These exercises are done voluntarily but need to be programmed to occur subconsciously. Contraction of the transversus is the first component of many exercises in an effort to stabilize the core of the body.

The abdominals must be exercised in both the shortening and elongating directions.

Figure 20.35.
Abdominal Muscles
Retraining with curl-up
1. Patient lies supine with hips and knees flexed.
2. Patient extends arms in front and slowly curls up beginning in the cervical spine and up to the upper back while reaching toward the knees.
3. Position is held for 5 to 7 seconds and then the spine is slowly lowered segmentally to the starting position.
4. Placing the hands behind the neck increases the difficulty.
Note: This mainly exercises the rectus abdominus with concentric and eccentric contraction.

b

c

d

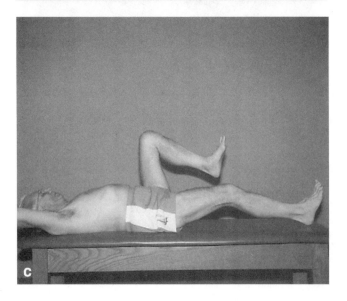

Figure 20.36.
Abdominal Muscles
Retraining
Heel slides and Norwegian
1. Patient lying with knees and hips bent and feet on the table or floor.
2. Patient contracts the transversus abdominus and slowly slides one leg down on the table or floor without losing the neutral lumbar lordosis and returned to the starting position. Each leg is alternately extended with six to 10 repetitions (Fig. 20.36a).
3. An alternative is to assume the 12-o'clock position for the lumbar spine and pelvis and slide the heel as far as possible without allowing the lumbar spine to extend and repeat on each side for six to 10 repetitions. The leg does not extend as far as in the first in this variation.
4. The Norwegian exercise begins in the same starting position, both hips and knees are flexed, and one leg at a time alternately touches the table or floor (Fig. 20.36b).
5. The patient increases the difficulty by touching the heel with gradually more extension of the hips and knees (Fig. 20.36c).
6. The lumbar lordosis must be maintained throughout these exercises by the contraction of the transversus abdominus muscle. Keeping a hand under the lumbar spine monitors the lordosis.
7. The goal is to perform the Norwegian leg extension for 2 minutes while counting aloud to prevent holding the breath.

Figure 20.37.

Abdominal Muscles

Retraining with sit backs

1. Patient sits with hips and knees bent, the heels digging into the table or floor, and the toes plantar flexed.
2. Patient maintains the lumbar spine in neutral mechanics and extends the arms over the knees (Fig. 20.37a).
3. The patient sits back from this position as far as possible without lifting the heels and while maintaining the neutral lumbar spine (Fig. 20.37b). This is held for 5 to 7 seconds and then returned to the starting position. This is repeated five to seven times (Step 1).
4. Patient places hands across the chest or behind the neck (Fig. 20.37c) to increase the difficulty of performing the same, sit back for five to seven repetitions with a 5 to 7 second hold (Step 2).
5. When proficient at Step 2, patient progresses but rotates the shoulders while maintaining the neutral lumbar spine and performing the sit back with the right elbow pointed to the left knee (Fig. 20.37d), then returning to the starting position, rotating with the left elbow pointing to the right knee and repeating. Again, five to seven repetitions of a 5 to 7 second hold are made on each side.

Note: This is the favorite abdominal exercise of the author because it automatically activates the transversus abdominus subconsciously, exercises both obliques and the rectus abdominus in the lengthened position, and maintains a neutral lumbar spine.

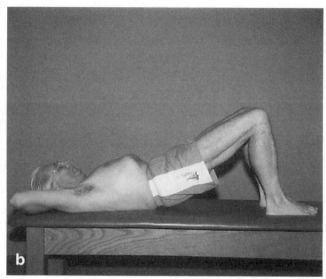

Figure 20.38.

Pelvic Seesaw (Lewit)

Trunk control exercise

1. Patient lies supine with knees bent and feet flat on the table or floor.
2. Patient contracts the erector spinae muscles introducing lumbar extension (Fig. 20.38a) and hip flexion.
3. Patient contracts the abdominal and gluteal muscles, flattening the lumbar lordosis and flexing one segment at a time from caudal to proximal until pelvis is lifted from the table introducing lumbar flexion and hip extension (Fig. 20.38b).
4. After a 5 to 7 second hold, the process is reversed by dropping the vertebral segments to the table one by one from above downward, introducing lumbar extension by contraction of the erector spinae muscles and hip flexion.
5. The process is repeated five to seven times to increase the control of lumbar flexion/hip extension and lumbar extension/hip flexion of the trunk.

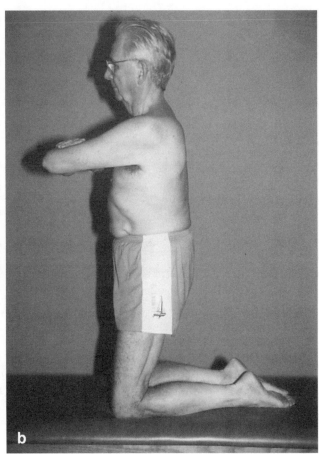

Figure 20.39.
Sitting to Kneeling (Lewit)
Trunk control exercise
1. Patient sits on heel with trunk erect and flexes and extends the lumbar spine until a neutral spine is identified (Fig. 20.39a).
2. While maintaining a neutral spine, patient lifts the body straight up to an erect kneeling position using the gluteal and thigh muscles (Fig. 20.39b).
3. Patient returns to starting position slowly and repeats five to seven times.
4. The exercise strengthens abdominal and gluteal muscles and provides trunk stability and trunk motor control.
5. A pillow under the knees and under the buttocks will reduce the stress on the knee.

Figure 20.40.

Trunk Lift Exercise

1. Patient kneels on one knee with the other leg flexed at the hip and knee to 90 degrees. The spine is held in neutral mechanics (Fig. 20.40a).
2. The toe of the leg in the kneeling position is placed on the floor.
3. Patient lifts the body so that the knee is 4 in. (10.16 cm) off the floor while maintaining the upper body posture in a neutral position and holds for 5 to 7 seconds (Fig. 20.40b).
4. Five to seven repetitions are performed.
5. This exercise is valuable for improving the patient's capacity to lift without adverse effect on the back.

EVALUATION AND TREATMENT OF THE UPPER QUARTER

In the upper quarter, the postural muscles that are facilitated, hypertonic, and short include the levator scapulae, upper trapezius, sternocleidomastoid, scalenes, pectorals, and flexors of the upper extremity. The dynamic muscles that are inhibited, hypotonic, and weak include the middle and lower trapezius, serratus anterior, rhomboids, supraspinatus, infraspinatus, deltoid, deep neck flexors, and extensors of the upper extremity.

Janda's upper crossed syndrome finds the upper trapezius, levator scapulae, and the scalene muscles shortened and hypertonic with weakness and inhibition of the lower trapezius and serratus anterior. The pectorals are short and tight and the interscapular muscles, the serratus anterior and rhomboids, are weak and inhibited. The sternocleidomastoid and suboccipital muscles functioning as neck extensors are short, whereas the deep neck flexors are weak and inhibited. The upper crossed syndrome pattern affects the functional capacity of the cervical spine and the upper extremities and results in a forward head posture, straightening of the lower cervical lordosis, extension of the upper cervical spine, increased kyphosis of the cervical thoracic junction, and internal rotation of the shoulder girdles. Resultant alteration in shoulder mechanics can contribute to strain of the shoulder joints.

IDENTIFICATION OF UPPER QUADRANT FAULTY MOVEMENT PATTERNS

Six tests are used to identify faulty movement patterns of the upper quarter.

Test 1

The first is the supine cervical flexion test (Fig. 20.41a–c). The patient lies supine and is asked to look down to the feet. In the presence of strong deep neck flexors, the chin tucks down and rolls forward, whereas in weakness of the deep neck flexors, the sternocleidomastoid and scalene muscles substitute and the head is carried forward before looking downward.

Figure 20.41.

Test 2

The second test is the bilateral shoulder abduction maneuver (Fig. 20.42). Particular attention is placed on the behavior of the scapula as it is asked to elevate and then return to normal. Symmetry is important, as is the absence of "winging" of the scapula, particularly as the arms are lowered. The firing pattern of the upper extremity is evaluated (Fig. 20.3). Weakness of the supraspinatus and deltoid results in substitution by the levator scapulae and upper trapezius muscles that excessively elevate the shoulder and is associated with loss of scapular stabilization by the lower trapezius and serratus anterior. This condition may result in impingement syndrome of the shoulder and place further strain on the cervical spine.

Test 3

The third test is for scapular stabilization. One method is to have the patient on the hands and knees with the spine level with the table and asking the patient to lift one hand and then the other off the table. Excessive winging of the medial border of the scapula occurs due to weakness and lack of stabilization by the

lower trapezius, serratus anterior, and rhomboid muscles (Fig. 20.43).

A second variation for testing scapular stabilization is having the patient perform a wall push-up (Fig. 20.44a). The operator observes the behavior of the scapula on the thoracic cage particularly for asymmetric "winging" (Fig. 20.44b).

Test 4

The fourth test is for scapular depression (Fig. 20.45). In the prone position, the patient is asked to push the inferior angle of the scapula in a medial and caudal direction against operator resistance.

Test 5

The fifth test is supine bilateral shoulder flexion (Fig. 20.46). Assessment is made of symmetry and the ability to maintain a neutral lumbar spine. Lumbar exten-

Figure 20.42.

Figure 20.43.

Figure 20.44.

Figure 20.45.

Figure 20.46.

sion is to be avoided and adequate bilateral shoulder flexion is the normal.

Test 6

The sixth test is for pectoralis minor length. The patient is supine and the operator observes the symmetry of the anterior aspect of the shoulders (Fig. 20.47). One may be carried more anterior due to tightness of the pectoralis minor muscle or tightness of the posterior shoulder capsule.

ASSESSMENT OF MUSCLE LENGTH AND TREATMENT BY MANUAL STRETCHING

The tight muscle groups of the upper quadrant can be treated in a fashion similar to those in the lower quarter and include static stretch of 20 to 30 seconds with two to three repetitions or postisometric relaxation after a 5 to 7 second contraction. Muscles to be assessed, manually stretched, and self-stretched include the levator scapulae and splenius capitis, upper trapezius and sternocleidomastoid, scalenes, pectoralis major and minor, and latissimus dorsi (Figs. 20.48–20.61).

Figure 20.47.

Figure 20.48.
Latissimus Dorsi Muscle
Length Test and Manual Stretch Position
1. Patient supine with operator at head of table.
2. Patient's knees are flexed and operator grasps both wrists and introduces upper extremity flexion.
3. Asymmetric arm elevation indicates tight latissimus dorsi muscle (Fig. 20.48a).
4. Operator resists patient's arm extension for 5 to 7 seconds with five to seven repetitions until arm flexion is symmetric (Fig.20.48b).
5. If another operator is available, a pumping on-and-off maneuver of hip and pelvic flexion, while traction is held on both arms, enhances the latissimus stretch.

Figure 20.49.

Latissimus Dorsi Muscle

Self-stretch, thoracic spine elongation position

1. Patient kneels with elbows together and placed on a stool or chair.
2. Patient separates the scapulae by externally rotating the arms and maintaining the elbows together.
3. Operator drops chest to the floor, elongates the lumbar spine by a 12-o'clock position, and sits back toward the heels.
4. The stretch is held for 30 seconds and repeated twice.
5. It is advisable to perform this exercise after any trunk rotational exercise to restore trunk elongation.

Figure 20.50.

Pectoral Muscles

Length test and manual stretch position supine

1. Patient supine with operator standing at side of table.
2. Operator controls patient's upper arm at the wrist and extends the elbow.
3. Operator's other hand monitors tightness in the pectoral region as the upper arm is abducted and horizontally extended until barrier is reached.
4. Comparison is made with the opposite side.
5. Stretching for shortness and tightness has patient perform a series of five to seven contract–relax efforts for 5 to 7 seconds with the operator engaging new barrier after each effort.
6. Operator modifies amount of abduction and horizontal extension to meet the fiber direction of the pectoralis major and holds sternum and clavicle for stability of pectoral attachment. For the pectoralis minor, operator's medial hand stabilizes third, fourth, and fifth ribs.

Figure 20.51.
Pectoral Muscles
Length test and manual stretch position prone
1. Patient prone with operator standing at the side of the table.
2. Operator stabilizes the scapula and clavicle with one hand with the metacarpophalangeal joint of the second finger overlying the posterior aspect of the head of the humerus.
3. Operator grasps wrist, extends elbow, and horizontally extends arm, assessing range. The normal range is 90 degrees of horizontal extension.
4. Comparison is made with the other side.
5. Stretching for shortness and tightness can be obtained by a sustained operator stretch supplemented by 5 to 7 second contract–relax patient efforts.
6. This position can be used to stretch the anterior shoulder capsule. Operator puts traction on the arm with one hand while the other rolls anteriorly against the humerus and provides a series of mobilizations.
7. Caution must be used with a history of anterior dislocation.

Figure 20.52.
Pectoral Muscles
Self-stretch position
1. Patient stands facing the wall and places both hands on wall at shoulder height.
2. Patient turns the body away from the involved side, keeping the shoulder from elevating until a stretch is felt in the pectoral region.
3. Using the other hand as a stabilizer, patient leans the body toward the wall increasing the pectoral stretch.
4. Patient maintains a neutral spine throughout the stretch.
5. Stretch is held for 10 to 15 seconds and is repeated three to five times. The shoulder should be able to be perpendicular to the wall.
6. The opposite side should be stretched to balance.

Figure 20.53.
Posterior Shoulder Capsule
Test and manual stretch position
1. Patient in the lateral recumbent position with the head on a pillow and the involved shoulder down.
2. Operator flexes the elbow and abducts the involved shoulder to 90 degrees (Fig. 20.55a).
3. Operator internally rotates arm to barrier (Fig. 20.55b). Normally the internal rotation should allow the long finger of the flexed hand to touch the table.
4. Stretch is performed in one of three ways: The patient provides five to seven repetitions of a 3 to 5 second contract–relax effort with operator engaging new barrier after each effort; the operator holds the arm at the barrier and rolls the patient's body forward in an on-and-off manner; or the operator applies an on-and-off short-range pumping action.

Figure 20.54.
Posterior Shoulder Capsule
Self-stretch position
1. Patient lies in the lateral recumbent position with head on a pillow and the involved shoulder down on the table.
2. Patient grasps at the wrist, flexes the elbow, and carries the shoulder to 90 degrees of abduction.
3. Patient internally rotates the arm to the barrier and applies a stretch by rolling the body forward in an on-and-off fashion with a gradual increase in the internal rotation.
4. A second stretch method has the patient apply an on-and-off pumping maneuver with the opposite hand gradually increasing range against the barrier.
5. A third stretch method is to perform five to seven repetitions of a 5 to 7 second muscle contraction against the barrier and to reengage the barrier after each effort.

Figure 20.55.
Levator Scapulae Muscle
Test and manual stretch position
1. Patient in the lateral recumbent position with the involved side up and with no pillow allowing the head to fall away from the involved side.
2. Operator grasps medial angle of the scapula in the web of the thumb of one hand and stabilizes the upper cervical spine with the other (Fig. 20.55a).
3. Operator moves the scapula into (a) upward rotation around an anteroposterior axis, (b) external rotation around a vertical axis, and (c) dorsal tilt around a transverse axis, then depresses it caudally to the barrier.
4. Stretch is performed by the patient's attempting to lift the head toward the ceiling against operator resistance for five to seven repetitions of a 5 to 7 second muscle effort. Operator engages a new barrier after each effort.
5. The opposite side is compared and stretched to balance.
6. The same patient position can be used as a self-stretch with the patient holding the position for 30 seconds and repeating two times (Fig. 20.55b).

Figure 20.56.
Levator Scapulae Muscle
Self-stretch position sitting
1. Patient sitting with hand on side to be treated holding the chair.
2. Patient flexes, side bends, and rotates the head away and supports the head position with the other hand.
3. Patient leans trunk away for stretch. The contact hand does not pull the head and neck.
4. The stretch can be enhanced by a contraction of the lower trapezius muscle on the same side.
5. The stretch is held for 10 to 15 seconds and repeated three to five times with increasing side bending away each time.

Figure 20.57
Upper Trapezius Muscle
Testing and manual stretch position
1. Patient supine with operator sitting at head.
2. Operator's lateral hand stabilizes patient's scapula and clavicle on the side being tested.
3. Operator's medial hand controls the occiput of the skull and introduces flexion, side bending away, and rotation toward the side being tested.
4. If range is asymmetric, shortness and tightness are present.
5. To stretch tightness and shortness, patient attempts to elevate the shoulder toward the ear against operator resistance for 5 to 7 seconds with five to seven repetitions. Operator increases the flexion and side bending after each effort.

Figure 20.58.

Sternocleidomastoid Muscle

Test and manual stretch position

1. The sternocleidomastoid and upper trapezius muscles are synergistic and can be tested and treated together.
2. Patient supine with operator sitting at head of table.
3. Operator's lateral hand stabilizes the scapula and clavicle.
4. Operator's medial hand controls the occiput of the skull and introduces flexion, side bending away, and rotation to the side being tested.
5. Comparison is made with the opposite side. If asymmetric, shortness and tightness are present.
6. Stretching of the shortness and tightness is performed by asking the patient to chin tuck and elevate the shoulder against operator resistance for 5 to 7 seconds and five to seven repetitions.

Figure 20.59.
Upper trapezius and Sternocleidomastoid Muscles
Self-stretch position sitting
1. Patient sitting with hand on treated side holding chair.
2. Patient flexes, side bends away, and rotates head and neck toward side being treated. The patient's other hand holds the head in this position but does not pull.
3. Patient leans body away until a stretch is felt. A chin tuck increases the stretch on the sternocleidomastoid.
4. Stretch is held for 10 to 15 seconds and is repeated three to five times.
5. The other side should be stretched to balance.
6. Do not stretch one side only; it may adversely affect symmetric temporal bone movement.

Figure 20.60.
Scalene Muscles
Test and manual stretch position
1. Patient supine with shoulders at edge and operator sitting at head of table supporting patient's head.
2. Operator's proximal hand supports the occiput and the forehead is placed in the axilla.
3. Patient's distal hand controls the patient's thoracic inlet, particularly the first and second ribs (Fig. 20.60a).
4. Operator depresses the head toward the floor, assessing range (Fig. 20.60b).
5. Comparison is made with the other side. If asymmetric, shortness and tightness are present.
6. Asking the patient to lift the forehead toward the ceiling against operator's resistance by the axilla for 5 to 7 seconds with five to seven repetitions stretches shortness and tightness. A complementary action is having the patient attempt to side bend the head toward the side being treated for 5 to 7 seconds and five to seven repetitions.

Figure 20.61.
Scalene Muscles
Self-stretch position sitting
1. Patient sitting with hand on treated side holding chair.
2. Patient's other hand is placed over the clavicle and upper ribs stabilize the first and second ribs.
3. Patient side bends the head and neck away, rotates back and forth to find tightness, and chin tucks until stretch is felt.
4. A sustained 10 to 15 second hold is repeated three to five times, fine-tuning the rotation and side bending after each stretch.

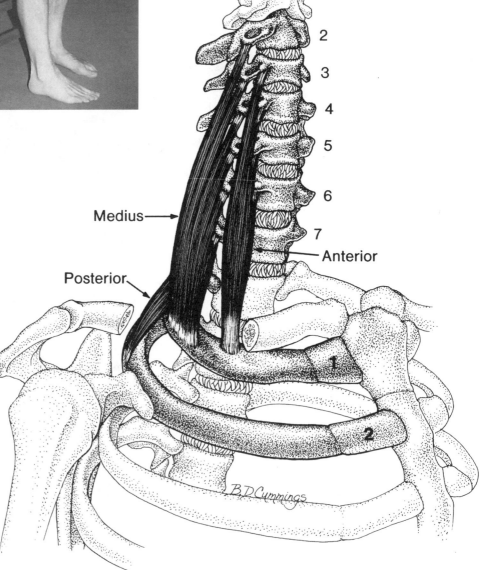

UPPER QUARTER RETRAINING

Upper quarter retraining is similar to that described for the lower quarter and includes modification of the testing procedures and repetitive action of the inhibited muscle group. These procedures are shown in Figs. 20.62 through 20.75.

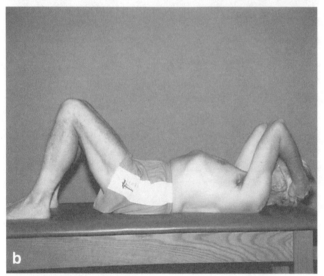

Figure 20.63.
Cervical Flexor Muscles
Assisted eccentric strengthening supine
1. Patient supine with hands behind the head passively flexes head and tucks chin to the chest, stretching the posterior cervical muscles (Fig. 20.63a).
2. After holding for 10 seconds, the head is slowly lowered, keeping the chin tucked, until head returns to the table (Fig. 20.63b).
3. As neck flexors become stronger, less assistance is provided by the hands on the head.
4. Repeat five to seven times.
5. Patient should be capable of performing this exercise before proceeding to unassisted strengthening.

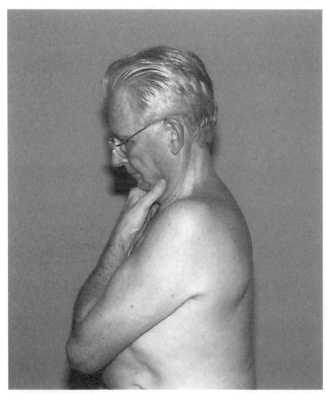

Figure 20.62.
Cervical Flexor Muscles
Retraining in sitting position
1. Patient sits and palpates superficial anterior cervical muscles.
2. Patient nods head forward, using deep neck flexors by a chin tuck and without contracting superficial muscles.
3. Patient holds for 5 to 7 seconds with five to seven repetitions.
4. Patient should be capable of performing this exercise before proceeding to the supine position.

Figure 20.64.
Cervical Flexor Muscles
Unassisted eccentric strengthening supine
1. Patient supine on table (Fig. 20.64a) and rolls head forward by a chin tuck, lifting the head from the table to look down at the feet (Fig. 20.64b).
2. Position is held for 5 to 7 seconds and the head is slowly returned to the table, attempting to touch one vertebra at a time (Fig. 20.64c).
3. Repeat five to seven times.

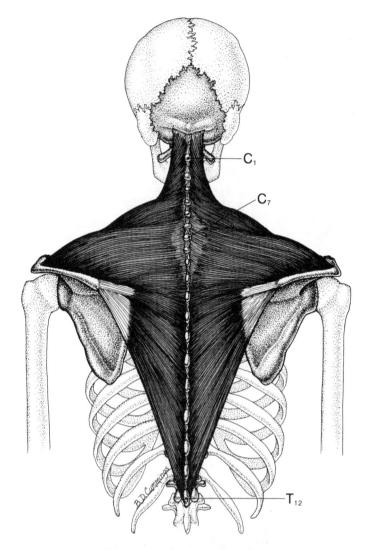

Figure 20.65.

Lower Trapezius Muscle

Testing and retraining prone

1. Patient prone on table with operator on side opposite of that being tested.
2. Operator puts monitoring hand on lower trapezius muscle and asks patient to activate by pulling scapula inferiorly and medially (Fig. 20.65a). Comparison is made with the other side.
3. If inhibited, retraining begins by asking patient to lift hand from the table, activating lower trapezius (Fig. 20.65b).
4. When activated, retraining is by the patient repeating lifting of hand and then lifting elbow for 5 to 7 seconds and repeating five to seven times.

Figure 20.66.

Lower Trapezius Muscle

Retraining position hands and knees

1. Patient on hands and knees, resting head on the table, sits back on heels.
2. Patient pulls the scapula in a medial and caudad direction without pulling the scapulae together,
3. Position is held for 5 to 7 seconds with five to seven repetitions.

Figure 20.67.
Lower Trapezius Muscle
Retraining position prone
1. Patient prone with arms extended above head (Fig. 20.67a).
2. Patient lift arms from table and pulls the medial border of the scapula caudally and holds for 5 to 7 seconds (Fig. 20.67b).
3. Repeat five to seven times.

Figure 20.68.
Rhomboids and Lower Trapezius Muscles
Isometric strength retraining position sitting
1. Patient sitting with feet on floor.
2. Patient grasps fingers together with hands in front of upper sternum and arms parallel to the floor (Fig. 20.68a).
3. Patient attempts to pull elbows backward to the wall for a 5 to 7 second isometric contraction and repeats five to seven times to strengthen rhomboids.
4. Patient grasps fingers together with hands over top but not in contact with head (Fig. 20.68b).
5. Patient attempts to pull elbows down to the floor for a 5 to 7 second isometric contraction and repeats five to seven times to strengthen lower trapezius.
Note: Figure 20.68c shows rhomboid muscles.

c

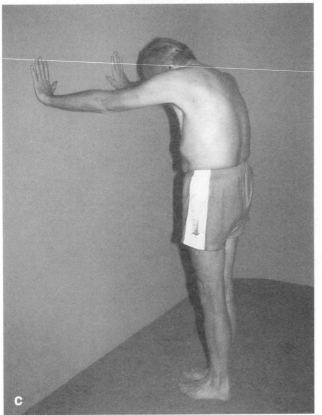

Figure 20.69.

Serratus Anterior Muscle

Retraining position standing

1. Patient stands with hands on the wall at shoulder height, arms extended, and spine in neutral (Fig. 20.69a).
2. Patient touches nose to wall while keeping the scapulae depressed (Fig. 20.69b) and holds for 5 to 7 seconds.
3. Patient performs a standing push-up while dropping the head toward the floor with cervical flexion and pushing the upper thoracic spine posteriorly without elevating the scapulae (Fig. 20.69c) and holds for 5 to 7 seconds.
4. Exercise is repeated five to seven times.

Note: When proficient when standing, serratus anterior strengthening can be performed in the prone position in the same manner.

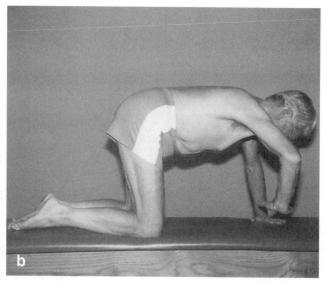

Figure 20.70.

Serratus Anterior Muscle

Retraining position hands and knees

1. Patient on hands and knees with elbows flexed so that spine is parallel to the table and in neutral position (Fig. 20.70a).
2. Patient raises one hand 1 to 2 in. (2.5 to 5 cm) off the table while maintaining trunk position (Fig. 20.70b).
3. Position is held for 5 to 7 seconds with five to seven repetitions.
4. Both sides are strengthened to balance.

Note: If excessive winging of the scapulae occurs, this exercise may be too strenuous and should be preceded by the wall push-up method.

Figure 20.71.

Shoulder Abduction

Retraining position supine

1. Patient lies supine with hands at side, palms up, and slowly abducts arms keeping back of arms on floor.
2. If one shoulder elevates higher than the other (Fig. 20.71a), patient has gone too far and arms are brought back to the side.
3. Exercise is repeated only as far as arms can be abducted without elevating the shoulders (Fig. 20.71b), and the patient reaches out with the restricted side several times, brings arms back down, and repeats five to seven times.
4. Care is exercised so that the abduction is symmetric on both sides.

Figure 20.72.
Shoulder Circle Integrator
Lateral recumbent position
1. Patient in lateral recumbent position, knees flexed, and both arms extended straight in front of body (Fig. 20.72a).
2. Patient further extends upper arm and starts reaching overhead, keeping the hand on the floor (Fig. 20.72b).
3. When arm is over the head, the hand is turned over and the back of the hand stays on the floor (Fig. 20.72c) as the patient continues the circle movement.
4. Patient's thorax rotates backward and the arm extends further behind the body (Fig. 20.72d) as far as possible.
5. Patient reverses the process and brings arm back around to the starting position.
6. Three to five repetitions are performed.
7. If patient has difficulty keeping hand on the floor, patient stops the circle, initiates repetitive arm extension movements, reverses the circle, and repeats.
Note: Difficulty in performing shoulder circles is frequently related to restricted rib mobility.

Figure 20.73.
Shoulder Circle with Rib Mobilization
Lateral recumbent position
1. Patient in lateral recumbent position with arms in front, upper arms extended furthest and with thorax rotated forward.
2. Operator places thumbs on upper posterior rib angles, shafts, or thoracic spine transverse processes and mobilizes anteriorly (Fig. 20.73a).
3. Operator repeats mobilization without impulse on mid to lower ribs (Fig. 20.73b).
4. Patient rotates thorax posteriorly and operator applies thumbs to the anterior costochondral articulations and mobilizes posteriorly (Fig. 20.73c).
5. Operator mobilizes mid- to lower anterior ribs (Fig. 20.73d).
6. Shoulder circle is repeated after rib mobilization.

SELF-MOBILIZING EXERCISES FOR SPECIFIC JOINT DYSFUNCTION

The patient can use exercise to maintain correction of joint dysfunction or to self-treat in the presence of recurrence. This assists patients in taking control of their musculoskeletal systems. In the pelvis, the symphysis pubis can be self-mobilized with isometric activation of the hip adductor musculature (Fig. 20.74). Appropriate balancing of the abdominal musculature above and the hip adductor musculature below the symphysis pubis should follow (Figs. 20.28 and 20.37).

Sacroiliac dysfunctions are frequently associated with asymmetric tone of the piriformis muscles. Self-correction for a forward sacral torsion is the same exercise as that for stretching a tight piriformis (Fig. 20.18f). In the presence of a posterior sacral torsion or unilateral posteriorly nutated sacrum (extended), a unilateral prone press-up is used. Frequently, it is necessary to mobilize this dysfunction adequately before the patient is able to perform this exercise (Fig. 20.75). Because the trunk's backward bending in the presence of a posterior nutated sacral base and flexed, rotated, and side-bent (FRS) dysfunctions of the lumbar spine are frequently painful, this procedure must be done cautiously and begun under strict supervision.

For the correction of iliosacral rotational dysfunctions, the self-correction procedures are as follows. In the presence of an anterior hip bone dysfunction, the patient lies supine and posteriorly rotates the right hip bone (Fig. 20.76). For a posterior hip bone, the spine-lying patient drops the dysfunctional leg over the edge of the table and uses muscle contraction to extend the hip on the side of the dysfunction (Fig. 20.77).

The Clock diagnostic exercise for trunk and pelvic control (Fig. 20.78) can also be useful in the diagnosis and self-management of lumbar spine dysfunctions. The patient is taught how to assess the lumbar spine by touching each number of the clock sequentially, both clockwise and counterclockwise. The inability to symmetrically touch each number of the clock identifies the presence of dysfunction. Inability to touch 1 and 2 o'clock identifies an extended, rotated, and side-bent left (ERS_{left}) dysfunction; 4 and 5 o'clock, an FRS_{left} dysfunction; 7 and 8 o'clock, an FRS_{right} dysfunction; and 10 and 11 o'clock, an ERS_{right} dysfunction. If the patient cannot move from 3 to 9 o'clock and from 9 to 3 o'clock easily and has some discomfort in trying, there is usually a sacroiliac dysfunction present. The inability to go to 3 o'clock identifies restricted left rotation of the sacrum. Inability to go to 9 o'clock relates to restricted right rotation of the sacrum. These restrictions

Figure 20.74.
Symphysis pubis.
Self-correction position supine.
1. Patient supine with the feet together.
2. Patient abducts knees and places a non-compressible object between them.
3. Patient performs a symmetric 5 to 7 second isometric activity of both legs trying to bring the knees together.
4. Repeat five to seven times.

Figure 20.75.
Posterior nutated (extended) sacrum.
Self-correction position prone.
1. Patient prone with involved leg slightly abducted and externally rotated on the table and opposite foot placed on the floor.
2. Patient performs a push-up and maintains a sagging abdomen while forcefully exhaling.
3. Five to seven respiratory cycles are made with an attempt to increase the push-up with each effort.

Figure 20.76.
Anteriorly rotated hip bone.
Self-correction position supine.

1. Patient supine on the table with involved hip and knee flexed.
2. Keeping the opposite leg straight, patient grasps both hands below the knee and attempts hip extension by a 5 to 7 second muscle contraction.
3. After each relaxation, patient increases hip flexion and repeats five to seven times.
4. After each relaxation, patient increases hip flexion and repeats five to seven times.

Figure 20.78.

Figure 20.77.
Posteriorly rotated hip bone.
Self-correction supine.

1. Patient supine with involved leg off the edge of the table or bed.
2. Patient flexes the opposite hip and knee bringing the knee to the chest.
3. At full exhalation, patient contracts the gluteal muscles to further extend the leg and holds for 5 to 7 seconds.
4. Five to seven repetitions are made with increasing amounts of hip extension.

are most commonly due to a posterior sacral base on one side, either a posteriorly nutated sacrum or a backward torsion. Useful self-mobilizing procedures are of two types. One is release by position wherein the patient assumes a body position exactly opposite the number of the clock denoting restriction, for example, if unable to touch 5 o'clock, the patient moves as far toward 11 o'clock as possible and holds that position for 60 to 90 seconds, using a counterstrain principle. Then the patient slowly returns to neutral and again attempts 5 o'clock. The second procedure for the same dysfunction calls for moving all the way to 11 o'clock, then to 5 o'clock as far as possible, then back again to 11 o'clock, and repeat as a mobilizing without impulse self-mobilization. With each repetition an attempt to go further into 5 o'clock is made until symmetry is achieved. Other self-correction procedures for lumbar spine dysfunctions of the FRS type are modifications of Mackenzie's procedure to reduce the lateral shift and then incorporate extension. Procedures that have been found useful include standing and side gliding into the wall (Fig. 20.79) and while facing the wall (Fig. 20.80). This procedure allows fine-tuning of the amount of lateral shift and extension. Prone press-ups (Fig. 20.81) and backward bending while standing (Fig. 20.82) are then used to enhance trunk extension. Lumbar spine rotational strengthening and control can be performed with trunk rotational reeducation (Fig. 20.83).

Figure 20.79.
Hip shift.
Self-correction standing.
1. Patient standing about 2 ft (60 cm) away from the wall with one shoulder, upper arm, and elbow against the wall.
2. Patient translates the pelvis toward the wall but avoids side bending of the spine.
3. Patient's other hand can assist by pushing the pelvis to the wall.
4. Position is held for 5 to 7 seconds and repeated five to seven times.
5. This exercise deals with the side-bending component of a flexion, rotated, and side-bent lumbar dysfunction.

Figure 20.80.
Lumbar spine flexed, rotated, and side-bent dysfunction.
Self-correction position standing.
1. Patient stands facing wall with feet acetabular distance apart and hands on wall at shoulder height.
2. Patient shifts hips laterally from side to side toward restriction four to five times with increasing movement into the restrictive barrier (**a**).
3. Patient introduces extension by sagging the trunk forward while maintaining the arms straight (**b**).
4. The side shifting and extension components are gradually increased with five to seven repetitions.

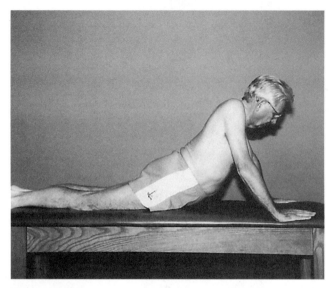

Figure 20.81
Lumbar spine extension restriction.
Self-correction position prone.
1. Patient prone with hand on table or floor.
2. Patient straightens elbows and extends trunk from above downward.
3. Spinal muscles are relaxed, and the stretch should be felt in the front of the chest and abdomen.
4. Position is held for 5 to 7 seconds and repeated five to seven times.

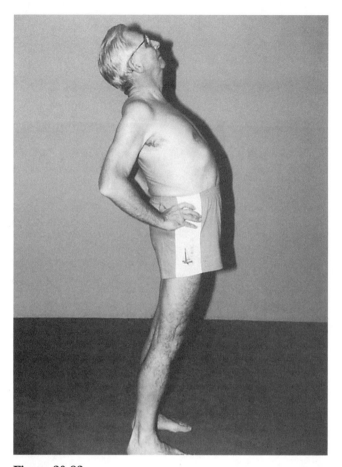

Figure 20.82.
Lumbar spine extension restriction.
Self-correction position standing.
1. Patient standing with hands on posterolateral buttock, feet acetabular distance apart and slightly externally rotated.
2. Patient extends trunk from the head and neck downward and the hips shift anteriorly.
3. Repeat five to seven times with increase in trunk extension each time.
4. This exercise can be added to the hip shift (Fig. 20.79) to correct the extension component of a flexed, rotated, and side-bent lumbar dysfunction.

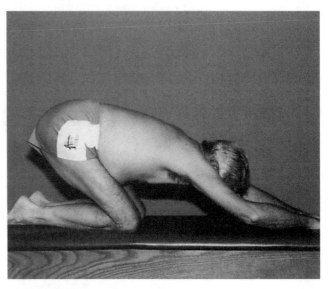

Figure 20.84.
Lumbar spine "prayer stretch."
Self-correction position prone.
1. Patient begins in the hands and knees position with feet and knees hip-width apart.
2. Patient sinks back, attempting to touch buttocks to the heels.
3. Patient's head and neck are dropped into flexion, allowing the spine to flex and the chest to drop to the floor.
4. The hands remain in contact with the floor.
5. Stretch is held for 10 to 15 seconds and is repeated three to four times.
6. This stretch deals with the flexion component of lumbar nonneutral dysfunctions.

Figure 20.83.
Trunk rotation.
Reeducation position supine.
1. Patient lies with knees and hips flexed, with feet together and flat on the table or floor. Arms are extended with the palms down.
2. Patient's knees are slowly dropped to one side and held for a 5 to 7 second stretch (**a**).
3. Knees are slowly brought back to neutral by touching each spine segment from above downward to the table or floor. Hip and thigh muscles are passive; the motion comes from the trunk muscles (**b**).
4. The other side is exercised in a similar manner. Repeat five to seven times.
5. This exercise is good for the rotational component of lumbar nonneutral dysfunctions.

Self-correction for ERS dysfunctions first needs to restore flexion. Single and bilateral knees to the chest in the supine position can achieve flexion. Another very effective exercise is a prayer stretch in the hands and knees position (Fig. 20.84). To restore flexion, rotation, and side bending together, the diagonal hip sink in the hands and knees position has been effective (Fig. 20.85). This exercise is also useful for stretching the quadratus lumborum and strengthening the gluteus medius and minimis muscles. Forward bending in step standing (Fig. 20.86) is also effective in self-correcting ERS lumbar dysfunction.

In the thoracic spine, stacked ERS and FRS dysfunctions are common. These should be successfully treated so that the patient can maintain correction at home. In the thoracic region, exercises to elongate the spine are always helpful. One exercise that is most useful is the wall stretch (Fig. 20.26). Another helpful elongation exercise is the kneeling prayer latissimus dorsi stretch (Fig. 20.87). For correction of restric-

Figure 20.85
Lumbar Spine Extended, Rotated, and Side-bent Dysfunctions.
Self-correction Position "Diagonal Hip Sink."
1. Patient begins in hands and knees position.
2. Patient sits back diagonally, (toward the dysfunctional facet) introducing flexion, side bending, and rotation.
3. Position is held for 5 to 7 seconds and repeated five to seven times.
4. With each repetition, an increased amount of "hip sink" is done, increasing the mobility of the dysfunctional facet.
5. This exercise also strengthens the gluteal muscles. The operator may offer resistance alternately to the buttocks and opposite shoulder as the gluteal muscles are asked to work eccentrically and concentrically.
6. This exercise is useful for self-correction of the anteriorly nutated sacrum, which is combined with an extended, rotated, and side-bent dysfunction at L5. Deep inhalation respiratory activating force is combined with the stretch position.

Figure 20.86.
Lumbar Spine Extended, Rotated, and Side-bent Dysfunction.
Self-correction Position Standing. (ERS_{right} example)
1. Patient stands and places one foot on a chair or stool with the other leg straight.
2. Patient places both hands on the sides of the knee and bends forward, drawing chest toward the knee as the hands slide down the leg to the ankle.
3. Position is held for 5 to 7 seconds and repeated five to seven times with increased trunk flexion with each effort.

tions of extension, a hands and knees rocking procedure (Fig. 20.88) and a supported extension during kneel stand (Fig. 20.89) are effective. For correction of restrictions of flexion, a variant to the classic cat back exercise is used (Fig. 20.90). The specific location of flexion can be isolated and flexion motion enhanced. A wall press-up exercise promotes flexion in the upper thoracic spine as well as neuromuscular reeducation of scapular control, particularly weakness of the serratus anterior and lower trapezius muscles

(Fig. 20.91). To restore rotation, the procedure identified for the lumbar spine (Fig. 20.83) is useful particularly in the lower thoracic region. A seated trunk rotation exercise uses respiratory assist as part of the rotary maneuver beginning from above downward or from below upward, to isolate the region most in need of rotary enhancement (Fig. 20.92). In the cervical spine, FRS and ERS dysfunctions, which are found in the typical cervical segments, can be treated as individual segments. Exercises for FRS (Fig. 20.93) and ERS dysfunctions (Fig. 20.94) are useful. The long restrictors of the cervical spine should be stretched prior to attempts at self-mobilization. In the C1 to C2 area, the primary motion to be restored is rotation. This is accomplished in the seated position with neck in full flexion and rotated to the restricted side (Fig. 20.95). At the occipitoatloid junction, the primary motion of flexion/extension is specificity enhanced to one occipitoatloid joint by rotating 30 degrees and introducing flexion and extension to the side to be mobilized (Fig. 20.96).

Figure 20.87.

Thoracolumbar and lumbar spine.

Self-correction position kneeling.

1. Patient kneels with elbows together on a stool or chair.
2. With the lumbar spine in neutral, patient sits back with the buttocks toward the heels.
3. Position is held for 30 seconds and repeated twice.
4. Patient performs a series of deep inhalation/exhalation efforts to mobilize vertebral segments while in the elongated position.
5. This is the same as the latissimus dorsi stretch (Fig. 20.49a) but is included here as a self-correction stretch to be used after any self-correction procedure for flexed, rotated, and side-bent or extended, rotated, and side-bent lumbar dysfunctions.

Figure 20.88.

Thoracolumbar and lumbar spine.

Self-correction position for extension restriction.

1. Patient on hands and knees and shifts weight over the hands while sagging the abdomen to extend the lumbar spine (**a**).
2. While maintaining extension, the weight is transferred over the hips, increasing extension into the thoracic spine (**b**).
3. Each extreme of the position is held for 5 to 7 seconds and repeated five to seven times.
4. This "hands and knees rocking" procedure is used after treatment for flexed, rotated, and side-bent dysfunctions to enhance extension movement.

Figure 20.89.
Thoracolumbar and lumbar spine.
Self-correction position for extension restriction.
1. Patient kneels with back to stool or chair and places hands on stool.
2. Patient extends hips with strong gluteal contraction.
3. Patient pushes down on hands and lifts the sternum by bringing scapulae down and back. (Hands may point forward or backward.)
4. Spinal extension is enhanced by anterior translation and lifting of the trunk.
5. Position is held for 5 to 7 seconds and repeated five to seven times.

Figure 20.90.
Thoracolumbar spine
Self-correction position (cat back).
1. Patient on hands and knees.
2. Patient arches back at location of segmental restriction and rocks forward and backward, enhancing flexion movement.
3. Patient lifts segment to the ceiling and holds for 5 to 7 seconds and repeats five to seven times.

Figure 20.91.
Upper thoracic spine.
Self-correction position (wall press).
1. Patient stands facing the wall with hands at shoulder height and maintains a neutral lumbar lordosis (**a**).
2. Patient retracts and depresses scapulae and touches the nose to the wall (**b**).
3. Patient holds position for 5 to 7 seconds and then pushes back slowly from the wall, dropping the head and neck into flexion, protracting the shoulders, and lifting the upper thoracic spine toward the ceiling (**c**).
4. Patient holds the position for 5 to 10 seconds and repeats the procedure five to seven times.

Figure 20.92.
Thoracic spine.
Self-correction position for rotation restriction.

1. Patient sits sideways in a chair holding the back with both hands.
2. Patient inhales deeply, straightens the spine, and during deep exhalation introduces rotation from above downward for three to four segments. Position is held for 5 to 7 seconds and repeated with increased rotation each time.
3. The arms assist in the rotational effort.
4. As the rotation get lower in the thoracic spine, the weight is shifted to the buttock opposite to the rotation.
5. Repeat three to five times on each side for symmetric balance.

Figure 20.93.
Cervical spine flexed, rotated, and side-bent dysfunction.
Self-correction position sitting.

1. Patient sits and grasps the articular of the lower vertebrae of the dysfunctional segment.
2. While stabilizing lower pillar, patient extends, side bends, and rotates the cervical spine to the right and looks up with the eyes.
3. Position is held for 5 to 7 seconds and repeated five to seven times.

Figure 20.94.
Cervical spine extended, rotated, and side-bent dysfunction.
Self-correction position sitting.
1. Patient sits and grasps the articular pillar of the superior vertebrae of the dysfunctional segment.
2. Patient flexes, side bends, and rotates the cervical spine to the right and looks down with the eyes.
3. Position is held for 5 to 7 seconds and repeated five to seven times.

Figure 20.95.
Cervical spine (atlantoaxial).
Self-correction position sitting.
1. Patient sits and grasps stool or chair with both hands.
2. Patient flexes neck to 45 degrees and introduces rotation in the direction of motion loss.
3. Position is held for 5 to 7 seconds and repeats five to seven times with increased rotation after each effort.
4. Inhalation/exhalation effort at the barrier assists in the correction.

Figure 20.96.
Cervical spine (occipitoatloid).
Self-correction position sitting.
1. Patient sitting with both hands grasping chair or stool.
2. Patient turns head 30 degrees.
3. Patient nods head while translating backward, introducing flexion movement to the condyle **(a)**.
4. Patient translates head forward, leading with the chin, introducing extension movement of the condyle **(b)**.
5. The position engaging the restriction is held for 5 to 7 seconds and repeated five to seven times.

This author's enthusiasm for exercise results from personal experience. With a more than 40-year history of recurrent back and right lower extremity pain and with significant pathology identified on radiographs, the best control of these symptoms has occurred after using the exercise principles identified in this chapter. Figure 20.97 shows plain films that demonstrate significant spondylosis, degenerative disc disease, lateral recess stenosis, and second-degree

Figure 20.97.
a: Anteroposterior erect lumbar spine. **b:** Lateral lumbar spine. **c:** Lateral spot film lumbosacral junction. **d:** Left oblique lumbar spine.

Figure 20.97.
e: Right oblique lumbar spine.

spondylolisthesis with isthmus defect bilaterally at L-5. Despite this osseous pathology, the author has demonstrated many of the exercises advocated in this chapter, highlighting the functional capacity of significant osseous pathology in the lumbar spine. In the clinic, the author challenges his patients to perform exercises as he can demonstrate. It is a powerful motivational tool.

THE EXERCISE PRESCRIPTION

Each patient needs an individualized exercise prescription. For this prescription to be effective, the patient must be compliant with the program and be willing to assume responsibility for his or her own health. If the practitioner continues to see the same dysfunctional pattern in the patient, several issues need be addressed. First, the patient may not be doing the exercises or may be doing them improperly. Second, some dysfunctional pathology has been missed. Third, the exercise prescription needs modification.

The prescription should include four elements: proprioceptive balance training, stretching of tight muscles, retraining of inhibited muscles, and aerobic training. They are prescribed in that sequence as well. Proprioceptive balance training is given to help restore correct muscle firing patterns. Then stretching, first manually by the operator and then followed by self-stretches, is performed until symmetry is achieved. When symmetry has occurred, inhibition of the antagonist is lessened and the retraining of inhibited muscle can begin. When the patient's capacity for an aerobic program has arrived, an appropriate aerobic exercise is given.

A home program should not contain more than five or six exercises. When one objective has been achieved, that exercise can be replaced by another depending on the progress being made. The basic program of balance training, stretching, and retraining should be accomplished in 20 minutes per day. When an aerobic program is added, it should be gradually increased until 20 minutes daily. The aerobic exercise should be one that the patient enjoys whether it is a "pep" walk, treadmill walking, Airdyne exercycle, Nordic trac, or swimming. Jogging and running are usually not recommended because they perpetuate tightness of the hip flexors.

SUMMARY

Exercise is a powerful tool in the management of patients with chronic musculoskeletal disorders and enhances the effectiveness of manual medicine interventions. The principles enumerated here focusing on centrally mediated and controlled motor balance, followed by stretching, and subsequently with strengthening (retraining), have been most effective. A properly designed and executed exercise program gives patients control of their level of musculoskeletal health and is very cost-effective.

SUGGESTED READINGS

Bullock-Saxton JE, Janda V, Bullock MI. The influence of ankle sprain injury on muscle activation during hip extension. *Int J Sports Med* 1994;15:330–334.

Evjenth O, Hamberg J. *Muscle stretching in manual therapy. a clinical manual: vol. 1 and 2.* Alfta, Sweden: Alfta Rehab Forlag, 1984.

Hodges PW, Richardson CA. Inefficient muscular stabilization of the lumbar spine associated with low back pain: a motor control evaluation of transversus abdominis. *Spine* 1996;21:2640–2650.

Hodges PW, Richardson CA. Altered trunk muscle recruitment in people with low back pain with upper limb movement at different speeds. *Arch Phys Med Rehabil* 1999;80:1005–1012.

Janda V. Muscle and motor control in cervicogenic disorders: assessment and management. In: Grant R, ed. *Physical therapy of the cervical and thoracic spine, clinics in physical therapy.* New York: Churchill Livingstone, 1994:195–216.

Janda V. Muscle weakness and inhibition (pseudoparesis) in back pain syndromes. In: Grieve GP, ed. *Modern manual therapy of the vertebral column.* Edinburgh, UK: Churchill Livingstone, 1986:197–201.

Janda V. Muscles as a pathogenic factor in back pain. In: *The Treatment of Patients. Proceedings of the 4th Conference on International Federation of Orthopedic Manipulative Therapists,* Christchurch, New Zealand, 1980:1–23.

Janda V. Muscles: central nervous motor regulation and back problems. In: Korr I, ed. *The neurobiologic mechanisms in manipulative therapy.* New York: Plenum Publishing, 1977:27–41.

Kendall FP, McCreary EK, Provance PG. *Muscles: testing and function,* 4th ed. Baltimore: Lippincott Williams & Wilkins, 1993.

Lewit K. *Manipulative therapy in rehabilitation of the motor system,* 2nd ed. Oxford: Butterworth, 1991.

McKenzie RA. *The lumbar spine, mechanical diagnosis and therapy.* Waikenae, New Zealand: Spinal Publications, 1981.

Richardson C, Jull G, Hodges P, et al. *Therapeutic exercise for spinal segmental stabilization in low back pain: scientific basis and clinical approach.* Edinburgh, UK: Churchill Livingstone, 1999.

21

ADJUNCTIVE DIAGNOSTIC PROCEDURES

The manual medicine practitioner primarily uses the structural diagnostic process to determine the presence or absence of somatic dysfunction, and its clinical significance, before instituting a manual medicine treatment. Adjunctive diagnostic procedures are frequently of assistance in determining the presence or absence of organic pathology of the musculoskeletal system in addition to the dysfunction. It is helpful to know whether the symptom presentation is due to organic pathology, dysfunction, or a combination of both. In most instances, it is a combination of both and the practitioner needs to address all components of the patient's presentation. Manual medicine must be practiced within the context of total patient care.

IMAGING PROCEDURES

The appropriate use and inappropriate abuse of imaging procedures remain controversial within the health care system. Imaging procedures can be expensive, carry some risk, demonstrate both false-positive and false-negative results, and provide information that may be of little assistance in patient care. An admonition for all musculoskeletal medicine practitioners is to treat patients and not images. The following sections are not designed to be comprehensive but to share with the reader the opinions of this author on the assistance imaging procedures can have in manual medicine practice.

Plain Films

Plain films of the lumbar spine and pelvis are not necessary before performing a manual medicine intervention. If the history and physical examination lead the practitioner to a high index of suspicion of organic bone or joint disease, plain films are indicated, because they are relatively inexpensive, reveal osseous and joint anatomy, and can be of assistance in ruling out major traumatic, neoplastic, and inflammatory diseases. Plain films should include as a minimum anteroposterior (AP) (Fig. 21.1) and lateral projections (Fig. 21.2). Right oblique (Fig. 21.3), and left oblique (Fig. 21.4) studies, while not routinely performed, provide good visualization of

the zygapophysial joints and of the pars interarticularis. These views visualize the "Scottie dog" appearance of the posterior elements of the lumbar spine. The Scottie dog's eye is the pedicle, the associated transverse process is the nose, the superior facet joint is the ear, the inferior facet joint is the front leg, and the neck is the pars interarticularis. A defect through the pars interarticularis is identified as spondylolysis and separation of the defect is termed "spondylolisthesis." Another commonly used view is a spot lateral projection of the lumbar sacral junction, particularly

Figure 21.1.
Anteroposterior lumbar spine (supine).

Figure 21.2.
Lateral lumbar spine (erect).

Figure 21.4.
Left oblique lumbar spine.

Figure 21.3.
Right oblique lumbar spine.

Figure 21.5.
Sunshine view of the sacroiliac and lumbosacral joints.

to look at the L5 to S1 disc space. Preference is given to a 30-degree cephalic angled study (sunshine view) (Fig. 21.5) because it provides excellent visualization of the lumbosacral disc space and both sacroiliac joints and is of great assistance in the detailed assessment of transitional lumbosacral vertebrae. Note the bat wing transverse process with a pseudoarthrosis to the sacrum and to the ilium in Fig. 21.5. This structural variation is one of the few predictors of future pathology and disability within the lumbar spine. The disc above the transitional vertebra is statistically at risk for herniation and the development of discogenic radiculopathy.

Plain Film Postural Study. If the practitioner has suspicion of a short-leg, pelvic-tilt syndrome on the basis of the clinical finding of unleveling of the iliac crest and greater trochanter in the standing position, plain film postural study is useful in confirming the diagnosis and in determining the amount of the leg inequality and unleveling of the sacral base. The postural study includes an AP projection of the lumbar spine and pelvis with the patient standing (Fig. 21.6) and in the lateral projection (Fig. 21.2). Great care by the technician is necessary to obtain quality images for postural analysis. The important technical factors are as follows:

1. An upright Bucky level with floor or footrest of the table
2. Fourteen by seventeen inch (14 × 17) film loaded level in the cassette
3. Cassette loaded level in Bucky
4. Patient standing erect with equal weight distribution on feet 15 cm (6 in.) apart at the medial malleolus
5. One meter (40 in.) target-to-film distance
6. Vertical film centered at iliac crest
7. Central ray projected at center of film

Figure 21.6.
Anteroposterior lumbar spine erect for postural analysis.

The AP and erect films are measured in the following fashion:

1. AP projection
    A. A horizontal line is drawn across the top of each femoral head.
    B. A horizontal line is drawn across the sacral base. Three variations are provided in the order of their reliability.
        (1) Across the most posterior aspect of the posterior margin of S1 body;
        (2) Inferior aspect of sacral notch (transverse process S1);
        (3) Medial corner of S1 facet at junction with sacral body.
    C. Two vertical lines are drawn from the bottom of the film through the highest point of the femoral head to the line drawn across the sacral base.
    D. The difference in the distance from the femoral head to the bottom of the film is the leg length deficit.
    E. The difference in distance from the sacral base line and the bottom of the film on each side is the amount of sacral base unleveling.
2. Lateral projection
    A. A line is drawn across the superior aspect of the body of S-1 to meet a horizontal line drawn parallel to the bottom of the film at the level of the anterior aspect of S-1. The resultant acute angle is called the "sacral base angle." In the erect position, the normal sacral base angle is 40 degrees plus or minus 2 degrees.

B. The midportion of the third lumbar body is identified and a vertical line dropped from the mid-third lumbar body. Normally this line should strike on the superior aspect of S-1.

3. Lumbar scoliosis

A. Assessment is made of the lumbar scoliosis in the AP projection. The normal adaptive process should show a lumbar convexity toward the side of sacral base unleveling.

Experience has shown that interrater and intrarater reliability using this methodology is 1 mm of difference. Unless the history and physical examination require plain film study before the initiation of treatment, it is advisable to treat the lumbar spine and pelvis to maximum biomechanical balance before performing a postural radiographic study. Occasionally, dysfunction of the lumbar spine and pelvis, particularly dysfunction associated with major muscle imbalance, makes the study technically difficult and the measurements less than reliable. The study is best performed with the patient at maximum biomechanical function of the lumbar spine, pelvis, and lower extremities.

Dynamic Studies

Plain films are frequently supplemented by dynamic studies in the erect position performing AP right-side bending (Fig. 21.7), left-side bending (Fig. 21.8), backward-bending (Fig. 21.9), and forward-bending lateral projections (Fig. 21.10). Assessment is made of the dynamic changes in the AP and lateral projections and compared with the neutral AP and lateral views. In the side-bending dynamic films, assessment is made of the presence or absence of neutral or nonneutral lumbar vertebral coupling. Figure 21.7 demonstrates side bending to the right with rotation of the vertebrae into the concavity consistent with nonneutral vertebral mechanics in the lumbar spine. Figure 21.8 shows side bending to the left with rotation of lumbar vertebrae to the right, consistent with neutral vertebral motion in the lumbar spine. By overlying one film on another, it is frequently possible to identify which segment within the lumbar spine is resisting side bending to the right or to the left. In the forward-bending and backward-bending lateral projections, analysis is made of intersegmental mobility. Again, by overlying one film on the other, in reference to the neutral lateral projection, it is possible to identify the vertebral segment that resists forward or backward bending. Coupling the neutral or nonneutral behavior of the lumbar spine in side bending with interseg-

Figure 21.7.
Anteroposterior erect, right-side bending dynamic film.

Figure 21.8.
Anteroposterior erect, left-side bending dynamic film.

mental restriction of flexion or extension can assist in the evaluation of nonneutral vertebral dysfunction within the lumbar spine. The role of dynamic studies remains controversial because of difficulty in the biomechanical research of the methodology. Despite this concern, clinical experience has shown them to be of assistance in the collaboration of the structural diagnostic finding.

Special Imaging Studies

There are a number of special imaging studies that have use in musculoskeletal problems particularly in lower back and lower extremity pain syndromes. Before ordering a special imaging study, the practitioner should show care in selecting a procedure that will provide the information desired. Different imaging studies provide different information. Special imaging studies should be done to confirm impressions gained from the clinical examination.

Magnetic Resonance Imaging. Special images such as magnetic resonance imaging (MRI) should not be used as a screening tool to look for pathology in a patient presenting with back pain. MRI has many advantages in the diagnostic process and provides the best information about the soft tissues of the musculoskeletal system. It has become the imaging method

of choice for diagnosis of disc herniation, cord lesions, brain lesions, and many of the less common developmental variants like syringomyelia and tethered cord (Fig. 21.11). MRI can provide images that demonstrate the nucleus of the disc similar to those revealed in a discogram and outline the spinal canal and its contents similar to those of a myelogram. The procedure involves no ionizing radiation, is noninvasive, and has few contraindications, namely metal implants and pacemakers. MRI gantries are becoming larger so that the patient is less likely to become claustrophobic in the machine. One drawback to MRI studies is the difficulty in obtaining dynamic studies because of the dimensions of the gantry and the fact that the patient is in an unloaded position. With special technical effort it is possible to obtain some dynamic flexion and extension studies of the cervical spine. Dynamic studies of the lumbar spine are much more difficult. Upright MRI technology has recently been developed and is currently being used in research studies of spinal mechanics in the loaded position. In the future, this technology may become available for clinical use and is exciting to contemplate.

Computed Tomography. Computed tomography (CT) studies have a longer history than MRI. CT is the imaging method of choice when looking for morphology of the osseous system. It is also useful in identifying disc disease, including herniation with extru-

Figure 21.9.
Lateral backward-bending dynamic film.

Figure 21.10.
Forward-bending, lateral, dynamic film.

Figure 21.11.
Magnetic resonance imaging, lumbar spine, sagittal view.

Figure 21.12.
Computed tomography scan, lumbar spine, bone window.

sion of nuclear material into the central and lateral vertebral canals as well as lateral and interior herniations (Fig. 21.12). This technology is particularly useful in the assessment of central and lateral recess stenosis as seen in Fig. 21.12. CT can be combined with discography and myelography to provide additional diagnostic information (Fig. 21.13). Plain CT is noninvasive but does require the patient to be exposed to ionizing radiation. Metallic implants are not

Figure 21.13.
Lumbar spine, discogram computed tomography.

a contraindication but the images are frequently distorted by artifact. A discogram CT and myelogram CT require an accompanying invasive procedure.

Myelography. Myelography is one of the older special imaging methods in the diagnosis of spinal pathology. Historically, it has been used for localization of disc pathology, neural compression, blockage of cerebral spinal fluid, and intraspinal pathology such as cord tumor. It is an invasive procedure and some of the dye material used in the past was toxic and led to complications. There is a statistically significant increase in arachnoiditis with pantopaque myelography. Currently, water-soluble contrast materials are much less toxic, but they are contraindicated in a few individuals who are iodine-sensitive. False-negatives in myelography are common for disc disease at the L5 to S1 level. Myelography occasionally becomes a procedure of choice, particularly in association with CT imaging, in certain diagnostic challenges.

Discography. Discography continues to have its advocates and detractors. It is an invasive procedure with considerable technical difficulty. Radiopaque material is injected into the nucleus of the disc and images are made for assessment of intradiscal pathology (Fig. 21.14). Discography also provides the opportunity to assess whether a disc is a pain generator. An injection into a normal disc is usually not painful. Injection into a diseased disc is frequently painful and if it replicates the patient's pain complaint, gives some corroboration of the disc as the site of pain generation. In the presence of disc herniation there is commonly exacerbation of the associated radiculopathy. Like myelography, the procedure is invasive and requires the introduction of a foreign substance that carries some allergic risk. Another value of discography is the ability to perform the study with the patient

Figure 21.14.
Disc anteroposterior and lateral projections.

Figure 21.15.
L4 to L5 lumbar discogram, erect, forward bending and backward bending.

loaded and unloaded. In the erect loaded position, flexion and extension can be performed to further assist in the diagnostic process (Fig. 21.15). Note in Fig. 21.15 that there was additional extrusion of the opaque nuclear material in a posterior direction during trunk backward bending. Like discography, myelography can be performed in the standing loaded position, and the patient can be subjected to dynamic stress of forward bending, backward bending, and right- to left-side bending.

Diagnostic Blocks and Injections

On occasion, additional special studies can be of assistance in determining the location of the pain generator and the significance of altered anatomy. These procedures include zygapophysial and sacroiliac joint injections, selected nerve blocks, and the previously discussed discography. These procedures require fluoroscopic control, the use of contrast material, and the instillation of anesthetic agents to determine if the structure is painful and responds to a local block (Figs. 21.16 and 21.17). Figures 21.16 and 21.17 show the role of a zygapophysial injection in determining if the spondylolisthesis at this level was symptomatic. Note that the needle is placed in the L4 to L5 joint, but with instillation of contrast

Figure 21.16.
L4 to L5 joint block, anteroposterior projection.

Figure 21.17.
L4 to L5 zygapophysial joint block, oblique projection.

material there, the image shows delineation of the pars defect and the zygapophysial joint at L5 to S1. The procedure was pain-free for the patient and the conclusion was that this defect was not pain producing. The sacroiliac joint can be challenged and visualized by arthrography (Figs. 21.18–21.20). Under fluoroscopic control, the inferior margin of the synovial portion of the sacroiliac joint can be entered and contrast material injected. Like zygapophysial joint injection, if the joint is contributing to pain generation, the injection is painful to the patient. Instillation of local anesthetic with relief of concordant pain identifies this structure as a pain generator. Figures 21.18 through 21.20 show an example of anterior capsular diverticula in the presence of a joint that was positive to the challenge of injection. After instillation of local anesthetic, the patient experienced complete removal of the concordant pain. This confirmed the left sacroiliac joint as a pain generator contributing to the patient's presentation. Figure 21.21 is a special CT view of the sacroiliac joints in the case represented in Figs. 21.18 through 21.20. Note the asymmetric relationship of the anterior aspects of the sacrum to the posterior aspects of the ilium as shown by the horizontal lines. This finding was imaging confirmation of the palpatory assessment of sacral torsion in this patient. Occasionally, information can be obtained about the functional capacity of the anatomy that is so well displayed by such imaging techniques. Selective nerve blocks require fluoroscopic guidance and again seek to identify whether a specific nerve root and its sheath are contributing to pain generation. This technology has

Figure 21.18.
Left sacroiliac arthrogram, anteroposterior view.

greater value in the diagnosis of acute discogenic radiculopathy than it does in the dysfunctional pathology dealt with by manual medicine.

Special Magnetic Resonance Imaging Studies

MRI is an excellent technology for distinguishing differences in soft tissues. For the past 2 years, a special protocol for MRI imaging of the upper cervical spine has been used to identify selective fatty replacement of rectus capitis posterior minor and rectus capitis posterior major muscles. This fatty replacement is seen in 87% of patients presenting with posttraumatic cervical cranial pain syndromes and is not found in 100% in a normative population (Figs. 21.22 and 21.23). Figure 21.22 shows good definition

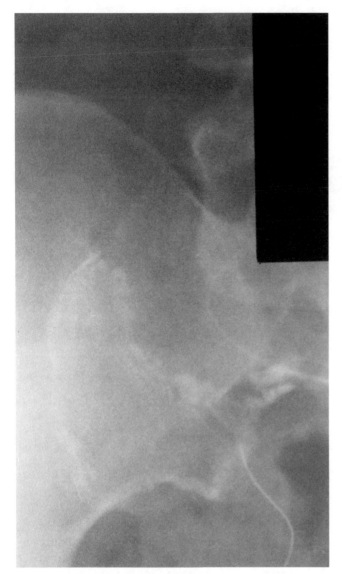

Figure 21.19.
Left sacroiliac arthrogram, right anterior oblique.

Figure 21.20.
Left sacroiliac arthrogram, left anterior oblique.

Figure 21.21.
Computed tomography scan of sacroiliac joints.

of both the rectus capitis posterior major and minor, with muscle densities identified with arrows, in an asymptomatic patient with no history of trauma. Figure 21.23 shows fatty replacement of rectus capitis posterior major and minor muscles (arrows) in a patient 2 years after a motor vehicle injury with flexion–extension of the cervical spine and resultant pain in the upper cervical region with radiation of head pain anteriorly from the cranial base. The cause of the fatty replacement is under study and its overall significance is yet to be determined. Intuitively one would assume that if muscle has been replaced by fat and has lost its contractile properties, this might contribute to persistent symptoms and the lack of response to manual medicine using muscle energy activating force.

Electrodiagnostic Studies

The use of electromyography and nerve conduction studies can be of assistance in the differential diagnosis of cervicobrachial and lower extremity pain syndromes to rule in or rule out the presence of signifi-

Figure 21.22.
Cervical spine magnetic resonance imaging in non-trauma, nonsymptomatic patient.

Figure 21.23.
Cervical spine magnetic resonance imaging in posttraumatic symptomatic patient.

cant radiculopathy from discogenic disease or other causes. Nerve conduction studies are particularly of value in documenting the presence of the carpal tunnel or tarsal tunnel syndromes. There are many sophisticated neurophysiologic tests available but they are seldom needed in the practice of manual medicine. Electromyography in the presence of acute radiculopathy is not diagnostic for the initial 3-week period: A negative study in an early presentation does not rule out the presence of radiculopathy. A positive electromyogram (EMG) with acute changes can help confirm the diagnosis of discogenic radiculopathy in a patient who presents with classic clinical findings when the positive findings are consistent with the diagnosis. This author uses confirmatory EMG studies before subjecting patients to surgical intervention for disc disease.

Electromyography of the rectus capitis posterior muscles identified by MRI (Fig. 21.23) has shown that they have denervation changes. The fatty replacement is not disuse atrophy, it is true neurologic change. The posterior primary division of C1 innervates the superior and inferior oblique muscles and the rectus capitis posterior major and posterior minor muscles. This leads one to wonder why fatty replacement of the obliques has never been seen and is rarely seen in the rectus capitis posterior major muscle. The rectus capitis posterior minor innervation is from the terminal branch of C1 and travels through the belly of the rec-

tus capitis posterior major. Perhaps the answer is that during the flexion–extension injury, the terminal branch is avulsed and the rectus capitis posterior minor is dennervated. It is interesting to note that during these EMG studies, the muscle is most active during anterior translation of the head and not during extension. The apparent role of the rectus capitis posterior minor muscle is to reduce forward translation of the occiput during flexion movement.

Surface EMG is of diagnostic assistance in the determination of normal or abnormal muscle firing pattern sequences. Janda has described normal muscle firing sequences for hip extension, hip abduction, and shoulder abduction (see Chapter 20). Surface EMG studies have been used in the research that has defined that major role of the transversus abdominus muscle in core stability. These aberrations can be documented by surface EMG study and the technology can be of assistance in documenting the response to treatment interventions.

Laboratory Testing

The practitioner has a vast array of laboratory diagnostic tests available. In musculoskeletal medicine, there are a few that can be of assistance, particularly in ruling out rheumatologic conditions and in identifying general systemic illness. It has been said that the sedimentation rate takes the temperature of the musculoskeletal system. It is a valuable screening test requiring additional laboratory testing if positive. Basic rheumatologic tests are found within the arthritic profile, and the findings may direct the clinician toward more extensive antinuclear antibody and DNA studies. Assessment of thyroid function is frequently of assistance in patients with chronic pain. Borderline hypothyroidism is frequently seen in patients with primary and secondary fibromyalgias. Not all patients who present with musculoskeletal pain syndromes are experiencing biomechanical dysfunction. The alert practitioner uses all tools available, including laboratory testing, to assess the total patient.

Psychological Evaluation

Psychological assessment of patients with musculoskeletal pain syndromes, particularly those with chronic pain, is frequently of assistance in patient management. Psychosocial factors play a large role in back pain disability. There are a number of standardized tests such as the Minnesota Multiphasic Personality Inventory test that have had extensive use in assessing the psychological and psychiatric status of a patient. A one-on-one psychological evaluation by a trained clinical psychologist conversant with musculoskeletal pain syndromes can be of great assistance. Psychological evaluation, particularly the neuropsychological examination, is of considerable value in identifying the presence and severity of traumatic brain injury. Traumatic brain injury is frequently seen in patients with chronic pain syndromes and is probably underdiagnosed. A probing history will frequently identify trauma resulting in transient unconsciousness and disorientation.

Occupational Therapy Assessment

A cognitive, perceptual, motor evaluation by a skilled occupational therapist is another test useful in the diagnosis of traumatic brain injury. Assessment of the work site, particularly in those patients presenting with repetitive strain injuries, can be very useful in total patient management. Work-site modification is frequently beneficial in the rehabilitation of disabled patients as well as in the prevention of injuries in the future.

Nutritional Evaluation

The services of a skilled nutritionist can be of assistance in the rehabilitation process. Many patients with musculoskeletal pain syndromes have poor nutrition with heavy use of caffeine, alcohol, and fast foods. A poor diet contributes to an unhealthy musculoskeletal system and interferes with normal neurologic control of motor system function. Obesity continues to be a societal problem particularly in patients with chronic musculoskeletal problems that reduce the patient's activity level. Smoking contributes to poor response to both nonoperative and operative care of spinal problems. Reduction in smoking, alcohol, and drugs, plus a well-balanced diet resulting in appropriate weight, can be of major significance in the recovery of patients with musculoskeletal problems.

CONCLUSION

The manual medicine practitioner should be aware of the role of adjunctive diagnostic procedures in patient assessment. Knowledge of the attributes and shortcomings of many of the aforementioned diagnostic procedures is necessary for their appropriate use. The practitioner should become acquainted with the expertise of other disciplines that can be included in the patient management process. Such knowledge will lead to the appropriate use and not the inappropriate abuse of medical technology.

SUGGESTED READINGS

Fisk JW. Clinical and radiological assessment of leg length. *N Z Med J* 1975;81:477–480.

Friberg O. Clinical symptoms and biomechanics of lumbar spine and hip joint in leg length inequality. *Spine* 1983;8:643–651.

Greenman PE. Lift therapy, use and abuse. *J Am Osteopath Assoc* 1978;79:238–250.

Hoffman KS, Hoffman LL. Effects of adding sacral base leveling to osteopathic manipulative treatment of back pain: a pilot study. *J Am Osteopath Assoc* 1994;94:217–226.

Irwin RE. Reduction of lumbar scoliosis by use of a heel lift to level the sacral base. *J Am Osteopath Assoc* 1991;91:34–44.

22

ADJUNCTIVE THERAPEUTIC PROCEDURES

Manual medicine is a powerful tool in the management of many health problems, particularly those involving the musculoskeletal system. In some cases, manual medicine is the primary therapeutic intervention. Other therapies may be used with manual medicine. When using manual medicine techniques, it is essential that it be done within the context of total patient care and the practitioner must determine that the manual medicine interventions are appropriate for the patient's physical condition.

The following are comments on a variety of other therapeutic interventions that this author has found to be most useful.

MEDICATION

In using an oral or injectable medication, the practitioner should be knowledgeable about the actions, reactions, and iatrogenic effects of any substance used. The medication protocol should be as simple as possible. A general observation is that the more potent the medication is for its effectiveness, the more common are its side effects and reactions.

Medication for pain control is of great importance in the management of musculoskeletal conditions. The longer the nociceptive process is ongoing, the more likely it is that sensitization of pain pathways and deprogramming of motor control will occur. The management of pain associated with acute tissue injury is quite different from the management of pain that has been present for months or years. Acute pain is characterized by its specific localization, lancinating quality, and associated tissue damage in a specific structure of the musculoskeletal system. Chronic musculoskeletal pain is quite different. It is characterized by being less well localized, more diffuse, and frequently a burning quality.

Analgesics and Narcotics

Analgesics and narcotics are most useful for the acute painful condition. In acute pain, it is advisable to see that the dose is adequate in strength and availability to control the painful perception. The persistence of nociceptive pathway stimulation has a negative effect on the patient's nervous system and can lead to chronicity.

The dose should be adjusted to avoid peaks and valleys of pain relief and increased pain perception.

It is unknown when acute pain changes to chronic pain. Some view chronicity as being related to time, with the changeover being from 3 to 6 months. Some believe that pain pathway stimulation for 30 days is sufficient to change central pain processing pathways. In chronic pain, the patient continues to perceive pain despite the lack of ongoing tissue damage. This is commonly frustrating for both the attending physician and the patient because of the absence of an identifiable cause of persistent pain. However, to the patient the pain is reality and it needs appropriate attention just as the more commonly recognized acute pain associated with acute tissue damage. Chronic pain in the absence of identifiable tissue damage is managed quite differently from the chronic pain of patients with associated diseases such as malignancy, inflammatory joint disease, and associated rheumatologic conditions. In these conditions, the appropriate mix of medications to assist the patient in the control of pain is clearly indicated. In the patient with chronic pain without ongoing tissue damage or disease process, medications are mainly contraindicated. Analgesics and narcotics seem to contribute to, rather than ameliorate, the chronic pain system. These patients need to be weaned off potent medications as rapidly as possible. During their rehabilitative process, particularly with increasing activity during an exercise program, there may be exacerbation of the tissue reaction, which results in short bursts of acute pain. Appropriate acute pain medication at this time is clearly beneficial, but needs to be discontinued as rapidly as possible. Acetaminophen in adequate doses seems to work well in these instances. The treatment of the patient with chronic pain syndrome requires an integrated team approach with only one physician being responsible for the medication prescriptions.

Antiinflammatory Agents

Another group of medications of great adjunctive use in the management of musculoskeletal conditions is the antiinflammatory agents. The nonsteroidal antiinflammatory drugs (NSAIDs) are quite popular and are available over-the-counter. The classes of NSAIDs differ primarily in the balance of analgesic and antiinflammatory effects and the length of action. Almost all are irritating to the gastrointestinal tract and caution must be used in prescribing these agents for patients with peptic ulcer disease, gastritis, and irritable bowel syndromes. Aspirin is the oldest and least expensive of this group; if tolerated by the patient, it is as good as any. In general, it is most effective to use short-acting NSAIDs in adequate antiinflammatory doses and then wean the patient off the medication as rapidly as possible. This author has found that 2,400 to 3,200 mg of ibuprofen in divided doses for 7 to 10 days is very useful for the patient with acute pain as well as for the acute exacerbation in the patient with chronic pain undergoing active manual medicine intervention and early exercise programming. Caution should be used for the longer acting NSAIDs because patients metabolize these drugs differently and toxic levels can be achieved with little warning. Injectable ketorolac tromethamine (Toradal) is frequently of value in achieving control of acute pain, particularly that associated with acute tissue injury and the acute flare following an active manual medicine intervention. In the long-term management of patients using NSAIDs, careful monitoring of gastrointestinal, hepatic, renal, and hematologic functions is prudent.

The newest of this group are the Cox-2 inhibitors (Celebrex and Veoxx are examples), which have longer action and are somewhat less irritating to the gastrointestinal tract when compared with NSAIDs, but recently there have been more reports of gastrointestinal problems with their long-term use. They are well worth considering in patients with arthritis, both osteoarthritis and rheumatoid disease.

Corticosteroids

Corticosteroids have a place in the management of musculoskeletal conditions, particularly during the acute phase. Oral and injection formulations are available and corticosteroids have particular value in the management of acute radiculopathy. Spinal and caudal epidural steroids have long been used in the management of acute radiculopathies and both have their advocates and their critics. The problem with caudal instillation is the difficulty in achieving levels high enough to affect radiculopathies above S-1. Spinal epidurals can be more precise in localization of steroid effect. Both of these invasive procedures should be done under fluoroscopic control to ensure correct needle placement and appropriate instillation of therapeutic material.

Oral Steroids

Oral steroid use in the presence of radiculopathy has been effective for many years. A regime beginning with 60 to 80 mg of prednisone in divided doses, decreasing daily by 10-mg increments, is effective and inexpensive. Again, caution must be expressed about the patient's tolerance to steroids, particularly from the perspective of the gastrointestinal tract. Cardiovascular and psychic alterations from long-term steroid use are always a risk, as is the danger of aseptic necrosis in the shoulder and hip joints. A guiding principle can be that steroids are useful in short-term application for acute conditions; they are much less useful in chronic conditions. Patients requiring long-term steroid use for the management of systemic disease should be monitored closely for deleterious side effects.

Antidepressants

Another class of drugs found to be useful in musculoskeletal conditions is those that deal with depression associated with chronic pain and in the restoration of the sleep cycle. The tricyclics benefit these patients. There are a number of tricyclic antidepressants, but this author has found amitriptyline (Elavil) to be useful if the patient can tolerate the drug. Doses from 10 to 150 mg may be necessary to restore a normal sleep cycle. There is some evidence that tricyclics have a positive effect on chronic pain pathways.

Muscle Relaxants

The muscle relaxants are very popular in the treatment of acute and chronic musculoskeletal conditions; however, this author has found their use to be quite disappointing. Many of them are central-acting depressants rather than local muscle relaxants. Oral and injectable diazepam (Valium) is somewhat useful in dealing with acute muscle spasm, and if a muscle relaxant is deemed necessary, it is probably the drug of choice.

Medication use requires that the patient understand the prescribed drug's beneficial effects, side effects, length of action, and allergy potential. Simpler medication programs are better. The prescribing physician must know what over-the-counter medications the patient is taking and the drugs prescribed by other physicians for other health problems. Iatrogenic drug interactions contribute greatly to health care cost and should always be on the physicians' mind when picking up a pen and prescription pad.

Injections

Different injection techniques have been useful in musculoskeletal conditions. These techniques have indications and contraindications and require that the practitioner be skilled in their use. Various injection techniques have both diagnostic and therapeutic indications. The use of epidural steroids in radiculopathy has been referred to in Corlicosteroids section. Concurrent selective nerve blocks are of assistance in identifying the nerve root involved with pain generation.

These procedures require adequate training and sufficient volume to maintain the skill for the procedure. They all require fluoroscopic control.

Acupuncture

One of the oldest injection procedures is classic acupuncture. There are a number of different schools of acupuncture that can all be classified as peripheral stimulating treatment. In selected cases, acupuncture has been very useful in assisting in pain control, particularly in patients experiencing postsurgical or dental pain. However, not all patients respond to acupuncture; appropriate selection of the patient, as well as the practitioner, is essential for success.

Trigger Points

Simon and Travell have long advocated the treatment of the primary and secondary trigger points. Some practitioners have found spray and stretch techniques useful. This author has found the injection technique of classic Travell triggers more effective than spray and stretch. A clear relationship between the presence of somatic dysfunction and myofascial trigger points has been observed. Adequate treatment of the somatic dysfunction frequently relieves the trigger points. In other instances, the trigger points persist despite adequate treatment of the somatic dysfunction. Appropriate treatment of the trigger points would then seem indicated. The reverse has also been found true. Primary treatment of trigger points has reduced observable somatic dysfunction in related parts of the musculoskeletal system, but it is not 100% effective. This author prefers to treat them in an integrated fashion and uses dry-needling or lidocaine hydrochloride (Xylocaine) injection to trigger points if they are present after adequate treatment of somatic dysfunction, or if they considered a primary contributor to the patient's presentation. It is interesting to note that trigger points are more common in phasic muscles. The two tonic muscles that seem to have the most persistent trigger points are the quadratus lumborum and the levator scapulae. This author's experience has been that these are the two muscles that may need treatment by injection for resolution. Follow-up treatment of trigger point therapy requires adequate and appropriate exercise, regardless of whether spray and stretch or injection technique is used.

Sacroiliac Injections

The use of injections in the sacroiliac syndrome is useful from the diagnostic and the therapeutic perspectives. Injection into the capsular portion of the joint requires fluoroscopic guidance and is best done from the inferior aspect of the joint. Both pain generation and arthrographic appearance can be used in diagnosing the painful sacroiliac joint. Occasionally, injection of the capsular portion of the joint demonstrates

extravasation of contrast material in an anterior direction outlining the L-5 and S-1 nerve roots. This mechanism may account for the lower extremity pain seen in the sacroiliac syndrome. From a therapeutic perspective, injection into the posterior ligamentous portion of the sacroiliac joint can be useful. If local analgesic infiltration of the posterior sacroiliac joint results in reduction or relief of the patient's pain, the sacroiliac joint is likely the pain generator. Steroid injection into the posterior sacroiliac ligaments for the antiinflammatory effect coupled with appropriate manual medicine and exercise programs have been useful in the management of the sacroiliac syndrome. Infiltration of the posterior sacroiliac ligamentous structures can be done without fluoroscopic control if one is familiar with the anatomy and skilled in the procedure. Instillation of steroids into the posterior sacroiliac ligaments is usually done no more than twice.

A similar, but less commonly used, procedure is the infiltration of local anesthetic and steroid into the posterior aspect of the zygapophysial joint in the lower lumbar spine. This is not classic facet injection that requires fluoroscopic control to ensure that you are in the posterior facet. Without fluoroscopy, it is possible to walk a spinal needle along bone to the base of the transverse process, and by moving slightly above and below, one can instill local anesthetic and steroid into the posterior aspect of the capsule of the joint. This can be useful in short-term management of an acute zygapophysial joint pain syndrome. Again, adequate training and practice are essential to successful performance of this procedure. Complications are exceedingly rare, but must always be considered.

Prolotherapy

A number of musculoskeletal medicine practitioners advocate the injection of proliferent solutions into ligaments. Gedney popularized this procedure in the osteopathic profession and Hackett in the allopathic medical profession. The principal concept is to inject material that stimulates proliferation of collagen in ligament to strengthen the ligament, particularly its attachment to bone, and to reduce ligamentous-related pain. Historically, a number of solutions have been advocated. The most popular current solution is that advocated by Ongley and consists of hypertonic glucose, glycerin, and phenol, diluted with water and then combined with lidocaine hydrochloride (Xylocaine) for injection. The reader is referred to the text *Injection Technique in Orthopaedic Medicine* by Dorman and Ravin for definitive information on this system. Prolotherapy, as it is currently called, has undergone basic and clinical research study and appears to have value in selected cases. As with all injection techniques, there is a learning curve and adequate instruction and practice are essential. This author has found prolotherapy useful in selected patients with recurrent sacroiliac syndrome, particularly those with hypermobility associated with hip bone shear dysfunction and chronic recurrent anteriorly nutated sacroiliac dysfunction with a significant inferior translatory component. Fluoroscopic control is not necessary but is advisable if available. Recently, some researchers have injected proliferent material into the intervertebral disc for the treatment of annular tear. This requires high-level skill and fluoroscopic control.

Recent experience in a small number of cases of fatty replacement of the rectus capitis posterior minor muscle using proliferent injection into the occipital attachments of the muscle and the zygapophysial joints at C1 to C2 has been effective in the relief of the classic occipital headache radiating toward the orbit in these patients.

Prolotherapy is quite uncomfortable for the patient and preinjection medication is frequently useful. Like many technologies, prolotherapy can be overused in the hands of an enthusiastic practitioner. For the right patient with the right diagnostic criteria, it is clearly a technology that can be useful.

ORTHOTIC DEVICES

There are numerous orthotic devices available to the manual medicine practitioner. The following are those that have been found most useful by this author.

Lumbar Corsets

There are numerous lumbar corsets and supporting belts. A contoured belt individualized to the patient by heating of the material can be useful in acute conditions. It stabilizes the patient's trunk during the acute phase, but should be replaced as rapidly as possible by an exercise program of trunk stabilization and control. Dependency on supporting corsets can easily occur. Patients should be cautioned that the corsets are for temporary use only and appropriate exercise is the long-term goal of the treatment plan.

Sacroiliac Cinch Belt

The orthotic device found most useful is the Hackett sacroiliac cinch belt manufactured by Brooks Company (Marshall, MI). These varying-sized belts without padding over the sacrum provide dynamic tension around the pelvis and assist in stability during the rehabilitative process (Fig. 22.1). All patients with hip bone shear dysfunction use them while weight bearing for a minimum of 6 weeks. If the hip bone shear does not recur within a 6-week period, the belt is discontinued except during strenuous exercise and long motor vehicle trips. Occasionally the same device is used for patients with chronic recurrent lower back pain syndrome associated with an anteriorly nutated sacrum, a posteriorly rotated hip bone, and a superiorly dis-

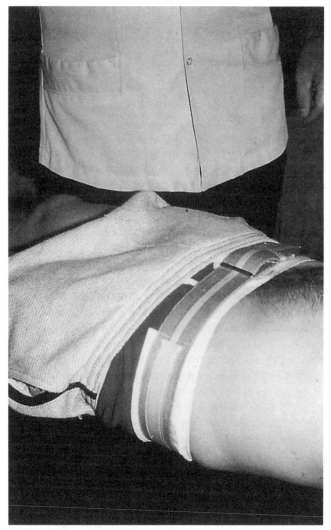

Figure 22.1.
Sacroiliac cinch belt.

placed pubic bone. This device allows free mobility of the pelvis during the walking cycle. Other devices that restrict the sacrum by a compressive pad have limited value in this author's experience.

Heel Lift

The most commonly used orthotic device is a heel lift for the long-term management of the short-leg, pelvic-tilt syndrome. The amount of shortness of a lower extremity and the amount of pelvic tilt that are clinically significant differ greatly from author to author. This author has found that sacral base unleveling of 6 mm or more is clinically significant in patients with lower back and lower extremity pain syndromes, particularly those recurrent in nature. The methodology for the diagnosis of the short-leg, pelvic-tilt syndrome has been described in Chapter 21. There are times when one does not wish to expose the patient to additional radiologic procedures. Clinical assessment of short leg and pelvic tilt can be quite accurate if plain films are available showing the shape and symmetry of the two hip bones and the sacrum. The practitioner can use a series of shims, which are placed under the supposed short lower extremity, to restore functional balance to the pelvis and lumbar spine. The $\frac{1}{8}$-, $\frac{1}{4}$-, $\frac{3}{8}$-, and $\frac{1}{2}$-in. shims are easily obtainable from a lumbar dealer. When the adequate manual medicine intervention has restored mobility to the lumbar spine and pelvis, the patient is evaluated in the erect position sequentially using shims to achieve a level of greater trochanter height, level iliac crest, and symmetric trunk side-bending behavior of the lumbar spine (Fig. 22.2). When the amount of lift needed has been identified, either by radiologic study or clinical assessment as described above, temporary lifts can be placed inside the heel of the shoe to be followed by permanent additions to the heel and sole to balance lumbopelvic

mechanics. In most cases, any shoemaker can add the appropriate amount of lift to the heel and sole. In some instances, a specialized prescription to an orthotist or pedorthist is necessary. Ideally, both heel and sole lifts should be used so that the device does not alter foot and ankle mechanics. Empiric reports indicate that most people can tolerate $\frac{3}{8}$-in. heel lift without additional sole lifting, but this must be individualized for each patient.

The following is a suggested prescription sequence for the use of lift therapy. If the desired lift is $\frac{3}{8}$ in. or less, a single addition of a heel lift to the side with short leg and pelvic tilt is sufficient. Despite past recommendations that lifts be increased in $\frac{1}{8}$-in. increments, most patients tolerate $\frac{3}{8}$ in. in a single application. If the sacral base angle is more than 42 degrees or clinical assessment shows an increased lower lumbar lordosis, it is advisable that the heel on the

Figure 22.2.
A: Iliac crest height. **B:** Trunk side bending left.
C: Trunk side bending right.

long leg be reduced by the appropriate amount, rather than adding to the short leg. One does not want to increase the anterior tilt of the pelvis more than necessary. If the lift needed is more than ⅜ in., but less than ¾ in., it should be applied in two stages. First, add half the amount needed to the heel of the short leg, followed in 3 to 6 weeks by reducing the other half from the heel of the long leg. If the amount of lift needed is more than ¾ in., it should be staged in a maximum of ⅜-in. increments, ultimately resulting in heel and sole lifts of the required amount. It is rare that a patient cannot tolerate lift therapy if the condition is appropriately diagnosed and treated. Caution must be used in the presence of significant degenerative joint disease, particularly of the hip, and in the presence of pelvic girdle osseous asymmetry when using a lift to the long leg to level the sacral base declination. In the latter case, this places additional stress on the hip joint and the lateral stabilizers of the hip, particularly the gluteus medius and minimus muscles. The lumbar spine usually adapts to the short-leg, pelvic-tilt syndrome by scoliosis convex to the side of sacral base declination and short lower extremity. Appropriate lift therapy reduces the severity of the adaptive scoliosis and assists in restoring neutral lumbar mechanics that are more normal. Complications of lift therapy are rare but occasionally occur. These are usually related to the foot and ankle. Lifting a heel changes talotibial mechanics and potentially increases instability of the joint. Appropriate sole lifting in addition to the heel can prevent this. The second complication involves the plantar fascia and results in heel pain caused by stress on the plantar side of the calcaneus. This is alleviated by appropriate heel and sole lift or using the lift with a foot orthotic device. It usually takes 6 to 8 weeks for a patient to adjust to lift therapy. Appropriate stretching exercises should be prescribed to assist the patient in achieving myofascial balance. The patient must be cautioned that lift therapy use is continuous and must be incorporated into all footwear. The amount of lift does not change unless there is subsequent fracture or rapidly progressive degenerative joint disease in a lower extremity.

Foot Orthotics

Foot orthotic devices can be used to assist the patient in restoring musculoskeletal balance. A podiatrist can individually customize appropriate orthotic devices for foot mechanics. Orthotic devices should never be prescribed until the joints and fasciae of the foot and ankle have been treated maximally by appropriate manual medicine. Great care must be exercised when using lift therapy with an orthotic device. Incorporation of the appropriate amount of lift to the orthotic device is frequently sufficient. Occasionally it is necessary to change the outside of the shoe to correct the requirement of the short-leg, pelvic-tilt syndrome and to use appropriate orthotic correction inside of the shoe for foot mechanics.

MODALITIES

Several treatment modalities are extensively used in the health care delivery system despite the paucity of research evidence for their effectiveness. The opinions expressed here are based on the author's clinical experience.

Ice

Ice packs are frequently used for acute soft-tissue injuries. The classic athletic medicine principle of RICE (**R**est, **I**ce, **C**ompression, and **E**levation) is appropriate for many conditions. Ice packs are used after treatment to reduce the inflammatory response after stimulating chronic dysfunctional musculoskeletal tissues. Frequent short-term applications are most effective. Caution must be used to not chill the skin.

Heat

External heat has wide acceptance by most patients and, while comforting, is frequently abused. A frequent history for a patient with an acute lower back injury is to continuously apply a heating pad overnight while asleep and find it impossible to get out of bed the next day. Short-term application of heat does enhance circulation to the body part and can be effective in mobilizing the inflammatory process. However, too much heat applied for too long a period can overly congest a part and contribute to the inflammatory process. Hot packs, particularly moist heat, are very useful prior to extensive manual stretching. For home use, the patient is advised to apply heat, either moist or dry, for no longer than 15 minutes and no more frequently than every 2 hours, with a maximum of six applications per day.

Ultrasound

Ultrasound is used to provide deep "heat" to tissue by its "stimulation." It is used mainly in the shoulder region in preparation for more extensive stretching and rehabilitation exercises.

Traction

The application of external traction, by static devices or machines, is used extensively in musculoskeletal medicine. Research evidence of the effectiveness of traction in the literature is sparse, but the empiric use of traction in certain conditions has been deemed valuable. Pelvic traction at 90 degrees of hip flexion and 90 degrees of knee flexion in acute lumbar discogenic disease can be helpful. In this instance, the patient's body weight provides the appropriate amount of traction and distraction of the lower lumbar spine in a flexed position.

The Natchez Mobil-Trac system is a mechanical table that allows the patient to self-position and apply muscle contraction to provide distraction and mobilization of the spine in the presence of discogenic disease. If this equipment is available, with expertise in its use, it is certainly worth a short-term trial. Traction is more frequently used in the cervical spine, particularly in home programs.

Head-halter cervical traction is an effective adjunctive intervention. The patient needs adequate instruction in positioning the head halter to avoid compression on the jaw and irritation to the temporomandibular joint. The recommended weight is 5 to 8 lb (2.25 to 3.6 kg) and should be maintained up to 20 minutes twice daily. Small increments of flexion–extension and rotation right–left exercises while unloaded seem to assist in the management of acute and chronic conditions of the cervical spine. The Gravity Lumbar Traction system (Camp International, Jackson, MI) provides more extensive use of traction and is available for both hospital and home use. A body jacket is applied and the patient's body weight is the activating force at various levels of inclination from horizontal to semivertical. A variation on this theme is to use the same body jacket to unload some of the patient's weight and then perform exercises, particularly walking on a treadmill. This system has been useful in the management of acute lumbar discogenic radiculopathy.

TENS (Transcutaneous Electric Nerve Stimulation)

TENS units are quite popular with health professionals and the laity. This author has been personally disappointed in their effectiveness. Electrical stimulation therapy has also been helpful to some practitioners. For this author (like the TENS unit) the results have been disappointing.

Surgery

Spinal surgery has two major objectives. The first is decompressing neural structures compromised by trauma or degenerative disease. The second is to stabilize hypermobile and unstable vertebral segments. There is a vast array of options available for both decompression and stabilization. A successful surgical outcome depends on identifying the right procedure for the right patient at the right level at the right time and performed by the right surgeon. The goal of any surgical intervention is to assist in the restoration of maximal functional capacity of the musculoskeletal system in postural balance. Before any surgical intervention is performed, the patient should have adequate and appropriate diagnostic studies and nonop-

erative care. The diagnostic studies should reveal a surgical pathology that contributes to or causes the patient's pain complaint. Appropriate nonoperative care should be aggressive and comprehensive and not consist of bed rest, modalities, and analgesics.

Most discogenic radiculopathies will respond to aggressive nonoperative care such as appropriate manual medicine, antiinflammatory agents, analgesics, short-term rest, and exercise. If the patient does not respond to nonoperative care and shows evidence of progressive neurologic deficit, surgical consultation and intervention should be obtained as soon as possible. The neurologic deficits of most concern are the cauda equina syndrome and progressive muscle weakness or increasing dural tension signs despite appropriate nonoperative care. The diagnostic workup should identify a surgical pathology consistent with the patient's presentation and should be confirmed by electrodiagnostic studies.

For successful surgical outcome, the patient should receive both prehabilitation and rehabilitation. Adequate nonoperative care before surgery should prepare the patient's musculoskeletal system for the surgical intervention. Postsurgical rehabilitation occurs as soon as possible. Even in the presence of a stabilization procedure, early isometric stabilization exercise can be done before ambulation. Restoration of mobility, muscle control, and balance is the goal of postoperative rehabilitation. A successful surgical outcome is based on the preparation of the patient for the anticipated outcome. Many patients expect total pain relief and restoration of a normal back following a surgical intervention. They should be cautioned that is not the case. The pathology for which the surgery is performed, coupled with the surgical procedure itself, results in alteration of the anatomy that can never be restored to "normal." Unwarranted patient expectations should be avoided.

The surgical intervention should be the least invasive possible. Every attempt should be made to maintain the integrity of the anatomy. Postsurgical magnetic resonance imaging studies show fatty replacement infiltration of the deep fourth-layer muscles of the spinal complex. Following fatty replacement, muscles no longer provide the proprioceptive information essential for muscle control and a good functional outcome. It is for this reason that the postoperative patient performs an intensive exercise program.

Exercise

Of all of the adjunctive therapeutic procedures, the one of most value to this author has been exercise. Exercise is fundamental to maintaining the therapeutic effectiveness of manual medicine intervention. The principles identified in Chapter 20 are applicable to all patients and are worth the effort of the practitioner to master.

SUMMARY

Manual medicine practitioners should avail themselves of any adjunctive therapeutic procedure that assists in patient management. The broader the physician's armamentarium, the more likely is success. Each patient must be individually evaluated and the devised treatment plans unique to that individual. Adjunctive therapeutic procedures, like manual medicine, should not be prescribed in a cookbook fashion.

SUGGESTED READINGS

Burton CV. The Sister Kenny Institute, *Gravity Lumbar Reduction Therapy. In: Lower Back Pain 2nd ed.,* Finneson BE, ed. Philadelphia: JB Lippincott. 1980:277–280.

Burton CV. *Low Back Care: The Gravity of the Situation. In: Managing Low Back Pain,* 3rd ed., Kirkalchy-Willis. WH, Burton CV, eds. Churchill Livingston: New York. 1992:329–336.

Dorman TA, Ravin TH. *Diagnosis and injection techniques in orthopedic medicine.* Baltimore: Williams & Wilkins, 1991.

Gedney EH. Hypermobile joint. Osteopathic Profession, 1937; 4:30–31.

Hackett GS. *Joint Ligament Relaxation Treated by Fibroosseus Proliferation.* 2nd ed, Springfield: Charles C. Thomas, 1957.

Natchev, E. *A Manual on Auto-traction Treatment for Low Back Pain,* Tryckeribolaget: Sundsvail, 1984.

Ongley MJ, Klein RG, Dorman TA et al. *A new approach to the treatment of chronic back pain.* Lancet, July 1987:143–146.

23

Practitioners of musculoskeletal medicine have experienced patients with similar clinical presentations. Those who use the structural diagnosis and manipulative treatment aspects of manual medicine will notice that many of these patients present with similar structural diagnostic findings. Appropriate treatment of the areas of somatic dysfunction in some instances results in total symptom resolution, whereas another patient's recurrence and persistence occurs. Included here are some of the common presentations seen in manual medicine practice.

COMMON COMPENSATORY (UNIVERSAL) PATTERN

Numerous authors have referred to a common "universal" pattern. It is commonly noted that patients are notoriously asymmetric in the functional behavior of their musculoskeletal systems. Symmetric function is the ideal but is seldom identified. The universal pattern consists of a cluster of findings including a pronated right foot, an anteriorly rotated right hip bone, a posteriorly rotated left hip bone, a right inferior pubis, a left superior pubis, a left-on-left forward sacral torsion, a lower thoracic scoliosis convex to the right, a left lumbar scoliosis, an anterior and inferior right shoulder girdle, and a left cervical scoliosis. A number of theories have been postulated to account for this pattern, including the Coriolis force of gravity. It was originally postulated that this pattern was common in the northern hemisphere and that the reverse would be identified in the southern hemisphere, similar to the differences noted in the way that water runs down a drain. This author has been privileged to assess patients in the southern hemisphere in New Zealand and Australia and finds the same universal pattern as found in the northern hemisphere. Obviously the Coriolis effect is not the cause. Another theory is that it results from right-handedness. Because right-handed people represent a high percentage of the population, this may have some credibility. Our society is dominated by tools and equipment that are made for a right-handed and not a left-handed person, so that even left-handed individuals must live in a right-handed world. Perhaps repetitive movement in this right-handed environment contributes to this universal pattern. This author has often wondered if the fact that most children are delivered in a vertex presentation with the left occiput anterior might be a factor in the development of the functional asymmetry of the musculoskeletal system. The dilemma remains a subject for future research. It is true that this pattern is frequently seen in symptomatic and asymptomatic patients. The question is what is the clinical significance of this common pattern? Observation shows that if the patient's dysfunctions are out of this pattern, they are more clinically significant. A structural diagnostic finding that does not fit the pattern should alert the diagnostician that the presentation is unusual.

In addition to the articular restrictions noted in the universal pattern, there are consistent patterns of asymmetric muscle function with some muscles becoming tighter and others becoming inhibited and weak. These patterns have been described in Chapter 20 and warrant study. It is amazing how the muscle pattern fits the articular dysfunction as well as causing the ever-present question of which came first and which contributes to the persistence of the other. Is it joint or muscle? In all probability, it is a combination of both.

The presence of the common universal pattern can result in practitioners treating patients in a cookbook fashion to restore motion to the segments in this universal pattern. That is poor practice. Patients should be viewed from their individual pattern and how it deviates from that which is more common. Again, dysfunctions out of pattern have been found to be more clinically significant.

THE "DIRTY HALF DOZEN" IN THE FAILED LOWER BACK SYNDROME

Disability from lower back pain continues to be a major societal problem. The cost of care to the patient with industrial back pain continues to escalate and frustrates the health care delivery system, the insurance industry (both public and private), and employers. For the patient, it can be catastrophic with loss of income, reduced activities of daily living, loss of self-esteem, and dependency. The prevention of the failed lower back syndrome and the rehabilitation of its sufferers are indeed challenges.

Structural diagnostic and manual medicine practice has demonstrated a clustering of findings in patients presenting with the failed lower back pain syndrome. This cluster has been designated the "dirty half dozen." The dirty half dozen consists of dysfunction within the lumbar spine, pelvis, and lower extremities. They are:

1. Nonneutral dysfunction within the lumbar spine, primarily flexed, rotated, and side bent (FRS) dysfunctions in the segments of the lower lumbar and thoracolumbar spine;
2. Dysfunction at the symphysis pubis;
3. Restriction of anterior nutational movement of the sacral base, either a posterior (backward) torsion or a posteriorly nutated (extended) sacrum;
4. Hip bone shear dysfunction;
5. Short-leg, pelvic-tilt syndrome; and
6. Muscle imbalance of the trunk and lower extremities.

This author studied 183 patients (79 men and 104 women) with an average age of 40.8 years who were disabled for an average of 30.7 months. All patients had disability with 53% working less than full-time and disabled for some activities of daily living, 42% were not working and had disability of most of the activities of daily living, and 5% were totally disabled and needed assistance for activities of daily living. Eighteen percent had previous surgical treatment suggesting that most cases of failed lower back syndrome are a failure of previous nonoperative care. The 18% surgical failure rate is close to the national average of 15%. In these patients, the primary presentation was of back pain with some radiation to the buttock and thigh and in 38% some radiation below the knee. None of the patients presented with leg pain alone. The primary presentation was back, buttock, and thigh pain. The yield from standard neurologic and orthopedic testing was low. Ten percent had some reflex change at the patellar or Achilles levels. Less than 5% showed evidence of significant muscle weakness. Seven percent showed some sensory loss. The classic straight leg raising with positive dural response was only identified in 2%. None had the classic crossed, straight leg raising sign pathognomonic of discogenic radiculopathy. Assessment of the dirty half dozen found 84% to have FRS or extended, rotated, and side bent (ERS) dysfunctions in the lumbar spine clustered at the L4 and L5 levels. Seventy five percent had un-

leveling of the symphysis pubis. A total of 48.6% had restriction of anterior nutation of the posterior sacral base. Sixty percent of the failed surgical patients had a posterior sacral base. This high incidence leads one to consider that this functional pathology may be associated with the structural pathology or that the original symptoms were not due to the structural but the functional pathology. In the past, laminectomy was done with the patient in a flattened lumbar lordosis, but today the preservation of a functional lumbar lordosis is the goal of a spinal surgeon. Twenty-four percent showed the presence of hip bone shear with a female to male ratio of 2:1. The short-leg pelvic-tilt syndrome was found in 63%. This is consistent with a number of previous studies showing two of three people with back and lower extremity disability having inequality of leg length as compared to 8% to 20% of the asymptomatic population. Muscle imbalance was found in almost all of the patients.

Only five patients (2.7%) failed to demonstrate any of the dirty half dozen. Fifty-five percent of the population showed three or more of the dirty half dozen. Despite an average of 2.5 years of disability, 75% of this population returned to full employment and active activities of daily living following a treatment plan directed toward the findings.

CHRONIC RECURRENT LOW BACK PAIN SYNDROME (COCKTAIL SYNDROME)

Patients who are victims of this problem present with chronic recurrent disabling back pain with minimal radiation to the lower extremity below the buttocks. They find it difficult to stand for any period because the back pain progressively increases while standing without being mobile. Hence the term "cocktail party syndrome." It is of major significance in patients who must stand in a confined area for long periods such as workers on assembly lines or cashiers at checkout counters. The pain is lessened by walking activities or by sitting. Victims of this problem are frequently one-legged standers who do not bear weight symmetrically on their lower extremities resulting in chronic postural imbalance.

The structural diagnostic findings in this population usually consists of the problem on the left side with the left pubis being superior, the left sacrum being anteriorly nutated (flexed), the left innominate posterior, and an L5 with ERS dysfunction to the left with tight erector spinae muscles and weak abdominals. Treatment of these patients is difficult and frequently frustrating. Recurrent exacerbations are common. They require appropriate manual medicine treatment for the dysfunctions described and a lifelong exercise program to maintain trunk and abdominal muscle control. The patient must learn not to be a one-legged stander and to maintain balanced standing posture. Modifications of the work activity may be necessary to provide the patient with the opportunity to move on a frequent basis and to minimize standing in the nonmobile posture.

SPINAL STENOSIS

Spinal stenosis is becoming an increasing problem as our society ages. Central canal and lateral recess stenosis resulting from spinal spondylosis and spondylarthritis can be seen at all vertebral levels but particularly in the lumbar spine. The classic presentation is a patient who is in a flexed position with difficulties in spinal extension and in walking in the upright position for any period of time or distance. Frequently the patient will relate that he or she is more comfortable walking behind a shopping cart. Persistent forward-bent posture for comfort leads to many secondary dysfunctions and muscle imbalances. The neurogenic claudication experienced by these patients may be due to perineural and endoneural passive congestion rather than compression. A manual medicine treatment plan that maximizes the lumbopelvic mechanics, particularly intersegmental motion, may reduce

the inflammatory reaction to the passive congestion and give the patient some relief. Manual medicine will not change the osseous pathology of spinal stenosis.

CASE HISTORY

A 64-year-old woman presented in October 1988 with disabling lumbar and bilateral leg pain worse on walking and relieved by sitting. She could not walk from her house to the one next door without disabling lower extremity pain. Physical examination failed to determine any vascular deficits of the lower extremities. The greater trochanters were level, but the left iliac crest was low and there was a long C-curve with convexity to the left in the thoracolumbar spine. Global trunk extension restriction was present. Neurologic examination findings were within normal limits. Plain film radiography (Figs. 23.1–23.6) of the lumbar spine, including erect films for postural study and flexion–extension dynamic studies, revealed unleveling of the sacral base plane that was inferior on the left side by 1.9 cm. Oblique studies (Figs. 23.2 and 23.3) revealed significant degenerative disease of the zygapophysial joints at L4 to L5. Lateral view in the

Figure 23.1.
Lumbar spine, erect anteroposterior projection.

Figure 23.2.
Lumbar spine, left oblique projection.

Figure 23.3.
Lumbar spine, right oblique projection.

Figure 23.4.
Lumbar spine, erect lateral projection.

erect position revealed a sacral base angle of 36 degrees, a slightly anterior mid-third lumbar perpendicular, and a first-degree degenerative spondylolisthesis at L4 on L5 (Fig. 23.4). The dynamic studies (Figs. 23.5 and 23.6) showed some increase in the translatory component of L3 on L4 during the flexion–extension process (Figs. 23.7 and 23.8).

Magnetic resonance imaging (MRI) showed significant stenosis of the spinal canal at the L4 to L5 level with other changes consistent with degenerative disc disease.

The patient was placed on a treatment plan consisting of manual medicine of the muscle energy and mobilization without impulse type directed toward maximizing intersegmental mobility to all elements of the lumbar spine in neutral mechanics. Progressive lift therapy was started in the left shoe beginning with 6-mm (¼ in.) lift with the ultimate goal of 12-mm (½ in.) lift, which was accomplished without difficulty. An intensive exercise program, including sensory motor balance training and stretching to symmetry, was used culminating in a home exercise program that the patient performed daily. The acute treatment plan was completed in 3 months. At the end of that time, the patient was able to walk erect for 1 mile in 20 minutes. As she gradually gained functional capacity, she was able to walk 2 miles in 40 minutes without symptoms.

She was followed semiannually for the next 3 years and then annually without recurrent symptoms until she was lost to follow-up after 10 years. This patient is an example of the ability to increase functional capacity despite the presence of osseous pathology. The goal of manual medicine—providing maximum pain-free movement in postural balance—was attempted and achieved in this patient and many others with similar presentations. The inclusion of mobilization without impulse to the lumbar segments to restore symmetric zygapophysial joint motion in neutral mechanics is believed to enhance the decongestive process in the lateral spinal canal thus reducing the neurogenic claudication. Regardless of whether this is the mechanism, this treatment plan has been successful in many patients with spinal stenosis. This approach should be aggressively used in patients before subjecting patients to decompressive surgical procedures that may result in spinal instability.

INTERCOSTAL NEURALGIAS

Pain in the chest wall aggravated by respiration is a common patient presentation. These patients are

Figure 23.5.
Lumbar spine, erect lateral backward-bending projection.

Figure 23.6.
Lumbar spine, erect lateral forward-bending projection.

given a diagnosis of "intercostal neuralgia" or "pleurisy." The chest wall complaint may be primary or associated with other complaints within the musculoskeletal system.

The common structural diagnostic finding in these patients is a structural rib dysfunction frequently associated with a nonneutral dysfunction of the ERS type in the thoracic spine. External rib torsional dysfunction with an associated ERS dysfunction of the thoracic spine is the most common finding and is associated with exhalation restriction of the ribs superior to the torsional dysfunction. The anterior and posterior subluxations and anteroposterior or lateral compressions can likewise lead to symptoms simulating intercostal neuralgia. These structural rib dysfunctions are also characterized by exquisite tenderness and tissue reactivity at the costochondral junction, the so-called Tietze's syndrome. If the practitioner does not identify structural rib pathology in a patient with this presentation, the index of suspicion for organic neurologic disease should be high. Tumors of the thoracic cord, herpes zoster infection, and diabetic neuropathy are but a few of those entities in a differential

Figure 23.7.
Magnetic resonance imaging, lumbar spine sagittal view.

Figure 23.8.
Magnetic resonance imaging, lumbar spine axial view at L4 to L5.

diagnosis. Most "intercostal neuralgias" are the result of structural rib dysfunctions. If one is not found in a patient presenting with intercostal chest wall pain, call your friendly neurologist for consultation.

CERVICAL BRACHIALGIAS

Painful stiffness of the cervical spine and associated pain, numbness, and tingling in the upper extremity is a common patient presentation. There are a number of structures that can be involved with structural pathology, dysfunctional pathology, or a combination of both that need to be assessed. From the structural diagnostic process, the following assessment sequence should be performed to identify those dysfunctions amenable to manual medicine intervention that could cause the symptom complex. Obviously, standard neurologic and orthopedic testing should also be performed.

The process begins in the cervical spine to assess the mobility characteristics of the zygapophysial joints for their potential involvement in compressive or inflammatory entrapment of a cervical nerve root. Zygapophysial dysfunction of the cervical spine always involves the intertransversarii muscles through which the nerve root passes as it exits the lateral vertebral canal. The cervical roots forming the brachial plexus pass through and between the scalene muscles. Imbalance in scalene muscle length and tone is common. Hypertonicity of the scalene musculature might entrap and irritate the plexus contributing to shoulder and arm symptoms. Assessment of the first rib for superior subluxation should be made, because it ap-

parently influences the lower trunk of the plexus with symptoms that respond to restoration of function. The next rib dysfunction to be assessed is the presence of a laterally flexed second rib that can mechanically narrow the costoclavicular canal resulting in entrapment of the neurovascular bundle. This dysfunction causes major exhalation restriction and patients present with exquisite tenderness at the most lateral aspect of the second rib as it moves beneath the lateral clavicle. If the examiner identifies a superior subluxation of rib one, assessment for a laterally flexed second rib beneath is in order. This is particularly true in a superior subluxation of the first rib that does not respond to the usual treatment intervention. Another potential site for neurovascular entrapment is under the tendon of the pectoralis minor muscle. The pectoral muscles are notoriously short and tight and alter the relationship of the shoulder girdle to the thoracic cage. Appropriate assessment and treatment of these potential sites of dysfunction, working from medial to lateral, have been quite successful in the cervical brachialgia syndromes.

A similar approach of working from central to distal is also of value in patients with symptoms around the elbow and at the wrist. The classic presentation of medial or lateral epicondylitis will most frequently be associated to restriction of pronation and supination of the radial head at the radiohumeral and proximal radioulnar joints. Restoration of function of the radial head is frequently sufficient to treat "tennis elbow."

Symptoms related to the carpal tunnel have escalated in recent years and appear to be related to repetitive strain injury, particularly those associated with hand action at a computer terminal. Any repetitive motion of the hands and wrists can lead to complaints of wrist pain and associated numbness and tingling in the fingers. While many of these patients will show borderline delay in median nerve conduction, few demonstrate denervation potentials in the hand muscles, particularly the thenar eminence. Structural diagnosis and manual medicine treatment to the joints at the wrist should follow the previously described assessment and treatment processes from the cervical spine distally. The joint play procedures and others addressing dysfunction at the wrist region described in Chapter 18 can be of assistance in management of these patients.

CERVICAL CRANIAL SYNDROME

Of all of the areas in the musculoskeletal system and the spinal column, this author finds the craniocervical junction the most difficult to adequately assess and successfully manage. Patients presenting with pain in the cervical spine with stiffness and an associated headache, usually hemicephalalgic and running from the occiput to the retroorbital area, are all too common in clinical practice. Trauma is a frequent initiator of the symptom complex, but the pain can occur without a single trauma, such as a motor vehicle collision, by chronic postural imbalance affecting the upper cervical musculature. Structural diagnosis of the upper cervical complex is difficult because of the unique anatomy in the region (see Chapter 13). Diagnosis of restricted mobility in the upper cervical complex is easier than the assessment of hypermobility. Relative hypermobility on the opposite side of restricted motion is quite common and confusing to the examiner. If there is high suspicion and physical findings consistent with hypermobility, special imaging studies are in order. They should include plain film flexion and extension studies in the lateral projection and rotary stress films with axial views of the cervicocranial and upper cervical regions by computed tomography or MRI.

The common structural diagnostic findings in these patients are an ERS$_{left}$ dysfunction at C2 to C3, the atlas rotated to the right, and the occiput flexed side-bent right and rotated left. There is frequently an associated dysfunction of the left occipitomastoid suture.

Figures 23.9 and 23.10 show the MRI findings in a patient presenting with a 6-year history of cervical cranial pain syndrome following a major motor vehicle collision. Her injuries included fractures of the pelvis and a traumatic brain injury. She had been successfully treated and rehabilitated and had returned to full-time work, but persisted with recurring upper cervical painful stiffness and an associated hemicephalalgia. Her structural diagnostic findings were as described above, but were very difficult to manage and sustain in a maximal functional capacity. The sagittal views of the cervical cord and cervical spine (Fig. 23.9) are essentially within normal limits. The axial MRI views (Fig. 23.10) show major loss of muscle density in the region of the rectus capitis posterior minor and major muscles. This finding may account for the difficulty in responding to manual medicine procedures of all types. Patients with changes in the rectus capitis posterior major and minor muscles are difficult to treat. Their somatic dysfunctions recur easily and are refractory to manual medicine procedures. A number of exercise programs have been tried in these patients with mixed results. Recently, there has been some success with prolotherapy into the insertion of these muscles into the occiput and into the zygapophysial joints at C1 to C2 and C2 to C3. More research into this approach is needed.

CEPHALGIA ASSOCIATED WITH TRAUMATIC BRAIN INJURY

Many patients who have sustained a closed head injury resulting in minimal to mild to moderate brain dysfunction have an associated headache complaint that is very resistant to treatment. Major structural diagnostic findings of the craniosacral mechanism are found in such patients in addition to dysfunctions elsewhere

Figure 23.9.
Magnetic resonance imaging, cervical spine sagittal cuts.

Figure 23.10.
Magnetic resonance imaging, cervical spine axial cuts.

in the system. The craniosacral findings have been remarkably consistent in this population. They all appear to have reduction in the rate and amplitude of the cranial rhythmic impulse with an average in the 6 to 7 range. They all appear to have some level of sphenobasilar compression, particularly of the anteroposterior type. The sphenobasilar strain patterns most consistently found are the presence of a lateral and torsional strain restriction to the same side and an inferior vertical strain. Appropriate craniosacral manipulation can be useful in the rehabilitation of these patients (see Chapter 12). If the craniosacral system responds to treatment by an increase in the rate and amplitude of the cranial rhythmic impulse and balanced and enhanced mobility of the sphenobasilar junction, there is a correlation with a positive outcome for the rehabilitation process. Conversely, if the patient does not respond to craniosacral manipulation with an enhanced cranial rhythmic impulse rate and amplitude, the outcome of the rehabilitative process is less satisfactory. Caution is advised in the use of craniosacral manipulation in this population because it carries approximately a 5% iatrogenic complication rate.

RECURRENT ANKLE SPRAINS

Recurrence of ankle sprain is common with the weekend warrior and the high-level athlete. These patients do not provide a difficult diagnostic challenge but are difficult to treat. Structural diagnostic findings in this population consistently show dysfunction at the proximal tibiofibular joint and dorsiflexion restriction of the talus at the talotibial articulation. Altered subtalar gliding movement is common in these patients along with pronation of the cuboid on the same side. Muscle assessment will frequently reveal weakness of the tibialis anterior and the peroneal muscles. Adequate treatment for this dysfunctional pattern will frequently prevent recurrence of ankle sprain. Another very troublesome outcome of ankle sprains is difficulty with proprioceptive balance, particularly when standing on one leg. This appears to result in altered muscle firing pattern sequence and contributes to muscle imbalance throughout the total musculoskeletal system. For this reason, patients should continue with proprioceptive balance training, particularly if they are an involved in athletic activities considered to be high risk for such injuries, such as basketball and volleyball.

CONCLUSION

This chapter includes many of the common clinical syndrome findings from the structural diagnostic and manual medicine perspectives. While these are frequently seen, the practitioner is urged to assess each patient on an individual basis in a very comprehensive fashion to determine the exact dysfunctional pattern present and to develop an appropriate treatment plan. The higher the level of structural diagnostic skill and the more competent the practitioner is in multiple manual medicine interventions, the better will be the outcome. The manual medicine armamentarium is quite broad and the practitioner should be familiar with as many as possible. Remember the admonition that if you only have a hammer in your toolbox, most everything begins to look like a nail.

SUGGESTED READINGS

Andary MT, Hallgren RC, Greenman PE, Rechtien JJ. Neurogenic atrophy of suboccipital muscles after a cervical injury. *AM J Phy Med Rehabil*, 1998. 77:545–549.

Greenman PE. Syndromes of the lumbar spine, pelvis, and sacrum. *Phys Med Rehab Clin N Am* 1996;7:773–785.

Greenman PE, Tait B. Structural diagnosis in chronic low back pain. *Man Med* 1988;3:114–117.

Hack GD, Koritzer RT, Robinson WL, et al. Anatomic relation between the rectus capitis posterior minor muscle and the dura mater. *Spine* 1995;20: 2484–2486.

Hallgren RC, Greenman PE, Rechtien JJ. Atrophy of suboccipital muscles in chronic pain patients. *J Am Osteopath Assoc* 1993;93:871.

Hallgren RC, Greenman PE, Rechtien JJ. MRI of normal and atrophic muscle of the upper cervical spine. *J Clin Engineering* 1993;18:433–439.

Kirkaldy-Willis WH, Bernard TN. *Managing low back pain,* 4th ed. New York: Churchill Livingstone, 1997.

Becker RF, Wilson JW, Gehweiler JA: The Anatomical Basis of Medical Practice. Baltimore, Williams & Wilkins, 1971.

Figures 1.1 through 1.6 and 15.1 through 15.5

Kuchera ML: Osteopathic Considerations in Systemic Dysfunction. Kirksville, Kirksville College of Osteopathic Medicine, 1992.

Figures 7.53 and 7.54

Chaitow L: Positional Release Techniques. London: Churchill Livingstone, 1991.

Figures 10.1 and 10.2

Agur AMR, Lee MJ: Grant's Atlas of Anatomy, ed 9. Baltimore, Williams & Wilkins, 1991.

Figures 12.1, 12.2, 12.4, and 12.6

Anderson JE: Grant's Atlas of Anatomy, ed 8. Baltimore, Williams & Wilkins, 1983.

Figure 12.3

Clemente CD: Anatomy: A Regional Atlas of the Human Body, ed 3. Baltimore, Urban & Schwarzenberg, 1987.

Figures 17.1 and 17.2

Travell JG, Simons DG: Myofascial Pain and Dysfunction: The Trigger Point Manual. The Upper Extremities. Baltimore, Williams & Wilkins, Vol. 1, 1983.

Figures 20.42C, 20.51B, 20.52B, 20.58B, 20.59B, 20.60, 20.63B, 20.68B, 20.70C

Travell JG, Simons DG: Myofascial Pain and Dysfunction: The Trigger Point Manual. The Lower Extremities. Baltimore, Williams & Wilkins. Vol. 2, 1992.

Figures 20.15B, 20.16B, 20.19B, 20.20B, 20.21A, 20.25B, 20.29B, 20.31C, and 20.34C

Aprill C: New Orleans, Louisiana.

Figures 21.16 through 21.21

Page numbers followed by f refer to figures; page numbers followed by t refers to tables.